# Illness and Healing Alternatives in Western Europe

Despite the recent upsurge in interest in alternative medicine and unorthodox healers, *Illness and Healing Alternatives in Western Europe* is the first book to focus closely on the relationship between belief, culture and healing in the past. In essays on France, the Netherlands, Germany, Spain and England, from the sixteenth century to the present day, the authors draw on a broad range of material, from studies of demonologists and reports of asylum doctors to church archives and oral evidence.

These studies offer a fundamental and exciting rereading of the history of healing, challenging Weber's concept of the 'disenchantment of the world'. Although the attribution of illness to witchcraft and demons has clearly been losing ground ever since the seventeenth century, there has by no means been a complete disappearance of these beliefs.

Engaging rigorously with the relationship between medical science, popular beliefs and healing, with the concept of a 'medical market place', and with alternative medicine right up to the present day, *Illness and Healing Alternatives in Western Europe* will make an invaluable resource for undergraduate and postgraduate students of medical, social and cultural history.

**Marijke Gijswijt-Hofstra** is Professor of Social and Cultural History at the University of Amsterdam. She has published widely on the history of witchcraft and alternative healing. **Hilary Marland** is Wellcome University Award Holder at the Centre for Social History, Warwick University, and is an editor of *Social History of Medicine*. Among her many publications are works on the history of midwifery. **Hans de Waardt** is Lecturer in History at Erasmus University Rotterdam, and has published extensively on witchcraft, sorcery and preacher-healers.

## Studies in the Social History of Medicine
## Series Editors: Jonathan Barry and Bernard Harris

In recent years, the social history of medicine has become recognised as a major field of historical enquiry. Aspects of health, disease, and medical care now attract the attention not only of social historians but also of researchers in a broad spectrum of historical and social science disciplines. The Society for the Social History of Medicine, founded in 1969, is an interdisciplinary body, based in Great Britain but international in membership. It exists to forward a wide-ranging view of the history of medicine, concerned equally with biological aspects of normal life, experience of and attitudes towards illness, medical thought and treatment, and systems of medical care. Although frequently bearing on current issues, this interpretation of the subject makes primary reference to historical context and contemporary priorities. The intention is not to promote a sub-specialism but to conduct research according to the standards and intelligibility required of history in general. The Society publishes a journal, *Social History of Medicine*, and holds at least three conferences a year. Its series, Studies in the Social History of Medicine, does not represent publication of its proceedings, but comprises volumes on selected themes, often arising out of conferences but subsequently developed by the editors.

**Life, Death and the Elderly**
*Edited by Margaret Pelling and Richard M. Smith*

**Medicine and Charity Before the Welfare State**
*Edited by Jonathan Barry and Colin Jones*

**In the Name of the Child**
*Edited by Roger Cooter*

**Reassessing Foucault: Power, Medicine and the Body**
*Edited by Colin Jones and Roy Porter*

**From Idiocy to Mental Deficiency**
*Edited by David Wright and Anne Digby*

**Nutrition in Britain**
*Edited by David F. Smith*

**Health Care and Poor Relief in Protestant Europe 1500–1700**
*Edited by Ole Peter Grell and Andrew Cunningham*

**Migrants, Minorities and Health: Historical and Contemporary Studies**
*Edited by Lara Marks and Michael Worboys*

**Midwives, Society and Childbirth**
*Edited by Hilary Marland and Anne Marie Rafferty*

# Illness and Healing Alternatives in Western Europe

Edited by Marijke Gijswijt-Hofstra,
Hilary Marland and Hans de Waardt

ROUTLEDGE

London and New York

First published 1997
by Routledge
11 New Fetter Lane, London EC4P 4EE

Simultaneously published in the USA and Canada
by Routledge
29 West 35th Street, New York, NY 10001



Typeset in Garamond by Routledge
Printed and bound in Great Britain by Mackays of Chatham PLC, Chatham, Kent



*British Library Cataloguing in Publication Data*
A catalogue record for this book is available from the British Library

*Library of Congress Cataloguing in Publication Data*
A catalogue record for this book has been requested

ISBN 0–415–13581–8

# Contents

# Contributors

**Gillian Bennett** holds degrees in English literature, modern English language and folkloristics. She is editor of *Folklore* and an Honorary Research Associate of the Centre for English Cultural Tradition and Language at the University of Sheffield. She is co-compiler of *Contemporary Legend: A Folklore Bibliography* (Sheffield, 1990). Her other works include *Traditions of Belief* (Harmondsworth, 1987) and *Spoken in Jest*, Folklore Mistletoe Series, no. 21 (Sheffield, 1991).

**Albrecht Burkardt** studied history, German and philosophy at the Universities of Bochum, Berlin, Paris and Florence. He has taught in the Department of German at the Sorbonne (Paris IV), and currently teaches early modern history at the University of Lyon II. He is preparing a doctoral thesis on accounts of miracles in French canonization procedures in the seventeenth and eighteenth centuries. He has published several articles on intellectual and religious history, as well as on the history of mentalités in the early modern period, particularly in France and Germany.

**Stuart Clark** is a Senior Lecturer in History at the University of Wales, Swansea, where he teaches the cultural and intellectual history of early modern Europe. His research has concentrated on the history of European demonology between the fifteenth and eighteenth centuries, and his book Thinking with Demons: The Idea of Witchcraft in Early Modern Europe was published in 1997.

**Sarah Ferber** is a Lecturer at the University of Queensland in Brisbane, where she teaches European history and the history of bioethics and medical experimentation. Her doctoral thesis, entitled 'Mixed blessings: possession and exorcism in France, 1598–1654' (University of Melbourne, 1994), has formed the basis for a number of articles. She is currently researching the demonic possession of Marthe Brossier (1598–1600) and the case of a private exorcism which resulted in manslaughter in rural Australia in 1993.

**Willem Frijhoff** is Professor of Modern History at The Free University, Amsterdam, and a member of the Royal Netherlands Academy of Sciences. His publications deal mainly with the history of mentalités and historical anthropology, and his research fields include the history of education, cultural transfer and religious experience in early modern Europe. He is editor of several volumes, including (with Marijke Gijswijt-Hofstra) *Witchcraft in the Netherlands from the Fourteenth to the Twentieth Century* (Rotterdam, 1991), and has published a number of books of which the most recent is a contextual biography centred on religious experience and the construction of the self, *Wegen van Evert Willemsz: Een Hollands weeskind op zoek naar zichzelf* [Pathways of Evert Willemsz: a Dutch orphan child in search of himself] *(1607–1647)* (Nijmegen, 1995).

**Marijke Gijswijt-Hofstra** is Professor of Social and Cultural History, at the University of Amsterdam. She is author of *Wijkplaatsen voor Vervolgden: Asielverlening in Culemborg, Vianen, Buren, Leerdam en IJsselstein van de 16de tot eind 18de Eeuw* [Places of refuge: the granting of asylum in Culemborg, Vianen, Buren, Leerdam and IJsselstein from the sixteenth to the end of the eighteenth century] (Dieren, 1984). She has edited three collections of essays on witchcraft, one on deviance and tolerance, and, most recently, two on the social history of medicine: *Geloven in genezen: Bijdragen tot de sociaal–culturele geschiedenis van de geneeskunde in Nederland* [Believing in healing: contributions to the social–cultural history of medicine in the Netherlands] (Amsterdam, 1991) and, with Willem de Blécourt and Willem Frijhoff, *Grenzen van genezing: Gezondheid, ziekte en genezen in Nederland, Zestiende tot begin twintigste eeuw* [Boundaries of healing: health, sickness and healing in the Netherlands, sixteenth to the early twentieth centuries] (Hilversum, 1993). She is currently engaged in three projects: homoeopathy in the nineteenth century, cultures of misfortune and popular conceptions of witchcraft.

**Hilary Marland** is Wellcome University Award Holder at the Centre for Social History, University of Warwick, and Honorary Research Associate at the Wellcome Unit, Oxford. She has published on nineteenth-century medical practice in England, on infant welfare, women doctors and Dutch midwives. She has edited volumes on maternal and infant welfare, midwife history and early modern medical practice in England and the Netherlands, most recently *The Art of Midwifery: Early Modern Midwives in Europe* (London and New York, 1993), *The Task of Healing: Medicine, Religion and Gender in England and the Netherlands 1450–1800* (with Margaret Pelling; Rotterdam, 1996) and *Midwives, Society and Childbirth: Debates and Controversies in the Modern Period* (with Anne Marie Rafferty; London and New York, 1997). She is one of the editors of *Social History of Medicine*, and is currently working on two projects: Dutch midwives 1897–1941 and puerperal insanity in nineteenth-century Britain.

**Enrique Perdiguero** is Lecturer in the History of Science and Medicine at the University of Alicante. He wrote his doctoral dissertation on domestic medicine treatises published in Spain during the Enlightenment. His main research interests are the popularization of medicine during the eighteenth and nineteenth centuries, popular medical culture and the organization of the sanitary administration in Spain. He has published on popular healers, the relationship between popular and scientific medical knowledge, and sanitary services in Spain in the twentieth century.

**Matthew Ramsey** teaches history at Vanderbilt University in Nashville, Tennessee. He is the author of *Professional and Popular Medicine in France, 1770–1830: The Social World of Medical Practice* (Cambridge, 1988) and is completing a companion volume on the origins of professional monopoly in French medicine.

**Cornelie Usborne**, born in Munich, studied English and German at Munich University, and history, English and art history at the Open University in England. She is Senior Lecturer in History at the Roehampton Institute, London, and author of *The Politics of the Body in Weimar Germany. Women's Reproductive Rights and Duties* (London and Michigan, 1992), *Frauenkörper – Volkskörper. Geburtenkontrolle und Bevölkerungspolitik in der Weimarer Republik* (Münster, 1994) and articles on German social and feminist history. She is a member of the editorial board of *German History*, the journal of the German History Society, and committee member of the Society for the Social History of Medicine. She is currently working on a monograph on cultures of abortion in Germany, 1900–39.

**Hans de Waardt** is Lecturer in History at Erasmus University Rotterdam, where he also holds a research fellowship. He is the author of *Toverij en Samenleving* [Sorcery and society], *Holland 1500–1800* (Den Haag, 1991) and of a number of papers on sorcery and preacher-healers. He is currently engaged in two fields of research: the history of irregular healers in the Netherlands during the early modern period, and the relationship between the sense of honour and socio-cultural developments in the Netherlands between 1450 and 1650.

**Gary K. Waite** was awarded a PhD from the University of Waterloo in 1987, and is Professor of Medieval and Early Modern European History at the University of New Brunswick, Fredericton. He has completed numerous articles and two books on the Dutch Anabaptist David Joris, including *David Joris and Dutch Anabaptism, 1524–1543* (Waterloo, 1990) and, as editor and translator, *The Anabaptist Writings of David Joris* (Waterloo, 1994). He is also engaged in two other projects: a book on the reform drama of the Dutch chambers of rhetoric during the reign of Charles V and a study of the intersections between popular perceptions and official prosecutions of radical religion and witchcraft in the Netherlands between 1530 and 1648.

**Ineke van Wetering** is an anthropologist specializing in African Surinamese cultures. She has published on witchcraft, religious movements and migrant women's rituals. She was Senior Lecturer at Amsterdam's Free University and, in 1995, holder of the Exchange Chair at the Amsterdam School for Social Science Research.

# Acknowledgements

The articles in this volume are based on a selection of the papers given at the conference, 'Healing, magic and belief in Europe fifteenth–twentieth centuries: new perspectives', held at Woudschoten in the Netherlands in September 1994. We would like to take this opportunity to thank the following sponsors who gave financial support for the conference: Erasmus Universiteit Rotterdam; Huizinga Instituut; Koninklijke Nederlandse Akademie van Wetenschappen, Amsterdam; Koninklijke Nederlandse Maatschappij tot Bevordering der Geneeskunst, Utrecht; P.J. Meertens-Instituut, Amsterdam; Rijksuniversiteit Limburg; Universiteit van Amsterdam; Vereniging tegen de Kwakzalverij; and the Wellcome Trust, London.

The Huizinga Instituut, Research Institute and Graduate School of Cultural History, provided further financial assistance for the preparation of this volume. Our thanks are due to Rachel M.J. van der Wilden-Fall for correcting a number of the articles written by non-English authors. Lastly, we would like to thank the participants at the conference for their stimulating role and Jonathan Barry and Bernard Harris for their support and guidance as Series Editors.

Marijke Gijswijt-Hofstra<br>
Hilary Marland<br>
Hans de Waardt

# Introduction

## Demons, diagnosis and disenchantment

*Marijke Gijswijt-Hofstra, Hilary Marland and Hans de Waardt*

In their conceptions and explanations of illness and in their reactions to it, individuals and groups attempt, and expect, to be coherent. They try to present a view which makes sense to themselves and which is also clear to others who may find it difficult to understand why healers, patients and other interested parties follow a particular line of reasoning. When these arguments are seen by contemporaries to be well founded, this can often be taken as a sign of conformity to an acceptable form of reasoning which fits into a particular 'cultural repertoire'. Individuals have a degree of liberty in the way they construct their arguments and select the elements with which to build them, but when these elements are incompatible with the basic premises of contemporaneous culture – mainstream or subsidiary – their statements become incomprehensible to other people.

The essays in this volume explore the ways in which people have conceived and explained illness, and reactions to illness, in Western Europe from the sixteenth century to the twentieth century. They are concerned with what we want to label the 'cultural repertoires' of illness and healing. They investigate approaches to illness and healing by doctors and other healers, along with their (potential) clients: persons of 'high' and 'low' rank, men and women. Taken together, the essays contribute to our knowledge and understanding of continuity and change in cultural repertoires of illness and healing.

A central issue addressed in this volume is to what extent the approaches to illness and healing have become 'disenchanted' during this long period or, for that matter, have remained or become 'enchanted' and thus accepted as part of a cultural repertoire. Not surprisingly, it will be shown that the concept or, if one wishes, the myth of the 'disenchantment of the world' needs (further) debunking, or at least modification. This brief introduction draws out some of the findings with respect to this and suggests an agenda of issues which future historians of medicine may wish to explore.

To get a tighter grip on the concept of 'disenchantment', the selected essays in this volume cover a varied, though far from complete, range of subjects over a long period. They also represent different disciplinary backgrounds. While much of the history of cultural repertoires of illness and healing still remains to be uncovered, the aim of this volume is to demonstrate and suggest ways of looking for and at this history. It hardly needs saying that attempts at the reconstruction of repertoires of illness and healing and their (perceived) rationality can only hope to be successful by a creative use of the sources. The essays in this volume hope to set an example in this respect. The authors have drawn on a broad range of material: church archives and religious writings, the studies of demonologists and academic authors, medical literature, the publications of 'unorthodox' healers, patient records and the reports of asylum doctors, records of individual practices, government papers, town archives, newspapers, field studies and oral evidence.

## THE 'DISENCHANTMENT' OF ILLNESS AND HEALING?

The concept of the 'disenchantment of the world', as first conceived by Max Weber and adopted by many others, has both inspired and confused the historical debate. It has inspired historians to examine in greater detail the intellectual and broader cultural transformations between the sixteenth and eighteenth centuries as manifested in the spheres of religion, science and witchcraft, and to adjust or refute over-simple linear accounts of these transformations. It has also inspired them to further theorizing, of which Keith Thomas's *Religion and the Decline of Magic* remains the most outstanding example.[1]

At the same time the predominantly indiscriminate use of the disenchantment concept has tended to blur the historical debate. For what is meant by 'the disenchantment of the world'? In Weber's wake this concept has been generally understood as referring to the elimination of magic from human action and behaviour.[2] This *pars pro toto* explanation (the decline of witchcraft referring to the decline of magic in general) clearly transfers and complicates the problem;

for what is then understood by magic? This is where most confusion and controversy has arisen.[3] Rather than claiming universal and timeless boundaries for 'magic', as opposed to 'science' or 'religion', historians are becoming increasingly aware of the risks of anachronistic and ethnocentric labelling.[4] Indeed, historical understanding has much to gain by attempting to identify indigenous classifications and their meanings in specific contexts.[5] But in doing so, historians must be aware of the fact that they are constantly constrained by the limits of their own cultural repertoire. There is probably no other field of research in which traditional hypotheses tend to dominate the debate without serious contention. The persistency, for example, of the traditional idea that magic, religion and science should be treated as separate ways to interpret the world can be seen in Valerie Flint's magnificent study on the Christianization of early medieval Europe.[6] Although she clearly shows that it is impossible to separate the religious aspect from the magical in early Christian beliefs, she nevertheless retrieves this distinction in her final analysis.

If 'magic' is a problematical yardstick for measuring the 'disenchantment of the world', the question follows as to whether other less controversial yardsticks are available. An easy solution to the problem would be to continue relying on the more literal meaning of the concept and to select witchcraft, whether maleficent or not, as *the* criterion. But it then seems only a small step to also include beliefs about the evil workings of demons and how to counter them as a criterion. From demons, the logical step seems to be to religion as such. If the decline of Satan is accepted as an indicator of disenchantment, so should the decline of God and his holy helpers as far as their direct or indirect interference with human affairs is concerned. We might go even further and include (other) occult or esoteric interpretations of the vicissitudes of human life as provided by, for example, spiritualism and the whole conglomeration of New Age culture.

Obviously, a multi-dimensional approach to the 'disenchantment' concept as proposed here will need rethinking. In the meantime the concept represents at least a useful heuristic device, directing our attention to problems of change and continuity with respect to different, partly overlapping explanations of human fortune and misfortune over a long period of time. Following this device, the studies in this volume do not unambiguously support the assumption that the diagnosis of illness and the practice of healing have become increasingly 'disenchanted'. Although the attribution of illness to witchcraft and/or demons has clearly been losing ground from the seventeenth century onwards, this has by no means resulted in a complete disappearance of these beliefs. In the case of witchcraft this is confirmed in this volume by Hans de Waardt for eighteenth-century Holland, Matthew Ramsey for France in the eighteenth and nineteenth centuries, and Enrique Perdiguero for nineteenth- and twentieth-century Alicante in Spain.

We are moreover confronted with a considerable variety of old and new religious, occult, magical and (other) alternative repertoires of illness and healing up to the present day. In addition to Ramsey, de Waardt and Perdiguero, who also report on different forms of magical healing, Gillian Bennett and Ineke van Wetering present more examples of continuing 'enchantment'. Bennett examines the persistent belief in the ability of snakes and other noxious creatures to inhabit human bodily organs, an explanation which co-existed alongside more direct causal ones and which can be documented from the early sixteenth century up to 1990. Van Wetering analyzes the cultural transfer of the *Winti* healing tradition among Creole immigrants from Suriname to the suburbs of late twentieth-century Amsterdam. Stretching the concept somewhat further, Marijke Gijswijt-Hofstra investigates the 'enchantment' of nineteenth-century homoeopathy, as revealed by conversion stories and other reports describing the 'miraculous' healing powers of homoeopathy. To a certain degree, a process of re-enchantment set itself in motion, though, interestingly, the advocates of homoeopathy did not refrain from claiming a 'scientific' status for homoeopathy at the same time. Many more examples, not included in this volume, could be added: faith-healing and pilgrimages, Christian Science and anthroposophy in the religious sphere, mesmerism and its variants and types of paranormal healing and New Age healing forms, to mention but a few cultural repertoires of a more or less 'enchanted' nature, most of them not yet examined using this approach.

It is an important first step to display the multiplicity of notions of illness and practices of healing. It is another, though related, issue to consider their mutual similarities and differences, and to assess their possible continuity, persistence, change and disappearance. All of these have elements of continuity and change, and all similar notions and practices could have meant something different for different people and in different contexts. Patients may not have had the same understanding of illness as the doctors they consulted, not only because of their different position and education, but also because they may have been shopping around on the medical market and therefore not (yet) have developed an exclusive preference for a particular therapy. Doctors were likely to have had a preference or at least laid claim to one. Moreover, the same terms may have been used for a disease or a therapy while their meanings could have changed over time. Hysteria is but one of many possible examples of a term for a disease which has undergone important connotational shifts, as related by Sarah Ferber.[7] Likewise homoeopathy, as conceived by its founder and earlier practitioners, is not the same as the homoeopathy practised by some of the nineteenth- and twentieth-century Spanish healers described by Enrique Perdiguero. So, in which respects and to what extent do notions, practices and their meanings differ, and how far have they remained the same? Take, for example, the age-old stories of bosom serpents and alimentary amphibians, as retold by Bennett. On the face of it they have elements of a remarkable continuity, but does this also hold for the actual use and meaning of these notions and therapies? These are clearly important issues for future research.

Like any system of knowledge or belief, these different cultural repertoires of illness and healing have been subjected to criticism and labelling, both by contemporaries and by later reporters, historians, folklorists and doctors. Labels such as 'superstitious', 'magical', 'deceitful' and also, from the Enlightenment onwards, 'irrational' and 'unscientific' have enjoyed popularity among their critics. Matthew Ramsey opens this volume with an analysis of how educated eighteenth- and nineteenth-century observers successively reported on magical healing and witchcraft in France. Although in the eighteenth century practitioners of witchcraft and magical healing were depicted as cynical unbelievers – 'swindlers' – and their patients as 'dupes', this Enlightenment interpretation was in the nineteenth century joined by another, ethnological and more romantic view of 'popular medicine' as an autonomous domain where indigenous practitioners, themselves believers, enjoyed a relative legitimacy, as healer–believers rather than healer–deceivers. Another interesting late nineteenth-century French example is presented by Sarah Ferber. She shows how Jean-Martin Charcot and his colleagues translated seventeenth-century interpretations of demonic possession into explanations of hysteria among female patients at the Salpêtrière, thus exchanging one label for another.

In a sense the twentieth-century debate on the 'disenchantment of the world' has carried on the Enlightenment tradition of labelling in terms of rational and irrational, measured by what were considered to be the norms of science. Although by no means immutable these norms have been very much the expression of the predominant mechanistic world view. Attempts to marginalize and disqualify alternative conceptions of illness and healing as irrational and possibly detrimental deviations from academic medicine form part of this tradition. These concerns have been manifested in the crusades of the Dutch Society Against Quackery, founded in 1880 and active to this day, along with many similar organizations. However, labelling alternative medical conceptions as irrational has not only offended their adherents, but also increasingly worried their historians.

Concern with the issue of the rationality of past notions of illness and healing is reflected in this volume. As Stuart Clark explains, a belief or action is rational if reasons for it can be given 'which both the giver(s) and receiver(s) accept as well grounded, coherent and, in some sense, correct. Since standards of well groundedness, coherence and correctness change from context to context, so does reason giving and reason receiving and, thus, rationality'.[8] Clark shows that the belief that devils could cause disease was a rational belief in the context of university-generated learning in the later medieval and early modern period. In a similar way, Van Wetering demonstrates the rationality of *Winti* belief and ritual for female immigrants from Suriname to Amsterdam, a rationality which survived a huge geographical and cultural shift.

This being so, it should be said that what was considered rational in the one context – for example, a particular religious belief – could be rejected as being non-rational or irrational in another context, say learned medical discourse. There has certainly been no lack of contested issues in this respect, involving debate and conflict between different parties, and tensions and uncertainty for both healers and those seeking a cure. Gary Waite demonstrates this for Dutch spiritualists and Mennonites in the sixteenth and seventeenth centuries. They faced the dilemma of accepting the notion of diabolical interference in human affairs or a commonsense, naturalistic explanation of supposed magical events, including sickness. In their case the devil tasted defeat. Albrecht Burkardt and Willem Frijhoff each present in more detail spectacular seventeenth-century cases of sickness and healing, showing how the available explanatory repertoires were used and manipulated by the parties concerned, each case resulting in a dramatically different outcome for the leading figure. In one case the church authorities imposed their rationality, mingled with political ambitions, over what they labelled 'superstition', while in the other a shared rationality was developed between individual, community and church. Even where religion did not play a role, the cultural repertoires of patient and healer could coincide, as in the case of Cornelie Usborne's account of rational choice, when poor women in Weimar Germany sought abortion through lay practitioners rather than licensed doctors.

## THE CONSTRUCTION AND REPRODUCTION OF CULTURAL REPERTOIRES OF ILLNESS AND HEALING

Having thus far concentrated on *what* happened, we will now shift our attention to *why* things happened the way they did. By no means pretending to offer complete solutions, we will concentrate on a number of 'mechanisms' which can contribute to our understanding and explanation of past approaches to illness and healing.

Theoretical reflection as such has hardly been assigned a prominent place on the agenda of medical history or the social history of medicine.[9] Recent articles by Ludmilla Jordanova and John Harley Warner may, it is to be hoped, mark a turning point in this respect.[10] Much as they have to offer by way of theoretical reflection, they pay little attention to the formulation of questions from a methodological point of view. Warner rightly recommends comparison across national, regional, or class boundaries – and one might as well add religious, gender, and time boundaries – as a means to identify the issues which need to be explained.[11] But we should also be aware of the rather neglected problem of formulating sufficiently specific questions to explain past approaches to illness and healing and of designing a strategy for comparative research in order to offer answers or explanations.[12] Questions of a too general nature tend to be met by general answers.

Although the essays in this volume all focus on specific problems – and most of them go beyond the descriptive level – there is a common denominator, namely the interest in how and why particular people or groups came to conceive and explain illness, and reacted to it in the way they did. In other words: how and why have cultural repertoires of illness and healing been constructed and reproduced?[13] While this is certainly not a specific question, it does denote the field and the types of questions with which we are concerned here, though seeking answers to these questions is no simple matter. It is therefore important to discuss a number of 'mechanisms' – in the sense of how things work or rather how people function – which are described in this volume as crucial to our understanding and which provide possible explanations of continuity and change within these cultural repertoires. These 'mechanisms' are trust, language and the medical market. Trust, or for that matter distrust, is an important psychological mechanism for assessing knowledge claims; language is as an important instrument for conveying knowledge claims; while the medical market, conceived as an economic and a sociological construct, is an important forum for presenting and practically demonstrating knowledge claims.

## The mechanism of trust

Truth is very much a matter of trust, as has recently and very convincingly been shown by Steven Shapin for the world of gentlemen philosophers in seventeenth-century England.[14] What people believe to be true depends to a large extent on their trust in the people who make or support particular knowledge claims. Trust engenders states of 'belief', to be understood as assent to these claims.[15] How did trust function in relation to conceptions of illness and healing? Who trusted whom, with respect to what and why? Future research may profitably be directed to a more systematic analysis of these matters, considering past relations between trust and 'belief' as they can be found with, for example, different social strata, sexes or institutional domains.

The essays in this volume all contribute to this type of analysis in one way or another, some of them concentrating on learned or at least educated discourse (Ramsey, Clark, Waite, Burkardt, Ferber, Gijswijt-Hofstra), while others focus on the beliefs of ordinary people (Usborne, Perdiguero, Bennett, Van Wetering) or on a combination of the two (Frijhoff, De Waardt). These essays show that people to be trusted were often from one's own, or a (slightly) higher, social background. Why trust was placed or not with these individuals, or why they were considered no longer trustworthy – whether doctors or healers – is often difficult to determine. Obviously, professional success – 'seeing is believing' – could greatly enhance trust in a healer and the therapy used by him or her, as is shown with respect to irregular healers in eighteenth-century

Holland (De Waardt), nineteenth-century conversions to homoeopathy (Gijswijt-Hofstra), alternative healers in nineteenth- and twentieth-century Spain (Perdiguero) and twentieth-century abortionists (Usborne). The reputation of a successful healer could also become contested, as Burkardt demonstrates with the case of Sophia Agnes van Langenberg who was finally labelled as a witch by the church authorities.

The relationship between trust and 'belief' is not a simple one. Trust can be furthered by a common 'belief', whether religious or otherwise. Belief in 'tradition', for example, in the healing powers of *Winti* ritual (Van Wetering), directs trust towards those sharing and promoting this belief. Belief in demonic interference in human affairs, as generated at universities in the later medieval and early modern period (Clark), directed trust to those propagating this belief rather than to those who were sceptical. Belief in 'scientific' medicine as taught in the nineteenth and the twentieth centuries tended to block trust towards those who advocated alternative ideas and therapies. In fact, the mutual reinforcement of trust and 'belief' tends to result in continuity, while change implies first the development of new ideas or practices or the reinterpretation of older notions, and only after that an acceptance through mediation by those one trusts. It should be noted that the essays in this volume tend to contribute more to our understanding of the continuity of cultural repertoires of illness and healing than to our understanding of change. In particular, the abandonment of formerly favoured repertoires, such as witchcraft or demonology, deserves further attention.

## The mechanism of language

Language is an important instrument for conveying knowledge claims and, one might add, for contesting them as well. But language is more than just the tool to express what one feels; it also structures the perception of speakers because they are confined to the boundaries of the concepts which are imbedded in the words they use. Any speakers who want to go beyond these boundaries, will soon be in great difficulties with others who will be unable to understand them.

The essays cover a wide range of 'languages' to describe and explain sickness, from early modern demonology to 'bosom serpents' or the *Winti* of the twentieth century. Metaphors such as the bosom serpents (Bennett) or teething, a *cause* of infant death according to popular conceptions in late nineteenth-century Alicante (Perdiguero), obviously had a conservative function. Apart from these metaphors which represent *a* language of sickness, we are also confronted with *the* language of sickness, namely when sickness and health were themselves being used as metaphors, for example as metaphors of a spiritual destiny, suggested in the case of the conversion of the Dutch orphan boy Evert Willemsz in seventeenth-century Holland (Frijhoff). Of course language was also frequently used for labelling the ideas and practices of others as untrue or undesirable. Thus, language could be instrumental in legitimating one's own repertoire of illness and healing, and in rejecting what deviated from this. Healers often tried to strengthen their claim to knowledge by using jargon or Latin terminology. It must have been difficult for many of their patients to understand them, certainly if the healer was a stranger and addressed them in a foreign language, like the Englishman John Taylor who repeatedly toured the Netherlands in the eighteenth century (De Waardt).

Nevertheless, it appears that these linguistic difficulties were not a major problem so long as the healer's words were compatible with the basic notions of his audience, so the use of a common cultural repertoire was an important condition for trust towards the healer (Usborne, Perdiguero, Bennett, Van Wetering). Indeed, healers could feel compelled to adjust the formulation of their diagnosis to what their patients expected from them (De Waardt). That language is by no means an unambiguous instrument for conveying meaning is further demonstrated by the retrospective medicine of the Salpêtrière school, which claimed past possessions to be cases of hysteria. Further research into the different uses of language by the sick, their healers and other interested parties is called for if we wish to gain a better understanding of how illness and healing have been constructed and reproduced.

## The mechanism of the medical market

In its broadest economic and sociological sense the medical market, as a forum for presenting and practically demonstrating knowledge claims, refers to relations of exchange between healers and clients, and to competition between healers.[16] Economic factors were important in determining choices and actions but so were other considerations, such as the esteem one would get or the expectation of a service which could be offered in return. The concept of the medical market can be used as a heuristic device for mapping the interaction between the supply of and the demand for all kinds of medical services in a particular region and at a particular time.

The continuity and change of the cultural repertoires of illness and healing can be regarded in terms of the success or failure of competing knowledge claims. We therefore need to know who made which claims, to whom they were directed and how they were received. We need to understand the role of doctors and healers compared to other groups, primarily their potential clients, but also the church, secular authorities and representatives of scientific culture.

Although the medical market concept as such does not figure prominently in this volume, it has certainly inspired many of the authors to consider competing medical knowledge claims with this concept in mind. The success of such claims was partly a function of the dynamics of the medical market, which in its turn was subjected to varying degrees of regulation by the authorities. The case of irregular healers in eighteenth-century Holland (De Waardt) clearly shows the complex interplay between these irregular healers, their patients and the magistrates as they were advised by medical doctors and sometimes also by patients. The essay on abortion practices in Weimar Germany (Usborne) explains the relative popularity of female 'quack' abortionists as opposed to male doctors in terms of trust, based on gender, social and cultural distance, and behaviour. The success of particular medical knowledge claims could obviously in large part be determined by what may be called 'external' considerations. The medical market was the arena where the effectiveness and success of a bid for trust and of the language that was used to ask for trust, were put to the test. Whether a cultural repertoire of illness was accepted by other people could only be established at this meeting point between healers, patients and other interested parties.

## The problem of using separate mechanisms

It is a source of regret that gender as a criterion influencing the status of the practitioner and in steering choices for patients has not emerged more strongly in this volume. Ferber and Van Wetering, however, point to gender claims. Ferber highlights the subjective observations of the Salpêtrière medical men of their female hysterical patients, while Van Wetering discusses the rigorously female *Winti* culture, which strongly influenced interactions between patients and healers. Perhaps we should be wary of the difficulties and dangers of attempting to distil out and separate criteria. As Usborne shows, it may not be possible or meaningful to separate gender considerations from those of social class, geographical distance and shared culture. Bennett also indicates the close interrelation between gender and other cultural claims on patients in seeking healers. The dangers of distillation apply not just to gender, but to the other categories discussed; often we are not talking about the patients' view and the healers' tactics but a shared culture, a shared language, a shared view of the medical market, convenience and familiarity rather than an act of choosing.

Having begun this introduction with problems of enchantment and disenchantment and having ended with problems of interpretation, we only hope that the ways in which these are presented here will lead to further reflection and research. Whether the cultural repertoires of illness and healing have become disenchanted or not, so much is sure – that much of this past world is still hidden to us.

## NOTES

1 Keith Thomas, *Religion and the Decline of Magic: Studies in Popular Beliefs in Sixteenth- and Seventeenth-Century England* (London, 1971). See also Jonathan Barry, M. Hester and G. Roberts (eds), *Witchcraft in Early Modern Europe: Studies in Culture and Belief* (Cambridge, 1996).

2 Recently by Robert W. Scribner in 'The Reformation, popular magic and the "disenchantment of the world" ', *Journal of Interdisciplinary History*, 23 (1993): 475–94. See also Robin Briggs, *Witches and Neighbours: The Social and Cultural Context of European Witchcraft* (London, 1996), pp. 377–81.

3 See, for example, the discussion between Hildred Geertz and Keith Thomas in 'An anthropology of religion and magic', *Journal of Interdisciplinary History*, 6 (1975): 71–89, 91–109.

4 Scribner, 'The Reformation'; Richard Kieckhefer, 'The specific rationality of medieval magic', *American Historical Review*, 99 (1994): 813–36; Willem de Blécourt, 'On the continuation of witchcraft' and Robin Briggs, ' "Many reasons why": witchcraft and the problem of multiple explanation', in Barry, Hester and Roberts (eds), *Witchcraft in Early Modern Europe*, pp. 49–63, 335–52.

5 See De Blécourt, 'On the continuation of witchcraft', pp. 337–8.

6 Valerie I.J. Flint, *The Rise of Magic in Early Medieval Europe* (Princeton, NJ, 1991).

7 See also Mark S. Micale, *Approaching Hysteria: Disease and its Interpretations* (Princeton, NJ, 1995); Sander Gilman, Helen King,

Roy Porter, George Rousseau and E. Showalter, *Hysteria Before Freud* (Berkeley, CA, 1995).

8 See Stuart Clark's chapter in this volume, p. 46.

9 See Ludmilla Jordanova, 'Has the social history of medicine come of age?', *The Historical Journal*, 36 (1993): 437–49.

10 Ludmilla Jordanova, 'The social construction of medical knowledge', *Social History of Medicine*, 8 (1995): 361–81; John Harley Warner, 'The history of science and the sciences of medicine', *OSIRIS*, 10 (1995): 164–93.

11 Warner, 'The history of science', p. 183.

12 As R.M. MacIver wrote: 'It is sometimes nearly as difficult to define our problem as to solve it'; R.M. MacIver, *Social Causation* (Gloucester, MA, 1973), p. 376.

13 See Jordanova, 'The social construction' for a recent discussion of social constructivist approaches. However, the adjective 'social', or for that matter 'cultural', seems superfluous in this context.

14 Steven Shapin, *A Social History of Truth: Civility and Science in Seventeenth-Century England* (Chicago and London, 1994).

15 Ibid., pp. xxiii, 8.

16 See, for instance, Lucinda M. Beier, *Sufferers and Healers: The Experience of Illness in Seventeenth-Century England* (London and New York, 1987) and Matthew Ramsey, *Professional and Popular Medicine in France, 1770–1830* (Cambridge, 1988), who analyzes interactions between patients and healers primarily in terms of a network.

Chapter 1

# Magical healing, witchcraft and elite discourse in eighteenth- and nineteenth-century France

*Matthew Ramsey*

In his classic study of magistrates and witches in seventeenth-century France, Robert Mandrou describes how a growing reluctance to accept the demonic origin of witchcraft practices led in 1682 to a royal edict that virtually ended prosecutions for witchcraft in secular courts. Previously, following a tradition that remained entrenched in some provincial jurisdictions, persons suspected of causing harm through witchcraft could be brought before a royal magistrate and charged with *sortilèges* and *maléfices* (acts of witchcraft and the casting of evil spells). Even those who had performed seemingly more innocent actions, such as reciting incantations to lift spells or treat illness, might also be charged with using diabolical arts. What these practices had in common was that they were believed to depend on the intervention of the devil or his agents. To indulge in them was to defy God, and no less so than the acts described in the demonological literature which more explicitly involved commerce with the devil, such as an overt pact, sexual intercourse with demons or participation in a witches' sabbath – behaviours that the prosecutors in any case readily attributed to the defendants. Hence the charge, sometimes levelled in French courts, of divine *lèse majesté*.

Although the edict of 1682 was presented as a measure for punishing cunning folk, magicians, witches and poisoners, the body of the text never explicitly treated 'witchcraft' as an offence, nor did it even use the word. What had once been the crime of witchcraft was now only 'so-called magic'. Under the provisions of the edict and earlier French law, those who used spells and conjurations could still be prosecuted, as could those who purported to lift the spells cast by others. But they would be charged with offences such as fraud, sacrilege and blasphemy, poisoning, or possibly even unauthorized medical practice. Persons who brought accusations of witchcraft against their enemies might be charged with defamation. The edict reflected a world view in which the active presence of the devil had become vanishingly small and 'witches' were to be treated as the victims of delusions or as tricksters seeking to exploit the credulity of others.[1] The celebrated affair of the Jesuit priest Jean-Baptiste Girard, accused in 1730 of using sorcery to harm Marie-Catherine Cadière, who had been under his spiritual direction, was the last major witchcraft case in France and definitively confirmed that French jurisprudence no longer recognized witchcraft as a criminal offence.[2] Although the church continued to admit the real (though rare) possibility of commerce with the devil, the educated laity increasingly denied it together with divination, magical healing and other practices that putatively depended on the intervention of supernatural or preternatural forces.

The end of official prosecutions forms a major topic in the history of witchcraft in early modern Europe. With some variations, the standard narratives generally point to the process of 'disenchantment' associated with the scientific revolution and later with the Enlightenment in conjunction with other factors specific to the witch hunts, such as the judiciary's dissatisfaction with the methods of criminal procedure followed in the trials.[3] In addition to witchcraft, this large cultural transformation affected a wide range of other practices and beliefs, particularly the arts of astrology and what we would now call magical medicine – that is, the manipulation of preternatural forces by a human agent to prevent, diagnose, prognosticate or, above all, cure disease.[4] Because it shaped the thinking of the educated classes but left the greater mass of the population largely untouched, this shift in outlook contributed to the growing divorce between popular and elite culture in the seventeenth and eighteenth centuries.[5]

The conclusion of one story is the beginning of another: the evolution of elite discourse on witchcraft and magical healing in the period following what Mandrou calls the 'retreat of Satan'[6] and the withdrawal of the state from witchcraft prosecutions. The end of prosecutions did not mean that the population as a whole had ceased to believe in witchcraft and magic or to engage in magical practices intended to lift spells or cure disease. Nor did educated observers cease to reflect on these phenomena, even after the urgency of the trials had passed. They continued to debate the reasons for their persistence and the stance that non-believers should adopt towards them. The basic outlines of this story are familiar. We know the Enlightenment scepticism of Voltaire and the Benedictine monk Benito Feijóo, the romantic fascination with witchcraft and magic shared by Sir Walter Scott and Prosper Mérimée (to cite just four totemic examples), and the development in the middle decades of the nineteenth century of folklore studies which purported to present these practices and beliefs as objects of neither scorn nor exaltation but of scientific description and analysis. But the question of elite discourse in the period after the last trials has received less attention than the 'decline of witchcraft' and it is worth revisiting, not least because it may help us reflect on how we ourselves talk about both the believers and the sceptics.

In this essay, I will use the French example to highlight some of the remarkably static features of elite discourse on witchcraft and magical healing. These predated the seventeenth-century turn from witchcraft prosecutions and survived both the nineteenth-century rediscovery of the folk and the development of positivist ethnography. I will also briefly explore where we may stand in relation to this tradition. In so doing, I do not mean to challenge the basic framework (just summarized) for interpreting the decline of witchcraft and its aftermath. Let us instead take this as a point of departure, while recognizing that the last generation of scholarship on seventeenth-century science has developed a more nuanced and complex account of the relationship between the new mechanical philosophy and older traditions concerning the occult, the spirit world, witchcraft and magic.[7]

I also ask the reader, for the purposes of this exercise, to accept several other premises. First, the broad distinction between elite and popular culture, which has been widely and often convincingly criticized,[8] but which for present purposes works well enough as a convenient shorthand. The critics of witchcraft and magical healing associated them with 'the people', by which they meant the uneducated masses, though some noted that they had their adherents among the cultivated elites and that the term 'people' should be construed broadly enough to include the deluded of all ranks and stations. Second, the distinction between magical and natural forms of healing. The labels that we now often apply to various forms of folk medicine – 'religious', 'magical', 'empirical' – would have been almost meaningless to those who practised them. Prayers might accompany the application of an ointment; herbs might have to be gathered on an appointed day, following certain hallowed rituals.

All remedies were, in a sense, empirical; they happened to have curative properties known from experience. For the educated commentators who wrote about these practices, however, the distinction was often crucial. Third and last, the notion of a widely shared 'discourse' constructed from a shared fund of terms, concepts, arguments and rhetorical devices. The expression is not used here in a technical sense; as will be quickly apparent, this essay is an empirical account of a tradition rather than an exercise in Foucauldian discourse analysis.

The discussion will focus on magical healing and related practices, including counter-witchcraft, rather than diabolism or the putative causing of harm through *maleficium*. This choice perhaps requires a few words of explanation. It has been shown that 'black' and 'white' witchcraft were closely linked in the prosecutions carried out in the sixteenth and seventeenth centuries in such regions as Lorraine and the Jura mountains;[9] theologians and jurists commonly lumped together as witches and Satan's henchmen all those who used occult arts, including practitioners of magical healing and *devins-guérisseurs* (cunning folk) who claimed to counteract the spells that witches had cast on their patients. Sceptics, too, tended to conflate all such practices, not as evidence of diabolical agency but as delusions. In French usage, the same term – *sorcier* or *sorcière* – was applied indiscriminately to those who cast spells, those who lifted them and even magician–healers in general, also known in some regions as *maiges* or *mèges*. Even so the distinction pervaded popular culture, and if one takes the long view, a secular shift in emphasis becomes apparent.

The sixteenth- and seventeenth-century trials could not have sustained their momentum without a succession of witches who had publicly admitted to making a pact with the devil and casting spells, however one may judge the sincerity of confessions extracted under torture or the place of diabolism in popular culture as opposed to learned demonology.[10] In subsequent periods, however, though witchcraft accusations continued at the village level – despite the efforts of the authorities to discourage them – there were virtually no self-professed practitioners of 'black' witchcraft. Harm caused by witchcraft – for those who believed in it – was either secret or involuntary and unconscious.[11] There were still, however, acknowledged counter-witches and magical healers, many of whom claimed a gift not from the devil but from God, and whom the elites had to confront as a real social presence. They attracted particularly close attention from medical practitioners, who saw them as rivals, especially for rural patients, and an obstacle to their larger project of professionalizing health care. Physicians arguably replaced the clergy as the closest observers of magical healing, which they described and denounced in texts intended for colleagues, administrators and often a broader public among the educated laity.

## THE SCEPTICAL DISCOURSE ON WITCHCRAFT AND MAGICAL HEALING IN THE SIXTEENTH AND SEVENTEENTH CENTURIES

In the early modern texts that figure as the *loci classici* for discussions of the decline of witchcraft beliefs in elite culture, from Wier in the mid-sixteenth century to Spee, Cyrano de Bergerac, Malebranche, Bekker and Bayle, a central theme is the search for alternative explanations for the experience of feeling bewitched or possessed by demons, or the memory of having participated in commerce with the devil. Some writers, such as Spee, were equally preoccupied with the procedural defects of witchcraft prosecutions. Many continued (or professed) to believe in the influence of the devil – if only on the imagination – and even in the occasional existence of witchcraft. Here the devil appears essentially as deceiver and impostor.[12] However, it is the sceptical elements, which seem to adumbrate the later positivist account of the witchcraft phenomenon, that have given these texts their canonical status.

The application of Occam's razor led to several naturalistic explanations which we might now label psychological, physiological and sociological. The first included mental illness (the physician Wier stressed the role of melancholia) and an overactive imagination, whose powers Montaigne analyzed in a celebrated essay,[13] and which the Cartesian Oratorian Malebranche saw, together with an irrational human need to be frightened, as the driving force behind the whole witchcraft phenomenon. The second type of explanation pointed to physical disease, debility and the use of mind-altering drugs (mentioned by both Malebranche and Cyrano). The third adduced the ignorance and folly of the unlettered peasantry; Malebranche and Cyrano singled out silly shepherds as fomenters of witchcraft beliefs. Witchcraft, in short, was a delusion and its victims fitter objects for medical attention than legal prosecution – a first, and critical, step in the medicalization of elite discourse on witchcraft and magic as a whole. Physicians also contributed in another way to the demystification of witchcraft phenomena by offering medical explanations of conditions, such as sexual impotence, commonly attributed to spells.[14]

So, witchcraft delusions in themselves were an involuntary affliction to which those considered weak of mind were most susceptible. Most commentators reflexively cited peasants, children and women, though even educated men, it was believed, could be led astray – Monsieur Oufle, the protagonist of Bordelon's long novel of 1710 detailing the effects of a disordered imagination, is the victim of his compulsive reading of books on witchcraft, magic and the occult.[15] Such delusions, however, owed their strength and persistence to the voluntary actions of others. Bekker, for example, linked the vitality of popular superstition to the work of cunning folk and counter-witches who stood to profit from it. Whereas those who falsely believed themselves bewitched or possessed or imagined that they had commerce with the devil might best be deemed victims of their own illusions and *naïveté*, those who practised divining, counter-witchcraft and the like could more appropriately be considered criminals, guilty not of sorcery but of fraud.

Taken together, these arguments in a sense secularized the demonological model, with its dynamic of human weakness, temptation and imposture. Here, irrationality displaced sin and the human trickster supplanted Satan as the great deceiver. The sceptics' emphasis on the victims' heightened suggestibility may also remind us that the witch hunters similarly allowed for a psychological element: superstitious credulity opened the way for Satan to perform his false miracles. For example, the magistrate Pierre de Lancre, one of the most ferocious prosecutors of witches in early seventeenth-century France, accepted the opinion that no witch healer would be effective with a patient who had a poor opinion of him or his therapy.[16]

Sceptical analyses of witchcraft and magic drew more directly, however, on two other intersecting discourses, both clearly defined by the end of the sixteenth century and both closely related to medicine. These were the rhetoric against popular errors and against quacks. The literature on popular errors comprised two key sub-genres: post-Tridentine works on religious superstitions, which attempted to distinguish what the authors generally considered pagan beliefs and practices from orthodox doctrine and ritual;[17] and the series of treatises on vulgar errors in medicine inaugurated by

Laurent Joubert, dean of the medical faculty of Montpellier.[18] These works condemned many widespread beliefs and techniques, the latter typically applied by the people themselves rather than supplied as a service by persons claiming special expertise.

The same shift in outlook that led clergymen like Bekker to oppose witchcraft prosecutions produced a convergence of theological and medical rhetoric on superstition and popular error. Not just the devil as a real agency in the physical world, but even demonic influences on the imagination played a diminishing role. A fair representative of the theological genre in its earlier form is the treatise on superstitions by the abbé Thiers, first published a few years before the edict of 1682 and richly illustrated with material taken from personal observation as well as the scholarly literature. Although wary of unwarranted accusations of witchcraft and magic, Thiers readily accepted the intervention of the devil in human affairs. Many incantations did, indeed, work, through the medium of 'bad angels'; thus it might, in fact, be possible to make warts disappear by saying 'good morning' to them in the morning and 'good evening' to them in the evening. So convinced was he of the efficacy of such charms that Thiers, like many others who wrote on the subject, sometimes omitted part of a healing formula or the name of the disease for which it was recommended in order to defeat his reader's sinful curiosity.[19]

Thiers' work on superstitions continued to be reprinted at least until 1777. It came to be valued, however, more as a source of amusement than as a work of theology and it yielded pride of place to a treatise by the Oratorian Pierre Le Brun, a *critical* history of superstitious practices first published in 1702, which, according to a later editor, won approval from both theologians and philosophers.[20] Le Brun still accepted in principle that the devil could intervene in the physical world, but whenever possible he sought natural explanations of seemingly magical occurrences; his reputation owed much to the discussion of Jacques Aymar and his celebrated divining rod with which he opened his treatise and in which he displayed a good grasp of the principles of physics. If the convergence between theological and enlightened medical discourse remained incomplete in the eighteenth century, it was largely because the most radical of the sceptics stood the traditional critiques of superstition on their head so that revealed and established religion itself became an error, the prejudice or superstition *par excellence*. The extreme statement of this view appeared in the work of the baron d'Holbach.[21]

The second discourse, on charlatanism, excoriated quacks for depriving the people of their wealth, health, and very existence, and for infringing on the physicians' and surgeons' legitimate livelihood. The quack was a bad citizen, unwilling to accept his assigned social station and economic role. He was lazy, mendacious and generally immoral, with a talent chiefly for deceiving and exploiting the weakness of others to serve his own material interests. Elements of these complaints can be traced back to the late Middle Ages when medicine first began to emerge as an organized profession, but the first extended polemics date, like the corpus of writings on popular errors, from the late sixteenth century, when the word 'charlatan' first came into common use.[22] Their authors, predominantly physicians and surgeons, sought to use the new medium of print in the contest for control of the growing medical marketplace of the market towns and cities.

The discourse on charlatanism and the discourse on popular errors were closely linked. The first condemned quacks for, among other offences, leading the people into error (some of the earlier texts on charlatanism even called quackery diabolical).[23] Conversely, the errors corpus held that error flourished in large part because unscrupulous impostors exploited the credulity of the unfortunate populace. Although the texts on error typically focused on the peasantry (it is no coincidence that the word 'pagan' derives from the Latin word for rustic), whereas texts on quacks focused on the mountebank who peddled his wares in the urban marketplace, the two overlapped in crucial ways. With the withdrawal of the devil, magical healing was increasingly represented as an encounter between quackery and error, cynic and fool, in a space where urban and rural intersected.

## WITCHCRAFT AND MAGICAL HEALING IN THE ENLIGHTENMENT

The *philosophes* of the French Enlightenment defined themselves explicitly as the adversaries of superstition and charlatanism in the broadest senses of those terms. They helped inspire a practical campaign of reform that included, in the medical domain, efforts to regulate the trade in 'secret' remedies, to promote consultations with qualified practitioners and discourage recourse to empirics, and to foster more appropriate forms of self-help where the services of regular medical personnel were unavailable – such as by publishing 'enlightened' versions of popular medical handbooks.[24]

In this undertaking, the reduction of counter-witchcraft and magical healing to charlatanism-sustained-by-popular-error was a crucial rhetorical move; even now it remains most closely associated with the Enlightenment project and its self-proclaimed rational scepticism. Thus Jean d'Iharce's treatise on popular medical errors cynically described how *devins* avoided saying 'that they have, like the witches, a pact with the Devil, in order to discover the authors of the spells they wish to cure . . . but they make every effort to suggest it and never fail . . . They put into play all sorts of superstitions to entice those who are idiotic enough to consult them'.[25] To be sure, the medical elite found many such practitioners as coarse and ignorant as their patients. The Breton physician Chifoliau characterized the 'witch of Pontorson', a well-known healer in his district, as a 'silly old woman'; his colleague Gastellier, in Bas-Poitou, described a vintner–urinoscopist who claimed to have a gift from God as 'the coarsest and most inept sort of yokel, who barely knows his right hand from his left'.[26] But the commentators rarely conceded that the healers might themselves believe in their own practices; unlike their patients, they were fully cognizant of what they were doing and must have known that it was a sham.

The parallel with the marketplace mountebank did not end here. Like the quacks, it was said, village healers were both mercenary and dangerous, taking their victims' resources and undermining their health. Local physicians and surgeons regularly complained of popular practitioners who claimed to act charitably but in fact accepted money or gifts.[27] Moreover, the most active local *maiges*, who typically used potentially toxic herbal remedies, seemed as murderous as the urban hawker of noxious drugs. For one colleague of Chifoliau, the tisanes of the witch of Pontorson 'caused as much devastation in this canton as the plague in Turkey'.[28] Like quacks, healers were also called shiftless – too lazy to live by honest labour – and immoral.

A few medical men, it is true, closely observed popular healers at work and what they saw could challenge their preconceptions. The physician Jean-Emmanuel Gilibert, who became mayor of Lyon during the Revolution, had spent several years in the countryside early in his career and believed that his devotion to his calling compelled him to study popular medical practices. He found that some of the healers whom he came to know sincerely believed that they owed their powers to a gift from God.[29] One can also make out the beginnings of an approach to popular medicine that went beyond the synchronic analysis of error to a historical account of the sources of contemporary beliefs and practices. For many scholars, the rustic was also the primitive. For some physicians, the peasantry was like a museum that had preserved remnants of older medical systems: either the 'superstitious' medicine of Gallo–Roman times, or, for at least one writer with a Rousseauist bent, the truly philosophical medicine of natural man, Théophile de Bordeu, the celebrated physiologist and physician of the Paris Charité Hospital, thought he could hear the aphorisms of Hippocrates, which themselves expressed the voice of Nature, issuing from the mouths of peasants. They seemed to have more wisdom to teach him than his professors at Montpellier.[30]

At least some of the elements existed that would have made it possible to replace the old distinction between supernatural and natural healing with a new one based on cultural difference, but no novel discourse on magical healing emerged in the eighteenth century. It was the rare commentator who recognized that a local *maige* (unlike the itinerant empiric) might well flourish because she or he shared, rather than simply exploited, the local belief system. Indeed, unlike Joubert, who had extensively recorded proverbs as well as popular beliefs and practices, the majority of the enlightened physicians showed little curiosity about the details of peasant culture. Their motives were more utilitarian: they sought to avert the harmful consequences of error.

## THE NINETEENTH CENTURY

For the nineteenth-century heirs of the Enlightenment, the purported practice of magical healing remained a special case of charlatanism. The author of one work on medical 'abuses' published under the Restoration found the notions of charlatanism, on the one hand, and of magic charms and spells on the other, 'perfectly identical'.[31] An essay on medical errors that appeared during the July Monarchy suggested that 'these prejudices would have been forgotten long ago if the charlatans, witches, bonesetters and old wives who exploit them had not maintained and propagated them'.[32]

As the century matured, the development of positivism and of scientism as an ideology encouraged new explanations of how healers tricked their clients but little interest in going beyond the old moral explanations of why they behaved as they did. At the end of the century, a study of the Morvan region in the Massif Central treated healers as humbugs. Their fakery, the author suggested, had been exposed by physicians who had treated them as patients and won their confidence, or who had simply observed their techniques. According to a colleague, witches' magic formulas were not only a ridiculous superstition; in many cases, they did not actually know any and simply recited some unintelligible phrases. 'The stupider people seem,' he reported one of them as saying, 'the more I overdo it'.[33]

Occasionally, it is true, the remedy of the *maige* seemed to work, but this outcome could be attributed, as always, to the patient's confidence in it. This phenomenon, it was said, might be observed even among educated people.[34] Theories of psychosomatic medicine enabled physicians to explain with ever greater sophistication how magical formulas could cure warts through 'suggestion' or how prayer and the shared ecstasy of a mass pilgrimage could produce some of the dramatic cures seen at Lourdes. Charcot's reflections on hysteria and the role of belief in faith healing make fascinating reading.[35]

Positivism absorbed, adapted and perpetuated the old discourses on quackery and popular error. However, it is possible to trace the spread of a new ethnological curiosity among some members of the professional elites – though their stance was usually quite consistent with a *philosophe*'s contempt for the delusions of the uneducated. Physicians participated in the programme of ethnographic research, the origins of which are customarily traced in France to three great surveys carried out in the Revolutionary and Napoleonic eras: the abbé Grégoire's investigation of patois (1790–91);[36] the *statistiques des préfets* of the Year IX (1800–01), followed by the more ambitious *Statistique générale de la France*, a vast official collection of information on the different *départements*;[37] and the questionnaire published in 1807 by the fledgling Académie Celtique (1805–13; replaced by the *Société des Antiquaires de France*), which took as its mission to recover whatever evidence it could of a Celtic–Gallic–French past distinct from the Graeco–Roman tradition.[38] All these surveys elicited information on popular medical beliefs, although only the prefects showed much interest in the behaviour of individual healers. The prevailing tone was the by now familiar one of disabused scepticism.

Work of this sort inspired a rapid growth of descriptive ethnography and contributed to the emergence of what we would now call the folklore movement in France, though the term 'folklore', coined in 1846 by the British antiquarian William John Thoms, had no exact equivalent in French. Its mixed heritage is apparent in the sometimes incongruous language of the mid-nineteenth-century texts. Thus in 1856, the marquis de Chesnel could publish a *Dictionary of Popular Superstitions, Errors, Prejudices, and Traditions* which, despite its unfriendly title, was an ethnographic compendium written with considerable sympathy for its subject. Like the German Romantics and their French disciples, Chesnel hoped to spark an interest in the national past; French antiquities were as worthy of study as the fables of the ancients, and equally 'poetic'. The facts might be false, but the feelings were true. One hears echoes here, not of the dominant Enlightenment discourse on errors, but of Rousseau.[39]

In the medical field, the nineteenth-century output of works on popular beliefs and practices is impressive; by the time of the July Monarchy the topic had even become an accepted subject of theses for the medical doctorate. In 1831, for example, J. Borianne published one of the first dissertations devoted to the popular medicine of a region, a study of the department of the Haute-Vienne, in the old province of Limousin.[40] Nearly all these texts could be called derivative, having been written in the shadow of the major treatise entitled, significantly, *On Popular Errors Relating to Medicine*, published in 1810 by Anthelme Richerand, a disciple of the celebrated physician-cum-philosopher Georges Cabanis and professor of surgical pathology at the Paris Faculty of Medicine.[41] No work of equal stature was to appear afterwards. For decades, most writers on these themes were conscious of participating in a long tradition that reached back to Richerand and ultimately to Joubert, the sixteenth-century founder of the genre.[42]

To a larger extent than their eighteenth-century predecessors, the nineteenth-century authors published the results of systematic local observation; Richerand, for example, cited folk practices from his native department of the Ain. Some, like Borianne and J.-Charles Voisin, had trained in Paris and then set up a practice in their home provinces – Brittany, in Voisin's case – which they observed with the keen eye of the returned expatriate.[43] Like Joubert, physicians began to listen to the *vox populi*; one thesis, written in 1808, dealt entirely with medical proverbs.[44] By the beginning of the next century, the output included some ambitious studies – such as Darmezin's work of 1904 on Touraine and Kaufmann's 1906 treatise on Poitou – which displayed considerable intellectual curiosity and attention to ethnographic detail. Darmezin painstakingly noted parallels between ancient Italian popular medicine, as recorded by Pliny, and current practices in Touraine; for example, snails were still mixed with human milk to form a remedy, as Pliny had described. Kaufmann used local archives to document the antecedents of popular medical practices in Poitou.[45] The physicians were particularly fascinated by those aspects of popular medicine that were most alien to bourgeois propriety, such as remedies made from ear wax, urine and excrement, or popular attitudes towards sexuality. Kaufmann called attention to treatments for whitlow on the finger, which included wrapping the finger in a cloth steeped in human faeces, coiling an earthworm around it, and applying what he coyly called a 'vaginal cataplasm'.[46]

All of this may loosely follow from what Peter Burke has called the 'discovery of the people' in the late eighteenth and early nineteenth centuries.[47] However, it is not the romantic celebration of the popular, still less Michelet's radically democratic defence of a heavily mythologized witch healer as the people's champion against the depredations of the feudal nobility in the Middle Ages.[48] Nor should this surprise us. In their often doctored versions of peasant stories, proverbs, songs, dance and festivals, the Romantics generally sought an aesthetic alternative to Classicism and the cosmopolitan rationalism of the Enlightenment. In some places (chiefly in central and eastern Europe), they went in quest of the vestiges of a national past around which a modern nation could start to coalesce. A usually edulcorated version of traditional magic and witchcraft figured in all this as one inseparable aspect of the folk heritage, but for most educated Europeans mistaken beliefs about the natural world remained just that, even if some from their own social milieu consulted healers or astrologers or dabbled in spiritualism. A representative text, the *Françouneto* of Jacques Boé ('Jasmin') of Agen, written in 1840, derives from a local legend about an accused witch, and ultimately from an actual case, according to Emmanuel Le Roy Ladurie. It celebrates the language and traditions of Jasmin's native Gascony and bears many of the marks of romanticism. In the narrative, however, the accusations against Françouneto turn out to have been the result of trickery, concocted by a spurned suitor. Once the deception is revealed, her many disappointed admirers 'say to themselves: "Never again will we believe in sorcerers!" '.[49]

The less hostile treatments of popular medical practices were typically linked to the search for national antiquities, which presented a popular culture more archaic than stupid or depraved. Many commentators retained the notion of the peasantry as a sort of museum in which the medicine of another era was preserved. For Paul-Abraham Pesme, writing in 1855, certain beliefs and practices of the people recalled the 'ideas of the ancients', while for Edgar-Jean-Ernest Porcheron, writing after World War I, the popular medicine of Poitou was derived from the distant past, only 'a little changed . . . by its passage through the centuries'.[50] Amateur antiquarians among the physicians sought often largely mythical Gaulish roots for the practices they described. To one thesis writer, women in the Seine-et-Oise who danced around an oak tree muttering prayers as a cure for hernia recalled the tradition of the sacred oak among the Gauls. Although he speculated that the women might have earned money for performing this ritual, he seems to have accepted them as participants in a tradition, rather than swindlers who cynically exploited it.[51] Towards the end of the Restoration, Lecourt de Cantilly, a Breton physician who took a keen interest in local antiquities, produced an extensive analysis of possible archaic survivals in the local practice of scarification for a condition known as *les hunes*, the vague symptoms of which resemble those now associated with chronic fatigue syndrome. He suggested that the usage might derive from the Druid practice of scarifying the body and added a little excursus on human sacrifices made to the god Teutates.[52]

One indication of the less polemical tenor of such works was a semantic shift from the dyslogistic vocabulary of the Enlightenment ('prejudice', 'error', 'superstition') to more neutral terms such as 'popular medicine', 'popular remedies', and related phrases – though 'superstition' proved a particularly tenacious usage. 'Popular medicine' appeared in one isolated book title in 1824[53] and then sporadically during the first half of the Third Republic ('medical folklore' – *le folklore médical* – is a more recent coinage). By the end of the nineteenth century, a recent work squarely within the vulgar errors tradition might sit on the shelf next to a monograph in the spirit of a folklorist like Paul Sébillot.[54]

The overlapping discourses on popular error and popular medicine reflect, in part, the social experience of those who produced them. Texts in the latter vein often came from writers who saw traditional popular culture as having declined to the point of marginality. Practices that might once have seemed dangerous now seemed merely quaint; the obligation of the educated observer was less to condemn than to describe them as fully as possible in order to preserve for posterity some record of a fast-vanishing world. The veterinarian A. Jacqmart wrote in 1880 that errors now affected only 'weak minds' – a situation he attributed to a revolution in the countryside brought about by such agents of modernization as the press and the army.[55] In contrast, those rural physicians who saw their practice threatened by local traditions clung to the older way of talking about popular errors.

But we should not forget the overlap. The 'people' were different, but only in the sense that they represented a lower stage of development; they were, as one writer put it, like a 'grown-up child', easily deceived.[56] The explanations that the authors offered for the persistence of counter-witchcraft and popular healing were for the most part traditional: poverty, ignorance, weakness and fear of pain, combined with charlatanism. 'Popular errors' did not constitute a coherent culture; folk medical beliefs and practices were the fragmentary and often obscure remnants of older systems.[57] Chesnel could characterize witches as charlatans, while Lecourt de Cantilly, for all his fascination with Druid survivals, still described healers as 'exploiting public credulity', denying that more than a handful could themselves be 'blind enough' to believe that they were actually acting charitably and suggesting that healers for *les hunes* owed their reputation to the 'blind confidence of the people'. The Academy of Medicine's Commission on Medical Police adopted a report welcoming de Cantilly's paper on *les hunes* 'as one more fact to add to the history of popular errors, [which are] so fatal to humanity'.[58] Well into the Third Republic, most writers on popular medicine continued to regard the *maige* as a sort of confidence artist.

## A TWENTIETH-CENTURY PERSPECTIVE

This overview has suggested that the 'retreat of Satan' did not lead to a radically new discourse on witchcraft and magical healing. Drawing on rhetorical conventions reaching back to the

Renaissance, writers who embraced Enlightenment ideology routinely equated those who practised such techniques with the quacks who peddled worthless nostrums from stages in the markets and public squares. Both were essentially deceivers, with one difference, that the supposed *maige* exploited the vulgar errors of the most ignorant and superstitious part of the population, whereas the mountebank simply catered to the age-old human longing for cures for incurable diseases. On the question of the relationship between healing, magic and belief, Enlightenment discourse characteristically treated patients as believers ('dupes') and practitioners as cynical unbelievers ('swindlers'). For all their professed allegiance to the empirical method, commentators typically based their interpretation on an a priori line of reasoning: unlike those they treated, practitioners *must have known* that their methods did not work.

The Romantic conception of popular culture, without substantially weakening the scepticism of the educated elites, opened the way to the possibility that some healers, rather than cynically exploiting vulgar credulity, might themselves participate fully in a popular medical system – part of a cultural universe different from that of the Faculty, but equally coherent. As we now see it, to the extent that this alien culture offered a way of understanding the world and dealing with misfortune that made sense to those who shared it, the medical profession might have considered reaching an accommodation with it, rather than repressing it. The doctors might, in a word, have invented ethnomedicine. But, in the period that concerns us, they did not. At most, they offered the occasional suggestion that popular delusions might sometimes be indulged as a way of winning patients' confidence and their business, or of calming their anxiety. To think otherwise of magical healing required not simply more extensive observation of its practitioners, which tended to confirm pre-existing interpretations, but the development of an ethnological consciousness that could recognize a community of belief bound together by common ideas of illness and misfortune – a shared culture rather than the peculiar bond forged between the ignorant and the depraved.

In the twentieth century, as folklore studies have consolidated their position as an academic discipline, we have tended to embrace just such an ethnological consciousness: the 'true' folk healers are at one with their culture and must be understood on their own terms, not ours.[59] In the world of historical scholarship this approach substantially influenced the accounts of popular practices written 'from below', in the 1960s and 1970s, as well as some of the first attempts to create a feminist history of witchcraft, midwifery and women's health.[60] In the process, we have tended to exaggerate the unity of peasant culture and its radical separation from the world of the urban elites, borrowing too heavily from anthropological models based on smaller and simpler non-western societies. Witchcraft and magical healing, which lost their metaphysical authenticity three centuries ago, have regained a cultural authenticity that would have astonished Malebranche.

In our twentieth-century *fin de siècle*, we are perhaps witnessing the culmination of a more profound mutation of the ways in which we talk about these subjects than the transformations associated with the Enlightenment and Romanticism. Mutually reinforcing trends both in academe and in the larger culture militate against presenting the decline of witchcraft as an aspect of the progress of western civilization. In the university, various tendencies associated with the post-modern critique of the Enlightenment project – anti-foundationalism, multiculturalism, cultural anti-elitism and the democratic indictment of expertise, the campaign to recover suppressed voices – have progressively delegitimated the old discourses on quacks and error, while at the same time undermining any unified conception of popular culture. In many of these academic debates we can recognize some of the besetting preoccupations of western post-industrial culture in a post-colonial world. Educated elites have inverted and turned inwards the Enlightenment campaign against error, with intolerance and ethnocentrism supplanting ignorance and superstition as the cardinal sins of the intellectually and ethically aware. A much larger part of the population has become increasingly suspicious of science, technology and the medical profession, and increasingly attracted to alternative forms of spirituality and medicine.

This is not the place to comment directly on these too-familiar and much controverted signs of the times. Let me offer instead, by way of conclusion, several related reflections on the development of post-Enlightenment discourse on witchcraft and magical healing, which is as much and as little a story of progress as any other chapter in our cultural history. First, what might be called romantic ethnology undoubtedly rescued witch healers from a long tradition of condescension and accorded them the dignity of taking their own discourse seriously. But the healer regained authenticity only by virtue of becoming more radically other. The healer–deceiver had been, in a sense, the *philosophe*'s evil twin, himself a sceptic and immediately recognizable as the mirror image of the philanthropic champion of Enlightenment. The healer–believer belonged to another, generally quite static world, for which the writer could feel nostalgia or envy or even an aesthetic empathy, but which he could not directly enter or confront. Such an approach, embraced too enthusiastically, runs the risk of reducing its subjects from historical actors, like ourselves, with complex, dynamic and not always admirable motives, to static artefacts – museum pieces, really. We have history, they have culture.

Second, the ethnological discourse on believers, just as much as the Enlightenment discourse on swindlers, purported to offer a scientific account of unfamiliar and puzzling behaviour. Each, however, was grounded in an ideological subtext, arguing for or against modernity, and each depended on a characteristic distortion; one denied the very human capacity for faith while the other denied the equally human capacities for foolishness and the cynical pursuit of self-interest. Both could be called naïve.

Third and last, we have understandably tended to deplore the condescension implicit in the vulgar errors tradition and the rigid positivism of so many nineteenth-century commentators.[61] But we often bring to this process the same sort of presentist condescension that they visited on the practitioners of witchcraft and magic, and much the same teleological bent – with the cultural relativism born of the anthropological perspective supplanting the Enlightenment's cult of reason, and the learned error of our positivist predecessors replacing the popular error of our peasant ancestors. Perhaps the time has come to hear their voices, too, with sympathy and respect.

## NOTES

1 Robert Mandrou, *Magistrats et sorciers en France au XVII*[e] *siècle: une analyse de psychologie historique* (Paris, 1968).

2 On the significance of the Cadière–Girard case, see B. Robert Kreiser, 'The devils of Toulon: demonic possession and religious politics in eighteenth-century Provence', in Richard M. Golden (ed.), *Church, State and Society Under the Bourbon Kings of France* (Lawrence, KS, 1982), pp. 173–221.

3 See, for example, Julio Caro Baroja, *The World of the Witches*, trans. O.N.V. Glendinning (Chicago, 1965), part 4, 'The decline of witchcraft'; Jeffrey B. Russell, *A History of Witchcraft: Sorcerers, Heretics and Pagans* (London, 1980), chap. 7, 'The decline of witchcraft'; and Joseph Klaits, *Servants of Satan: The Age of the Witch Hunts*

(Bloomington, IN, 1985), chap. 7, 'An end to witch hunting'. For an analysis emphasizing the efforts of the highest levels of the judiciary to control abuses and 'lynchings' at the local level, see Alfred Soman, 'La décriminalisation de la sorcellerie en France', *Histoire, économie et société*, 4 (1985): 179–203. Soman traces the decriminalization of witchcraft back to the early seventeenth century and downplays the role of Cartesianism and the new science.

4 See Keith Thomas, *Religion and the Decline of Magic* (New York, 1971).

5 See Peter Burke, *Popular Culture in Early Modern Europe* (New York, 1978). Robert Muchembled gives a more political twist to this interpretation in his *Popular Culture and Elite Culture in France, 1400–1750*, trans. Lydia Cochrane (Baton Rouge, LA, 1985), which emphasizes the ramifying authority of the centralized state.

6 Mandrou, *Magistrats et sorciers*, p. 561.

7 See, for example, Charles Webster, *From Paracelsus to Newton: Magic and the Making of Modern Science* (Cambridge, 1982).

8 See, for example, Roger Chartier, 'Culture as appropriation: popular cultural uses in early modern France', in Steven L. Kaplan (ed.), *Understanding Popular Culture: Europe from the Middle Ages to the Nineteenth Century* (Berlin, 1984), pp. 229–53.

9 See Étienne Delcambre, *Le Concept de la sorcellerie dans le duché de Lorraine au XVI^e et au XVII^e siècle*, three fascicles (Nancy, 1948–51), 3, chap. 16; and E. William Monter, *Witchcraft in France and Switzerland: The Borderlands During the Reformation* (Ithaca, NY, 1976), chap. 7.

10 Something of the difficulty of the latter, much-vexed question is suggested by two essays in Robin Briggs, *Communities of Belief: Cultural and Social Tension in Early Modern France* (Oxford, 1989). The first, more general, essay – 'Witchcraft and the community in France and French-speaking Europe' – embraces the prevalent view that 'diabolism was never more than a secondary, even an imposed element in peasant belief' (p. 15), while a second, monographic essay on 'Witchcraft and popular mentality in Lorraine, 1580–1630' concludes that 'the pact was clearly a part of popular belief' (p. 68) and minimizes distinctions between elite and popular views of witchcraft in this region.

11 On the survival of witchcraft beliefs and counter-witchcraft practices in the absence of 'witches', see Jeanne Favret-Saada, *Deadly Words: Witchcraft in the Bocage*, trans. Catherine Cullen (Cambridge, 1980).

12 Johann Weyer (Wier), *De Praestigiis Daemonum et Incantationibus, ac Veneficiis* (Basel, 1563); [Friedrich von Spe(e)], *Cautio criminalis, seu de processibus contra sagas liber* (Rinteln, 1631); Savinien Cyrano de Bergerac, '[Lettre] contre les sorciers', in *Les Oeuvres diverses de M. de Cyrano de Bergerac* (Paris, 1654), letter 13; Nicolas de Malebranche, *De la recherche de la vérité*, 2 vols (Paris, 1674–75); Balthasar Bekker, *De Betoverde Weereld*, 4 vols (Amsterdam, 1691–93); Pierre Bayle, *Réponse aux questions d'un provincial*, 2 vols (Rotterdam, 1704). Mandrou, *Magistrats et sorciers*, provides a useful guide to the debates in the French context. See also G.J. Stronks, 'The significance of

Balthasar Bekker's *The Enchanted World*', in Marijke Gijswijt-Hofstra and Willem Frijhoff (eds), *Witchcraft in the Netherlands from the Fourteenth to the Twentieth Century*, trans. Rachel M.J. van der Wilden-Fall (Rotterdam, 1991), pp. 149–56.

13 Michel de Montaigne, *Essais*, book 1, chap. 21, 'De la force de l'imagination' (first published 1580).

14 See especially François de Saint-André, *Lettres de M. de Saint André . . . au sujet de la magie* (Paris, 1725).

15 Laurent Bordelon, *L'Histoire des imaginations extravagantes de Monsieur Oufle* (Amsterdam, 1710).

16 Pierre de Lancre, *Tableau de l'inconstance des mauvais anges et démons* (Paris, 1612), p. 332.

17 These publications formed part of the drive to rehabilitate popular culture that figured prominently in the Counter-Reformation. See Burke, *Popular Culture*, chap. 8, and Jean Delumeau, *Catholicism Between Luther and Voltaire: A New View of the Counter-Reformation*, trans. Jeremy Moisier (London, 1977). As Keith Thomas has emphasized, the Protestant Reformation distinguished still more sharply between religion and magic and tended to relegate many Catholic practices to the latter category. Nevertheless, the parallels between the Protestant and Catholic campaigns are at least as striking as the differences – as are the parallels between the persistence of magical beliefs and practices in the Catholic and Protestant worlds: Robert W. Scribner, 'The Reformation, popular magic, and the "disenchantment of the world" ', *Journal of Interdisciplinary History*, 23 (1993): 479–94.

18 Laurent Joubert, *Erreurs populaires au fait de la médecine et régime de santé* (Bordeaux, 1578) and *Segonde partie* (Paris, 1580). The title varied in later editions. For the publication history, see Gregory David de Rocher's introduction to his translation, *Popular Errors* (Tuscaloosa, AL, 1989). On the development of the subgenre and its significance for the larger question of the relationship between popular and elite culture in early modern Europe, see Natalie Zemon Davis, *Society and Culture in Early Modern France* (Stanford, CA, 1975), chap. 8, 'Proverbial wisdom and popular errors', esp. pp. 258–64.

19 Jean-Baptiste Thiers, *Traité des superstitions qui regardent les sacramens*, 4th edn, 4 vols (Paris, 1741), unpaginated preface and vol. 1, pp. 418 and 483. This edition brings together the *Traité des superstitions selon l'écriture sainte* (1679) in vol. 1, and *Traité des superstitions qui regardent les sacramens*, 2 vols (1703–04), in vols 2–4. On Thiers, see François Lebrun, 'Le "Traité des superstitions" de Jean-Baptiste Thiers, contribution à l'ethnographie de la France du XVIIe siècle', *Annales de Bretagne et des pays de l'Ouest*, 83 (1976): 443–65.

20 Pierre Le Brun, *Histoire critique des pratiques superstitieuses qui ont séduit les peuples et embarrassé les sçavans* (Rouen, 1702); 2nd augmented edn, 4 vols (Paris 1732–37, reprinted 1750–51). On Thiers as a source of amusement, see 'Au lecteur', preface to *Superstitions anciennes et modernes* (reprint of works by Thiers and Le Brun), 2 vols (Amsterdam, 1733–36). On reactions to Le Brun, see preface to 2nd edn, vol. 1, pp. xii–xiii.

21 Paul-Henri-Dietrich, baron d'Holbach, *Le Christianisme dévoilé* (London, 1756) and *Essai sur les préjugés* (London, 1770) – also attributed to César Chesneau Dumarsais.

22 On the origins of this discourse, see Alison Klairmont Lingo, 'Empirics and charlatans in early modern France: the genesis of the classification of the "other" in medical practice', *Journal of Social History*, 19 (1985–86): 583–603.

23 The *Discours de l'origine, des moeurs, fraudes et impostures des ciarlatans, avec leur descouverte, par I.D.P.M.O.D.R.* (Paris, 1622), p. 21, suggests that the devil and quackery work towards the same end and have the same character. Attributed to Jean de Gorris but also Jean Duret, this work is essentially a translation, with a few additions, of a work by the Roman physician and philosopher Scipione [Girolamo] Mercurio, *De gli errori popolari d'Italia, libri sette*, 2 vols (Venice, 1603), vol. 4, chaps 1–8.

24 On secret remedies and popular medical books, see Matthew Ramsey, 'Traditional medicine and medical enlightenment: the regulation of secret remedies in the Ancien Régime', *Historical Reflections/Réflexions historiques*, 9 (1982), nos 1–2: 215–32, and *idem*, 'The popularization of medicine in France, 1650–1900', in Roy Porter (ed.), *The Popularization of Medicine, 1650–1850* (London, 1992), pp. 97–133. On the broader role of medicine in the programme to modernize the peasantry, see Harvey Mitchell, 'Rationality and control in French eighteenth-century medical views of the peasantry', *Comparative Studies in Society and History*, 21 (1979): 82–112.

25 Jean-Luc d'Iharce, *Erreurs populaires sur la médecine* (Paris, 1783), p. 421.

26 René-Georges Gastellier, 14 March 1782, in Société Royale de Médecine, archives (Académie Nationale de Médecine, Paris), box 107; Jean-Guillaume Chifoliau, 'Préjugés opposés aux sages précautions du gouvernement, aux efforts des ministres de santé et à la voix de la Nature', 22 March 1780, in *ibid*, box 124.

27 This theme emerges in the survey of surgery conducted in 1790–91 by the health committee of the Constituent Assembly. See, for example, Archives Nationales $F^{1}7$ 2276, dossier 2, no. 271.

28 Louis Lépecq de la Cloture, *Collection d'observations sur les maladies et constitutions épidémiques* (Rouen, 1778), p. 540.

29 Jean-Emmanuel Gilibert, *L'Anarchie médicinale*, 3 vols (Neuchâtel, 1772), vol. 1, pp. 255–6.

30 Théophile de Bordeu, *Recherches sur le tissu muqueux* (Paris, 1790), pp. 157–60 (first published 1767). On rustics and primitives, see Davis, 'Proverbial wisdom', p. 264.

31 A[te] Treille, *Quelques réflexions sur les principaux abus en médecine* (Auch, 1823), p. 52.

32 V. Nivet, 'Essai sur les erreurs populaires relatives à la médecine et aux personnes qui exercent l'art de guérir', *Annales scientifiques, littéraires et industrielles de l'Auvergne*, 13 (1840): 93–213, p. 94.

33 Paul Bidault, *Les Superstitions médicales du Morvan*, Paris medical thesis (1898–99), no. 321 (1899), p. 22. This and the other French medical

theses cited below were published in the city where the faculty had its seat.

34 See, for example, J. Borianne, *Essai sur les erreurs en médecine répandues dans le département de la Haute-Vienne et sur leurs dangers*, Paris medical thesis (1831), p. 16.

35 Jean-Marie Charcot, *La Foi qui guérit* (Paris, 1897). See Sarah Ferber's article in this volume on the ways in which Charcot's circle applied the hysteria diagnosis retrospectively to early modern cases of demonic possession.

36 On Grégoire's investigation, see Michel de Certeau, Dominique Julia and Jacques Revel, *Une Politique de la langue: la Révolution française et les patois: l'enquête de Grégoire* (Paris, 1975). Grégoire's survey formed part of a project that aimed, in the spirit of the Enlightenment, both to collect information on popular error and to eradicate it; the patois were to be annihilated. On the connections between folklore investigations and the control of popular culture, see Michel de Certeau, Dominique Julia and Jacques Revel, 'La Beauté du mort: le concept de "culture populaire"', in Michel de Certeau, *La Culture au pluriel* (Paris, 1974), pp. 55–94.

37 On the *statistiques*, see Jean-Claude Perrot, *L'Âge d'or de la statistique régionale française. an IV – 1804* (Paris, 1977), and on their ethnographic content, Marie-Noëlle Bourguet, 'Race et folklore: l'image officielle de la France en 1800', *Annales: économies, sociétés, civilisations*, 31 (1976): 802–23.

38 *Mémoires de l'Académie Celtique, ou recherches sur les antiquités celtiques, gauloises et françaises*, 5 vols (1807–10), vol. 1, pp. 75–86 (list of questions). See Harry Senn, 'Folklore beginnings in France: the Académie Celtique, 1804–1813', *Journal of the Folklore Institute*, 18 (1981): 23–33, and Mona Ozouf, 'L'Inventeur de l'ethnologie française: le questionnaire de l'Académie Celtique', *Annales: économies, sociétés, civilisations*, 36 (1981): 210–30.

39 Louis-Pierre-François-Adolphe de Chesnel de la Charbouclais, *Dictionnaire des superstitions, erreurs, préjugés et traditions populaires* (Paris, 1856). On romanticism, history and folklore, see the interesting study by Charles Rearick, *Beyond the Enlightenment: Historians and Folklore in Nineteenth-Century France* (Bloomington, IN, 1974).

40 Borianne, *Essai sur les erreurs*.

41 Anthelme Balthasard Richerand, *Des erreurs populaires relatives à la médecine* (Paris, 1810; 2nd edn, 1812).

42 For example, Georges Foucart, *Des erreurs et des préjugés populaires en médecine*, Paris medical thesis (1893–94), no. 5 (1893) p. 6, invokes Joubert, Primerose, Browne, Tissot and Richerand. See Jean de Rostagny, *Traité de Primerose sur les erreurs vulgaires de la médecine* (Lyon, 1689), based on James Primerose, *De vulgi erroribus in medicina* (Amsterdam, 1644); Thomas Browne, *Essai sur les erreurs populaires*, 2 vols (Paris, 1733), trans. J.-B. Souchay from *Pseudodoxica Epidemica, or Enquiries into Very Many Received Tenents and Commonly Presumed Truths* (London, 1646); and Samuel-Auguste-André-David Tissot, *Avis au*

*peuple sur sa santé* . . . (Lausanne, 1761; and at least 47 subsequent French-language editions and printings).

43 Borianne, *Essai sur les erreurs*; J.-Charles Voisin, *De quelques préjugés relatifs à la médecine* (Paris, 1831).

44 G.-M. Couhé, *Essai sur quelques expressions proverbiales et sentences populaires relatives à la médecine*, Paris medical thesis (1808). Astonishingly, Couhé wrote that no one before him had ever gathered medical proverbs (p. vii). He was apparently unaware of Joubert's work.

45 Adolphe-Joseph-Hyacinthe Darmezin, *Superstitions et remèdes populaires en Touraine*, Bordeaux medical thesis (1904–05) no. 8 (1904) p. 43; Raphaël Kaufmann, *Pratiques et superstitions médicales en Poitou*, Paris medical thesis (1906).

46 Kaufmann, *Pratiques*, p. 59.

47 Burke, *Popular Culture*, p. 6.

48 Jules Michelet, *La Sorcière*, ed. Robert Mandrou (n.p., 1964; first published 1862).

49 Emmanuel Le Roy Ladurie, *Jasmin's Witch*, trans. Brian Pearce (New York, 1987). Includes translation from the 1842 French version of *Françouneto*; quotation p. 109.

50 Paul-Abraham Pesme, *De quelques erreurs en médecine*, Paris medical thesis (1855), no. 34, pp. 10–11; Edgar-Jean-Ernest Porcheron, *Les Braconniers de la médecine au pays de Poitou*, Bordeaux medical thesis (1923), p. 91.

51 A.-F.-Émile Bessières, *Étude sur les erreurs et les préjugés populaires en médecine*, Paris medical thesis (1860), no. 228, p. 15.

52 J. Lecourt de Cantilly, note on illegal medical practice, August 1827, in archives of Académie Nationale de Médecine, box 234.

53 P. Philippe Colon, *Essai sur la médecine populaire et ses dangers*, Paris medical thesis (1824).

54 See Paul Sébillot's magisterial *Le Folk-lore de France*, 4 vols (Paris, 1904–7).

55 A. Jacqmart, 'Erreurs, préjugés, coutumes et légendes du Cambrésis', *Mémoires de la Société d'Émulation de Cambrai*, 36 (1880): 315. Eugen Weber has attempted to chart how at the end of the nineteenth century the school and other forces of modernization gradually displaced the old beliefs in the French countryside and closed or at least narrowed the gap between popular and elite culture: *Peasants into Frenchmen: The Modernization of Rural France, 1870–1914* (Stanford, CA, 1976).

56 Darmezin, *Superstitions et remèdes*, p. 48.

57 On this theme, see, for example, Nivet, 'Essai sur les erreurs populaires'. Some later writers, while still treating popular medicine as archaic, considered it coherent. Porcheron, in his 1924 thesis on medical 'poachers', insisted that 'this therapeutics is not, as many believe, a jumble of disparate recipes; it is, on the contrary, a real, appropriate, homogeneous therapeutics . . . ': *Les Braconniers*, p. 91.

58 Lecourt de Cantilly, note on illegal medical practice; commission report to Academy, 5 July 1828, box 234.

59 For an overview of the ethnological approach to French medical folk-

lore, see Marcelle Bouteiller, *La Médecine populaire d'hier et d'aujour-d'hui* (Paris, 1987).

60 See, for example, Barbara Ehrenreich and Deirdre English, *Witches, Midwives and Nurses: A History of Women Healers*, 2nd edn (Old Westbury, NY, 1973). For a corrective, see David Harley, 'Historians as demonologists: the myth of the midwife-witch', *Social History of Medicine*, 3 (1990): 1–26.

61 For an example of how this can be done with modesty and sensitivity, see the conclusion to Davis, 'Proverbial wisdom', pp. 264–7.

Chapter 2

# Demons and disease

## The disenchantment of the sick (1500–1700)

*Stuart Clark*

### SICKNESS BY DEVILS

In early modern demonology – that is to say, among those intellectuals who took a broadly orthodox view of witchcraft, magic and demonism – the idea that devils could cause disease was a commonplace. The nature of the causation itself was a matter of some debate. The popular view that witches could inflict sickness on the bewitched had to be corrected in order to show that the witches themselves (unless they used natural means, like poisons) had no more power in this respect than anyone else, since their unnatural means (spells, charms and the like) lacked all efficacy. It was demons that brought the sicknesses 'caused' by witchcraft, with the spells and charms acting as the sacraments of their activity. Furthermore, demonic efficacy itself had to be circumscribed within the bounds of natural possibilities. Devils could bend nature's rules but never break them, acting preternaturally, not supernaturally. If they caused real diseases – as opposed to pretending to – this had to be done either by local motion or the application of actives on passives.

This left them plenty of scope. Armed with the speed of angels, the subtlety of spirits and six thousand years of experience, devils could play havoc with the minds and bodies of human beings. It was commonly said that the devil had more knowledge and skills than all human medical practitioners put together. The canon and civil lawyer and auditor of criminal cases in Arezzo, Paolo Grillando, reported that he was called 'the best philosopher, theologian, arithmetician, mathematician, dialectician, logician, grammarian, musician and the most excellent physician'.[1] According to Francesco Maria Guazzo of the Ambrosian Order in Milan, the devil could induce

> the melancholy sickness by first disturbing the black bile in the body and so dispersing a black humour throughout the brain and the inner cells of the body: and this black bile he increases by superinducing other irritations and by preventing the purging of the humour. He brings epilepsy, paralysis and such maladies by a stoppage of the heavier physical fluids, obstructing and blocking the ventricle of the brain and the nerve-roots. He causes blindness or deafness, bringing a noxious secretion in the eyes or ears. Often again he suggests ideas to the imagination which induce love or hatred or other mental disturbances. For the purpose of causing bodily infirmities he distils a spirituous substance from the blood itself, purifies it of all base matter, and uses it as the aptest, most efficacious and swiftest weapon against human life: I say that from the most potent poisons he extracts a quintessence with which he infects the very spirit of life, and . . . so establishes his devil-made disease that human skill is hardly able to find a remedy, since the devil's poison is too subtle and tenuous, too swift and sure in killing, and reaches to the very marrow of the bones.[2]

In a sermon of 1612, the French theologian and abbé, André Valladier, was equally explicit. The devil, he said, had full power over all the spirits and humours of the body to displace them, weaken or excite them, or otherwise disable them from working properly. He could produce anger, vengefulness, violence and murder by flooding the heart with blood, awaken venereal lust by inflaming the male sperm and genitals, and cause unbearable heaviness by acting on the melancholic humour: 'and so with the others, causing especially the strange raptures that one sees much of in the case of witches'.[3] There was, indeed, no medical disorder that the devil might not inflict on his victims, with or without the cooperation of witches – not even leprosy or epilepsy, said the Dominican authors of *Malleus maleficarum*, these being diseases arising usually 'from some long-standing physical predisposition or defect'. 'The natural power of devils', they wrote, 'is superior to all corporeal power.'[4] Among the other demonically caused ailments discussed in the literature of witchcraft were blindness, contortions and vomitings.

Such ideas have often been viewed as little more than rationalizations of witch hunting. Yet the idea that devils could cause diseases was as common in academic medicine as it was in demonology. It was made the subject of single treatises, like those of Giovanni Battista Codronchi, Pietro Piperno and William Drage, and it was dealt with in demonologies written by professors of medicine, like Andrea Cesalpino, whom Lynn Thorndike called 'the most distinguished Italian scientist' to write on witchcraft.[5]

It was discussed in many dissertations and disputations held in the medical faculties of the European universities[6] and the subject also appeared regularly as a topic in many general surveys of medicine. Some of the most important medical writers of the age committed themselves to the notion, including Thomas Browne, Jean Fernel, Jacques Fontaine, Jourdain Guibelet, Francisco Vallés (Vallesius) and Daniel Sennert.

Specialist areas of research, such as gynaecology, were drawn into the debate. There was scarcely a serious treatment of monstrous births that did not allow for the workings of devils (together with miscegenation between humans and devils), besides other non-demonic possibilities relating to the physical and mental conditions of the mothers. Substantial portions of Ambroise Paré's *Des monstres et prodiges* read like a conventional demonology, while Ulisse Aldrovandi, Martin Weinrich, Girolamo Cardano and Fortunius Licetus all felt it essential to consider this type of explanation.

Demonic causation was also a main issue in medical discussions of the conditions associated with fascination (bewitchment by sight), melancholy ('the devil's bath'), lycanthropy and ephialtes (nightmare). The expert on diseases of the brain, Jason a Pratis (Jasonis Pratensis), from Zierikzee in Zeeland, wrote in his chapter on 'mania' that devils were 'subtle and incomprehensible spirits' and could insinuate themselves into the bodies of men, attacking the health of the visceral organs and causing diseases, but also terrifying the mind with dreams and ravings so that attacks of madness were diagnosed.[7] As for the actual physical possession of the human body by devils, this was obviously a matter which doctors, and not merely theologians and priests, were frequently asked to confirm. Many did so.

Surveying this broader medical literature, one finds exactly the same views as those put forward by the writers on witchcraft. Codronchi assembled the same reasons for ascribing disease by bewitchment to the natural efficacy of devils, listing impotence, sterility, removal of the genitals, abortings, the drying up of milk and the retention of urine.[8] Fernel spoke of devils sometimes entering the human body, but also attacking it from outside 'either to disturb the body's beneficial humours, or lead the harmful ones into the principal parts, or obstruct the veins, and other channels, or change the nature of the supply, from which causes many illnesses arise. The devils are the authors of these'.[9] According to Sennert, 'the virtues, as well as the sympathies and antipathies of natural things are not unknown to the devil, and he best understands what is favourable and what is harmful to the health of each person, and what particular illness he is able to bring'. He was able to cause sicknesses by poisons, but also by stirring up the evil humours and corrupting the good ones to change their 'natural constitution'. Among the results were epilepsy, convulsions, paralysis, melancholy, insane love, hatred without reason, impotence and abortings.[10]

For Drage, a disease brought by witchcraft was 'a Sickness that arises from strange and preternatural Causes, and from Diabolical Power . . . afflicting with strange and unaccustomed Symptoms, and commonly preternaturally violent, very seldom or not at all curable by Ordinary and Natural Remedies'. Cases were strange vomitings, convulsions, 'Barrenness, Lameness, Madness, Sterrility, and *Impotentia coeundi* [impotence], Cholicks, Fainting and Sweating'.[11]

In 1703, Friedrich Hoffmann, who with Boerhaave and Stahl dominated medical thought in the early part of the eighteenth century, published a doctoral dissertation by a student named Bueching, which explained that the devil acted on the 'animal spirits' in the human body, thus interfering with the imagination, other mental functions and the motor activities, and inducing illusions, trances and convulsions. Various internal physiological factors, together with differences of sex, age and diet made some people more prone to this than others.[12]

On the subject of devils and diseases there was, then, a complete identity of belief between the specialist writers on witchcraft and a substantial portion of the medically orthodox. Guazzo was able to appeal with confidence to Codronchi, Cesalpino, Fernel, Vallés 'and other most learned physicians';[13] and Piperno, Drage and Sennert were familiar with the literature of witchcraft. There was a two-way intellectual traffic at work in which the medical monographs and disputations provided the scholarly underpinnings for belief in one particular facet of demonic activity, while academic demonology confirmed the expectations of the physicians and provided illustrative case-studies.

## OCCULT QUALITIES AND CAUSES IN MEDICINE

There is no reason to be surprised by this two-way traffic, once we give up any lingering resistance to the idea that demonology might have made sense. Both sets of authors were products of the same sort of university training, and whether they were graduates or members of faculties of theology, law or medicine, they shared assumptions that were common to all three. Nevertheless, there was one intellectual development of the later medieval and early modern period that brought them closer together still. This was the increasing attention shown to the 'occult' workings of the natural world, not merely by Neo-Platonists and what Frances Yates called 'Hermeticists' but also by scholastic natural philosophers (in whom I include medical academics) interested in 'natural magic'.

The very great significance of this intellectual development for demonology and witchcraft theory lay in the fact that demonic agency was associated, above all, with the manipulation of occult qualities and causes – and, in the case of demonic diseases, with the occult workings of the human body and of pathogenic substances. Thus, Sennert's substantial discussion of sicknesses brought by witchcraft occurred in the section of his *Practicae medicinae* devoted to *morbis occultis* [occult diseases]. When the Brescia physician Giovanni Francesco Olmo published his book on the role of occult properties in medicine (for example, the occult virtues in foods, medicaments, poisons and their antidotes, and the role of occult 'sympathies' and 'antipathies'), he was able to include a section on the injuries due to *veneficia*, dividing them into natural and demonic types. The latter were more difficult to remedy, but sulphur or musical harmony might be used to disturb demons by antipathy.[14] 'Sathan', wrote the English witchcraft author Henry Holland, citing Fernel in support, 'useth poisons that have hidden, unknowne, and straunge operations in the bodies of men, for he is an Empiricke of many yeeres experience'.[15]

What were 'occult' qualities and causes? The chief agents of change in sublunary things were the four principal qualities (hot, cold, wet, dry) and their secondary compounds. But whereas these were directly accessible via sensation, there were other qualities that could never themselves be apprehended by the senses, even though the results of their operations were manifest to all. In other words, sensation gave access to their effects but not to the causes of these effects. Such qualities and causes were, thus, the subjects of experience (even in the sense of experiment) but not of rational explanation, as this was understood. The behaviour of solid bodies in free fall was an obvious instance, so was the reaction of iron to the lodestone. Comparable examples from the field of medicine were the spread of contagions, the effects of poisons and their antidotes, the properties of narcotics, the behaviour of allergies and the relief of bodily ailments by purgatives – the last of which seemed, typically, to go beyond the workings of the ordinary qualities involved and the routine therapies associated with the doctrine of the temperaments. Since none of these local motions could be deduced from the perceptible qualities of the objects in question, they had to be treated contingently as the effects of hidden virtues whose power of acting might be experienced and described but never properly known.

A natural magic that tried to make the insensible intelligible could not, in later medieval scientific learning, be classed as a true form of knowledge. But Bert Hansen has written that its causality, at least, 'as its notions of being . . . flowed in the streambed of Aristotelian thought'. The doctrine of sympathies and antipathies, in particular, flourished in a natural philosophical tradition that gave prominence to final causes and the category of purpose. It did not have to rely on Renaissance Hermeticism for its credentials and should not be thought of as a uniquely 'Hermetic' idea. 'Medieval magic's view of the world', Hansen concludes, 'was fully that of scholastic natural philosophy.' And if natural magic did eventually contribute to the dramatic scientific changes of the next age, it did so, in part, with a scholastic weighting.[16] The pursuit of nature's innermost secrets and the production of wonders came to be safely acknowledged as important aspects of orthodox natural philosophy.

The specialist account of sympathies and antipathies most frequently cited in early modern Europe was by Girolamo Fracastoro. But he was a product of Padua, a physician to the early members of the Council of Trent, and in astronomy and medicine a committed Aristotelian and Galenist. Jean Fernel's widely noted study of the occult causes of diseases, *De abditis rerum causis*, was in many ways the work of a medical traditionalist;[17] so too was the Paris physician Jacques Grévin's *Deux livres des venins*, where natural magical causation and occult diseases were nevertheless acknowledged. Less illustrious medical philosophers, like Antonio Ludovico (Antáo Luis) of Lisbon and Giovanni Francesco Olmo of Brescia, approached the problems posed by occult properties as commentators on Galen.

Thomas Erastus might denounce natural magic in attacking Paracelsus, but, noted Marcus Friedrich Wendelin, the great weight of philosophical and theological opinion was against him.[18] Nor did the consideration of things occult necessarily commit natural philosophers and academic physicians to what Frances Yates called 'the occult philosophy'. Historians do not, therefore, have to adopt her interpretation of the history of early modern science and medicine in order to recognize natural magic's very considerable significance in intellectual circles at the time.

The overwhelming reason for its relevance during much of the sixteenth and seventeenth centuries was the attempt made *within* both Christian Aristotelianism and Galenic medicine to deal more satisfactorily with the epistemological difficulties created by occult qualities. This is a further indication of the flexibility, adaptability and eclecticism that enabled traditionalists to respond positively to fresh emphases in early modern science – of which the problem of occult causes was certainly one.[19] The 'manifestation' of the occult has accordingly been seen as a central component of the writings of prominent figures in the field of medicine, men like Pomponazzi, Fracastoro, Cardano, Fernel and Sennert.[20] But it had repercussions across the whole world of Aristotelian academic philosophy and medicine which can be illustrated in the works of many more anonymous individuals. As the pace of natural philosophical change quickened elsewhere, theorizing on occult qualities reached its summation not with an academic but with a court physician, the Coimbra-trained Duarte Madeira Arrais, who ministered to the medical needs of King John IV of Portugal and who published his *Novae philosophiae et medicinae de qualitatibus occultis . . . pars prima* in Lisbon in 1650.

The catholicity of the occult cause and its resistance to demonstration made it a *cause célèbre* in the debates between traditional and 'new' natural philosophers, and led to many contemporary charges of indulgence and scientific laziness against its proponents. But the onset of the 'mechanical' philosophy did not mean the immediate end of occult qualities – only further adaptation to new needs. For the moment, what is important is the endorsement that was given in the adaptable and, thus, changing circles in which demonology thrived to the idea of natural magic as a science of the occult – that is to say, to a branch of natural philosophy and medicine which specialized in precisely that type of causation that was the devil's own.[21]

## HEALING AND ITS RATIONALITY

These developments had obvious practical implications for healing, even if their immediate context was often academic and theoretical. Patients and healers everywhere had to consider at least the possibility that individual ailments might be traced to witches or demons.[22] Whether, and to what extent, the contents of texts of medical theory worked their way into the general world of sickness and healing are highly debatable questions. But Codronchi was the town physician at Imola near Bologna, Piperno practised in Benevento, Guibelet at Evreux and A Pratis at Zierikzee. Drage was an apothecary in Hertfordshire. They and their fellow authors drew up diagnostic programmes for distinguishing demonic from non-demonic sicknesses (or the precise ingredients of each) and they discussed a range of healing strategies.

One major issue was the balance between the use of natural remedies and the resort to religious ones. Since the devil worked by natural causes, naturalistic cures were perfectly in order. Cesalpino favoured amulets, alexipharmaca (poison antidotes), aromas and suffumigations, favouring, in particular, the use of theriaca (mithridatum).[23] Codronchi analyzed the use of vomiting, baths, suffumigations and liniments, and added a discussion of the herbal simples and compounds whose manifest qualities made them most effective against demons – rue, hypericum, vervain and the like.[24]

Since the devil was also an agent of God, spiritual curatives could be as important as herbs, or in some eyes, more so. Distinguishing between the two categories was easier for Protestant authors, than for Catholics; the exact medical benefits of wearing an amulet with both natural properties and religious symbols on it exercised the best theologians and casuists of the Catholic Reformation. This is because a second major issue was the drawing of boundaries between 'real' cures which had natural efficacy and could therefore work, at least in principle, and 'superstitious' ones, which were causally spurious and relied on precisely the demonic agency that had brought the sickness in the first place.

Discussions of these two issues are found throughout the literature of both Protestant and Catholic reform; they were not the monopoly of the medical theorists and certainly not of the 'demonologists'. Working them out involved potential conflicts of interest that were fundamental to the history of medicine and to early modern cultural history in general, above all, between the potentially rival therapies of the clergymen and the doctors, and between the proscriptions of both these groups of professionals, on the one hand, and the behaviour of those they sought to 'improve', on the other.

The demonology of disease also bears on the broader issue of the rationality of past healing beliefs. A rational belief or action is one for which reasons can be given – reasons which both the giver(s) and receiver(s) accept as well grounded, coherent and, in some sense, correct. Since standards of well groundedness, coherence and correctness change from context to context, so does reason giving and reason receiving and, thus, rationality. In the context of university-generated learning in the later medieval and early modern period the belief that devils could cause disease was a rational belief. The religious and natural philosophical grounds for believing in devils and their natural powers were overwhelming; the arguments for their intervention were presented with all the force that formal educational and rhetorical practices at the highest level could give them; and their truth was also ensured by their espousal by a great number of respected past authors.

Rationality, as well as the power to enforce it, is contingent on institutions and positions of authority and, in this respect, the medical 'establishment' was well represented among those authors discussed here. Cesalpino was professor of medicine at Rome and taught also at Pisa, Vallés taught in the medical faculty at Alcalá and was physician to Philip II, Fontaine was *médecin ordinaire* to the French king and the first medical professor at the royal university at Aix-en-Provence, Fernel was physician to Henry II, A Pratis was physician to Duke Adolph of Bevern, and Sennert was the most important medical academic at Wittenberg in the opening decades of the seventeenth century.

It used to be said that early modern healers and their clients resorted to a demonic explanation when they could account for an affliction in no other way, or simply out of general ignorance about the real causes of illness. Indeed, the view has been that it was one of the 'functions' of witchcraft beliefs to explain afflictions in communities that had no other way of accounting for them.[25] These are ways of talking about the beliefs and behaviour of the past that ought now to be revised. The diagnosis of demonic illnesses was done on the basis of *knowledge* (rational knowledge, I have argued) not on the basis of ignorance, with healers and patients making a choice between – or a mixture of – different explanations and therapeutic strategies. Guibelet was speaking for the majority of theorists of the demonic when he argued that tracing every unusual symptom to devils or insisting that every pathology had natural causes were equally unacceptable extremes.[26] It is, in any case, tautologous to talk of a belief being 'used' to explain what in fact constituted its meaning, as well as philosophically absurd to imply that it would not have meant anything at all if only people had known better.

## THE DEBATE ABOUT DEMONIC CAUSES

Nevertheless, there was no unanimity and competing rationalities were at work. Many healers did not diagnose bewitchment or demonism when invited to do so, and two of the most effective denouncers of witchcraft beliefs, Johan Wier and John Webster, practised as physicians. The arguments I am concerned with were invariably presented as contributions to a *debate*. This raises the further question of how the link between devils and disease could have been broken and sickness released from its 'enchantment'. From which intellectual direction might such a change have come? Not necessarily from the witchcraft sceptics themselves. Johan Wier, for example, needed more demonic intervention in human sickness, not less. He could only exonerate women from accusations of witchcraft by applying to them the full weight of a medical theory that gave the devil huge physical powers to cause delusions and sickness in the female mind and body. Those physicians who directly followed him, like Johann Ewich, were likewise committed.

One basis for taking a more radical step was the pure Aristotelianism of those who argued that Aristotle had not allowed for demonic agency in the natural world. Guazzo conceded that, strictly speaking, Avicenna, Galen and Hippocrates had also denied 'that it is possible for any diseases to be brought upon man by demons'.[27] This was the basis of Pomponazzi's celebrated analysis of the healing powers of incantations in terms of their psychosomatic properties. As Keith Hutchison has explained, there was a stark opposition between this kind of naturalism and traditional Christianity, which made the strict Aristotelians the least 'supernat-uralistic' of early modern natural philosophers.[28] The difficulty here, however, is that very few Aristotelians were prepared to be strict in this way, and Pomponazzi's contemporary reputation as an atheist helped further to dissuade them. Besides, the purpose of works like Cesalpino's *Daemonum investigatio* and Codronchi's *De morbis veneficis* was to argue either that Aristotle and the peripatetics had indeed acknowledged demonic agency after all or that this kind of agency was at least compatible with the Aristotelian natural philosophy.[29] Similarly lacking in impact were the innovations of the 'new' philosophy in their iatromechanical form. Of these, it has been said that they 'made no significant impact on the practice of medicine'.[30]

The strongest source of disenchantment has been said to be a cluster of ideas stemming from the very same tradition that, as I have already argued, fostered so much interest in occult and demonic causation in the sixteenth and seventeenth centuries – the 'natural magical' tradition. It has been suggested that invoking occult natural causes could *supplant* demonological explanations of phenomena rather than support them. In this view occult causation gave greater explanatory power over mysterious natural effects than demonology did and could account for them without bringing in the devil. It was thus no accident, according to Trevor-Roper's influential version of the argument,

> that 'natural magicians' like Agrippa and Cardano and 'alchemists' like Paracelsus, Van Helmont and their disciples were among the enemies of the witch-craze, while those who attacked Platonist philosophy, Hermetic ideas, and Paracelsian medicine were also, often, the most stalwart defenders of the same delusion.[31]

There is undoubtedly support for this view in instances like that in 1598–99, when some of the physicians of Paris, led by Michel Marescot, pronounced on the case of the demoniac Marthe Brossier. They concluded that she was a fraud on the grounds that her symptoms were not remarkable enough to warrant a demonic explanation. Many stranger things happened, they declared, that were nevertheless attributed 'to the hidden secrets of Nature', not to devils. The researches of the natural magicians had shown that the world was full of secretly produced effects. If all of them were attributed to devils, 'then, to unfolde the Questions of Naturall Philosophie and Phisicke, from the beginning to the end of these two Sciences, we should alwaies have recourse to Devils'.[32] A comparable example in England was that of Edward Jorden, a physician strongly influenced by Paracelsian and iatrochemical ideas, who, in 1603, explained the alarming symptoms of the supposed demoniac Mary Glover in terms of the hysterical condition known as 'the suffocation of the mother'.[33]

There is also evidence of unorthodoxy and scepticism regarding demonism and witchcraft among the leading exponents of natural magic. The Lyon physician Symphorien Champier, an editor of the Hermetic texts, whom Yates called 'a leading apostle of Neo-Platonism in France, and an admirer of Ficino', doubted the genuineness of witches' sabbats enough to say that 'rather often' they turned out to be (demonic) illusions. Anticipating Wier, he suggested that judges in witchcraft trials should consult experts in medicine and theology so that the accused could be treated for disorders and given religious guidance if necessary.[34] Paracelsus himself attributed the powers of witches, which he accepted as real, not to the demonic pact but to congenitally acquired personality traits and the sheer force of their imaginations, while at the same time narrowing the sphere of witchcraft altogether by ascribing much of their behaviour and that of their victims to non-demonic pathologies.[35] The history of the Paracelsian movement suggests that the only Paracelsians likely to show interest in demonic causation were those who were prepared to compromise with traditional medical views – men like Andreas Libavius and Daniel Sennert.[36] Later still, purely natural accounts of two characteristic witchcraft phenomena – the vomiting of strange objects by the bewitched and the harmful effects of enchantments – were offered by Joan Baptista Van Helmont.[37]

As for the other earlier natural magicians, Cornelius Agrippa defended a peasant woman accused of witchcraft at Woippy near Metz in 1519 and wrote a now-lost work *Adversus lamiarum inquisitores*.[38] Cardano's demonology was highly unorthodox, theologically speaking, since he restricted demonic activity to the aerial regions and spoke rather disparagingly of spirits as having few significant dealings with men and women and, in some matters at least, less knowledge. He was clearly reluctant to accept demonic explanations for strange phenomena when others would do.[39]

The classic natural magician of the whole period, Giambattista Della Porta, rejected the belief that witches induced flight by smearing themselves with an unguent, having tested it in a notorious experiment that was reported in the first edition of his *Magiae naturalis*. He and his colleagues physically assaulted an old woman after she had anointed herself and fallen into a trance, so that they could show her the bruises when she regained consciousness. The fact that she still insisted on having travelled to a sabbat proved that only dream experiences, produced entirely by the natural constituents of the ointment – of which Della Porta provided formulas – had actually occurred.[40]

In addition, witchcraft sceptics themselves turned to the findings of natural magic in order to explain away supposedly demonic phenomena. Wier had been servant and assistant to Agrippa in Bonn in the early 1530s and spoke of him as his 'revered teacher'. He was also indebted heavily to Cardano, using almost all the latter's chapter on witchcraft at some point or other in *De praestigiis daemonum*.[41] Reginald Scot recounted Agrippa's clash with witch hunters, cited Cardano on witchcraft with admiration, and appealed to Della Porta's experiment with the witch's ointment.[42] He undoubtedly knew and understood the natural magical literature and deplored condemnations of it as demonic by those who did not. Its secrets and marvels – Scot devoted many chapters to the usual examples – were nothing but the work of nature, even if deceit and trickery could corrupt their use.

There were other instances of critics of witchcraft beliefs and witch hunting who resorted to the alternative explanations proffered by the natural magicians, but the outstanding example is that of John Webster, who was something of a synthesizer of earlier views and who cited approvingly the entire early modern natural magical tradition from Lull and Roger Bacon onwards. Closest to Scot, Webster thought that 'witchcraft' was no more than either an 'active' delusion wrought by the tricks and cheats of impostors, or a 'passive' delusion in the minds of the ignorant, melancholic and credulous. Real *maleficium* could always be redescribed as some other condition, like the contagious poisoning that occurred in 'fascination', when infected women hurt their victims 'with the virulent steams of their breath, and the effluviums that issue from their filthy and polluted bodies'.[43]

Like Cardano, Webster stressed the severe limitations and weaknesses of demonic knowledge and power, and like Paracelsus he allowed for 'middle creatures' who

> because of their strange natures, shapes and properties, or by reason of their being rarely seen, . . . have been and often are not only by the common people but even by the learned taken to be Devils, Spirits or the effects of Inchantment and Witchcraft.[44]

Above all, he developed the fully sceptical implications of his own claim that there was 'no other ground or reason of dividing Magick into natural and Diabolical, but only that they differ in the end and use'. If both were worked (in the case of devils, allegedly) by natural agency, then men might do 'without the aid of Devils whatsoever they can do'; that is, they could apply actives to passives and produce wonders. The history of natural magic from King Pharaoh to Robert Boyle showed that this was true, and contemporary discoveries concerning the secret properties of many natural things and 'the strange and wonderful things that Art can bring to pass' meant that there would be even less reason to believe in demonic agency and witchcraft in the future.[45]

Nevertheless, we must be careful not to exaggerate. The Benedictine abbot Johannes Trithemius, who, according to Paola Zambelli, cooperated with Agrippa 'in the elaboration of the Hermeticism and natural magic of the Florentines in Germany', and to whom Agrippa presented a first draft of *De occulta philosophia*, entered the witchcraft debate on the opposite side. In two interventions dating from 1508, he wrote of the sins of witches and the range and gravity of their *maleficium* under four headings, each more serious than the last, with the fourth embracing full homage to devils and carnal dealings with them. The general tone and the sense of urgency regarding the punishment of witchcraft are reminiscent of the *Malleus maleficarum*.[46]

Champier's modern commentator, Brian Copenhaver, has said that Champier was so far from being a sceptic 'that he sometimes suggested that it was possible to make pacts or contracts with demons – even without knowing it'. Champier followed Augustine and Aquinas in regarding incubus and succubus devils as having actual physical dealings with humans and, by the transference of semen, assisting in real births.[47] There was also enough common ground between Paracelsus and his more orthodox contemporaries for him to prove, in Charles Webster's assessment, 'an enigmatic witness on the question of witchcraft and demonic magic'.[48]

Cardano finished his discussion of witchcraft by talking inconsistently about witches who persevered stubbornly with sabbats, despite the dangers, and who deserved death for their heresy and impiety. He was undoubtedly very scornful of traditional witchcraft beliefs but the criticisms he actually offered did not depend on a close application of natural magical principles to witchcraft phenomena. Instead, they were founded on more usual misgivings about the judicial process, on some fairly acute observations about the social and cultural deprivations of the accused, and, above all, on a clinical reduction of their confessions, thoroughly Galenic in its principles, to the humorial imbalances that led to melancholy. One could see that witches suffered from an excess of black bile, Cardano said, simply by looking at them.

When we look more closely at Van Helmont, too, we find that although the devil is dispensable as a physical agent, he is not in fact dispensed with – quite apart from acting as a powerful spiritual inciter to witchcraft.[49] Even Levinus Lemnius, like A Pratis a physician at Zierikzee in Zeeland in the middle years of the sixteenth century – who was reputed then and has been since as an outright sceptic in witchcraft and allied matters – did not exclude evil spirits from the physical world. In his much reprinted and translated *De miraculis occultis naturae* they contribute to pathology and to witchcraft (which Lemnius also acknowledges) by worsening natural disorders and increasing the virulence of sicknesses like melancholy.[50]

As for the scepticism of the specialist witchcraft authors themselves, this was not always based solely or even predominantly on natural magical arguments. The idea that effective criticism could only have come from something as 'hard' as science is a prejudice born of modern rationalism. Natural magic does not appear extensively in Wier, who despite his early dealings with and admiration for Agrippa, devoted an entire book of *De praestigiis daemonum* to a denunciation of the magical tradition from the Persians to the Paracelsians. In some incisive remarks on this episode, Erik Midelfort argues that Wier came away from his encounter 'unimpressed by Plato and appalled at learned magic'. The Agrippa he 'revered' was the author of *De vanitate*, not the author of *De occulta philosophia*.[51]

Reginald Scot followed Wier in this respect, but, ultimately, his own most subversive arguments stemmed from a radically unorthodox theology, not from an alternative natural philosophy. Of John Webster, too, it has to be asked whether his argument, like Scot's, depended as much on theology as on natural philosophy. More aware than ever of the dangers that might attach to a defence of the absolute incorporeality of spirits, he insisted that the fallen angels were corporeal. Nevertheless, he ruled out the physical contact presupposed by orthodox demonology, their 'leagues' with 'witches' and other evil persons being entirely spiritual in character.

This was because the bodies of devils were not like those of other corporeal substances. They were not affected by fire and they were not 'as solid and tangible as flesh and bones', being 'ethereal, airy and shadowy, and yielding and giving way to touch', subject to contraction and distention, changes of colour and so on. Thus, devils had 'pure and spiritual' bodies, and there was no need or capacity for them to assume ones made of the inferior elements in order to influence human behaviour.[52]

However satisfactory this compromise was, it did not derive from Webster's enthusiasm for natural magic, but from contemporary religious and political anxieties about the relationship between the material and the spiritual worlds. Eventually, and again like Scot, he may well have been most concerned to protect the idea of an anti-permissive deity: 'there is no one thing', he wrote, 'that hath more promoted this false and wicked Tenent of a kind of omnipotency in Devils, and the exorbitant power ascribed to Witches, than the misunderstanding of the true and right Doctrine of Divine Providence'.[53]

Above all, it is in any case artificial to contrast natural magical with Aristotelian explanatory powers when, as was explained earlier, Aristotelian physics itself embraced notions of occult causation and sympathetic and antipathetic action. The peripatetic philosophy that still dominated Europe's pedagogic circles was not, by and large, purist. Augustinian and Thomistic ingredients alone ensured the recognition of demonic causation in preternatural contexts. Demons were now emphatically within a nature that was not compromised by their inclusion. Aristotelians therefore had their own natural magic to complement their demonology, not undermine it. Since witchcraft beliefs were sustained largely by those with a traditional education and outlook, this was an important intellectual resource.

## SCIENCE, RELIGION AND DEMONOLOGY

It seems, then, that the most likely early source for the disenchantment of the sick, natural magic, did not always weaken demonology by implying some challenge to theories of the demonic causes of disease. On the contrary, it could provide important strengthening points of reference whenever there was a need to contrast or equate this agency with something comparably natural yet occult. Natural magic was, so to speak, epistemologically neutral in the great witchcraft debate. It could certainly be used to supplant demonological accounts of medical phenomena, but it was also employed to support them. Until its demise, it was impossible on natural philosophical grounds alone to make a clear choice between the conventional belief in witchcraft and the demonological scepticism most frequently directed against that belief. The scientific evidence, we might say today, was inconclusive since it could be made to work in either direction. Even with the demise of natural magic, a sufficient enough number of its features had by then been absorbed by the 'new' natural philosophy, especially in England, to continue making demonic magic, and with it witchcraft, scientifically credible.

All this suggests that the really crucial decision in witchcraft matters – whether to allow devils a presence in the physical world or exclude them from it – had to be initiated not on natural philosophical grounds but on religious and moral ones. We have just seen these at work in John Webster's account and they were later crucial to the arguments of Balthasar Bekker. When devils were excluded, in whole or in part, a whole range of phenomena then became available for natural magical or, later, 'new scientific' explanations to deal with. But it is not easy to see how these explanations themselves could involve this radical step. In the debates I have been tracing, they had a vital but ancillary 'mopping up' role; they explained witchcraft phenomena away once the need to do so had arisen from some other, more subversive, source.

Reginald Scot provides the classic instance of this pattern. Certainly, his radical scepticism was 'made possible' by his commitment to the natural magical tradition,[54] in the sense that this was one of its necessary ingredients. *The Discoverie of Witchcraft* is largely a book that tries to account for all the strange phenomena left stranded once a religious and moral decision has been taken to remove devils from material activity; and natural magic (together with 'juggling', 'cousening', 'popishness', melancholy and the rest) offered ways of doing this.[55] But it was not the origin of Scot's argument, nor sufficient to sustain it; in the history of demonology it cut both ways. This has not been the usual view of the matter, which has tended to pit 'science' – both as natural magic and 'new philosophy' – against demonology in a one-sided contest. And as long as we think of witchcraft theories as somehow intellectually weak and 'unscientific', their vulnerability in the face of better grounded versions of nature will command attention. However, in early modern Europe, natural and demonic magic were grounded in nature on the same terms. This is why it was rational to think about diseases in demonological terms until theology itself was made subject to reason.

## NOTES

1 Paolo Grillando, *Tractatus de sortilegiis*, in *Malleus maleficarum, maleficas et earum haeresim framea conterens, ex variis auctoribus compilatus*, 4 vols bound in 2 books (Lyon, 1669), vol. ii, pt. 2, p. 250.
2 Francesco Maria Guazzo, *Compendium maleficarum*, trans. E. A. Ashwin, ed. M. Summers (London, 1929), p. 106.
3 André Valladier, *La Saincte philosophie de l'ame* (Paris, 1614), p. 619.
4 [Heinrich Krämer (Institoris) and Jakob Sprenger], *Malleus maleficarum*, trans. and ed. M. Summers (London, 1928; repub. 1971), p. 297.
5 Lynn Thorndike, *A History of Magic and Experimental Science*, 8 vols (New York, 1923–58), vol. vi, p. 338.
6 For examples, see Oskar Diethelm, 'The medical teaching of demonology in the 17th and 18th centuries', *Journal of the History of the Behavioural Sciences*, 6 (1970): 3–15; Thorndike, *History of Magic*, vol. vii, pp. 338–71.
7 Jasonis Pratensis, *De cerebri morbis* (Basel, n.d. [epistle dated 1545]), p. 214; see also pp. 262 and 318.
8 Giovanni Battista Codronchi, *De morbis veneficis, ac veneficiis* (Venice, 1595), fos. 110$^{v}$–115$^{r}$.
9 Jean Fernel, *De abditis rerum causis* (Venice, 1550), p. 274; see more generally, pp. 270–9.
10 Daniel Sennert, *Practicae medicinae*, in *idem*, *Opera*, 3 vols (Paris, 1641), vol. iii, p. 1140; see also vol. ii, pp. 136, 157–8 and 220.
11 William Drage, *Daimonomageia: A Small Treatise of Sicknesses and Diseases from Witchcraft and Supernatural Causes* (London, 1665), pp. 3 and 10.
12 See Lester S. King, 'Witchcraft and medicine: conflicts in the early eighteenth century', in *Circa Tiliam: Studia historiae medicinae, Gerrit Arie Lindeboom septuagenario oblata* (Leiden, 1974), pp. 122–39, esp. pp. 127–8, discussing Friedrich Hoffmann, *praeses, Disputatio inauguralis medico–philosophica de potentia diaboli in corpore* (1703), repub. in *idem*, *Opera omnia physico–medica*, 6 vols (Geneva, 1740–53), vol. v, pp. 94–103. King fails to notice the utter conventionality of Hoffmann's demonology.
13 Guazzo, *Compendium maleficarum*, p. 105.
14 Giovanni Francesco Olmo, *De occultis in re medica proprietatibus* (Brescia, 1597), pp. 158–61.
15 Henry Holland, *A Treatise Against Witchcraft* (Cambridge, 1590), sigs. Hi$^{r–v}$.
16 Bert Hansen, 'Science and magic', in David C. Lindberg (ed.), *Science in the Middle Ages* (Chicago, 1978), pp. 483–506 (quotations pp. 490

and 495). See also Bert Hansen, 'The complementarity of science and magic before the Scientific Revolution', *American Scientist*, 74 (1986): 128–36.

17 For a detailed account of Fernel's pathology of occult diseases and their remedies, stressing his departures from Galenic orthodoxy in this area, see Linda Deer Richardson, 'The generation of disease: occult causes and diseases of the total substance', in A. Wear, R.K. French and I.M. Lonie (eds), *The Medical Renaissance of the Sixteenth Century* (Cambridge, 1985), pp. 175–94.

18 Marcus Friedrich Wendelin, *Contemplationum physicarum* (Cambridge, 1648), p. 23.

19 Here I follow Charles B. Schmitt, *Aristotle and the Renaissance* (London, 1983), esp. pp. 7, 10–33 and 89–109, together with Nancy G. Siraisi, *Avicenna in Renaissance Italy: The 'Canon' and Medical Teaching in Italian Universities after 1500* (Princeton, NJ, 1987), pp. 12, 279–89. Indispensable for the subject of occult qualities and its continuing role in Aristotelian physics is J.L. Heilbron, *Elements of Early Modern Physics* (London, 1982), pp. 1–89, esp. 11–22. I also rely heavily on Ron Millen, 'The manifestation of occult qualities in the Scientific Revolution', in Margaret J. Osler and Paul Lawrence Farber (eds), *Religion, Science and Worldview: Essays in Honour of Richard J. Westfall* (Cambridge, 1985), pp. 185–216. On occult qualities and causes in Galenic medicine, see Nancy G. Siraisi, *Medieval and Early Renaissance Medicine* (London, 1990), pp. 145–6; Lester S. King, 'The transformation of Galenism', in Allen G. Debus (ed.), *Medicine in Seventeenth Century England* (London, 1974), pp. 20–4; and Andrew Wear, 'Explorations in Renaissance writings on the practice of medicine', in Wear, French and Lonie (eds), *Medical Renaissance*, pp. 141–4.

20 Millen, 'The manifestation of occult qualities', pp. 191–7, 202–8.

21 To this limited extent, I accept Leland L. Estes's hypothesis that medical progressiveness was supportive of witchcraft beliefs (and, perhaps, of witchcraft prosecutions), rather than inimical to them: 'The medical origins of the European witch craze: a hypothesis', *Journal of Social History*, 17 (1983): 271–84.

22 For an especially sensitive account of witchcraft accusations and consultations in the context of 'health-seeking behaviour', see Ronald C. Sawyer, ' "Strangely handled in all her lyms": witchcraft and healing in Jacobean England', *Journal of Social History*, 22 (1988–89): 461–85.

23 Andrea Cesalpino, *Daemonum investigatio peripatetica* (Florence, 1580), fos. $24^{r}$–$25^{v}$.

24 Codronchi, *Morbis veneficis*, fos. $177^{r}$–$195^{v}$.

25 For the origin of this idea, see E.E. Evans-Pritchard, *Witchcraft, Oracles and Magic among the Azande* (Oxford, 1937), pp. 63–83, 99–106. See also Keith Thomas, *Religion and the Decline of Magic* (London, 1971), pp. 535–46.

26 Jourdain Guibelet, *Trois discours philosophiques . . . le troisième de l'humeur mélancolique* (Evreux, 1603), fos. $262^{r}$–$265^{v}$. On Guibelet, see

Jean Céard, 'Folie et démonologie au XVIe siècle', in A. Gerlo (ed.), *Folie et déraison à la Renaissance* (Brussels, 1976), pp. 135–43.

27 Guazzo, *Compendium maleficarum*, p. 105.

28 Keith Hutchison, 'Supernaturalism and the mechanical philosophy', *History of Science*, 21 (1983): 307–13.

29 See esp. Codronchi, *Morbis veneficis*, fos. $16^v$–$20^v$.

30 John Henry, 'Doctors and healers: popular culture and the medical profession', in Stephen Pumfrey, Paolo L. Rossi and Maurice Slawinski (eds), *Science, Culture and Popular Belief in Renaissance Europe* (Manchester, 1991), pp. 191–211 (quotation, p. 211).

31 Hugh Trevor-Roper, *The European Witch-Craze of the 16th and 17th Centuries* (Harmondsworth, 1978), p. 59, and see the long note on pp. 59–60.

32 Michel Marescot *et al.*, *A true discourse, upon the matter of M. Brossier of Romorantin, pretended to be possessed by a devill*, trans. A. Hartwel (London, 1599), p. 22.

33 See the full account in Michael Macdonald (ed.), *Witchcraft and Hysteria in Elizabethan London: Edward Jorden and the Mary Glover Case* (London, 1991). For Jorden's Paracelsianism, see Allen G. Debus, *The English Paracelsians* (New York, 1966), pp. 162–4.

34 Symphorien Champier, *Dyalogus . . . in magicarum artium destructionem* (Lyon, c.1500), trans. Brian P. Copenhaver and Darrel Amundsen, in Brian P. Copenhaver, *Symphorien Champier and the Reception of the Occultist Tradition in Renaissance France* (The Hague, 1978), p. 289, commentary on pp. 191–8. See also Frances A. Yates, *Giordano Bruno and the Hermetic Tradition* (London, 1964), p. 172.

35 I rely here on the excellent summary of Paracelsus's views on witchcraft in Charles Webster, *From Paracelsus to Newton: Magic and the Making of Modern Science* (Cambridge, 1982), pp. 80–5, and on the Paracelsian fragment 'De sagis et earum operibus', in *Philosophiae magnae* (Basel, 1569), pp. 214–39.

36 Allen G. Debus, 'The medico-chemical world of the Paracelsians', in Mikulás Teich and Robert Young (eds), *Changing Perspectives in the History of Science* (London, 1973), pp. 85–99.

37 Joan Baptista van Helmont, *Oriatrike or Physicke Refined*, trans. J[ohn] C[handler] (London, 1662), pp. 568–73.

38 Paola Zambelli, 'Scholastic and humanist views of hermeticism and witchcraft', in Ingrid Merkel and Allen G. Debus (eds), *Hermeticism and the Renaissance: Intellectual History and the Occult in Early Modern History* (London, 1988), pp. 137–8. See also Henry Cornelius Agrippa, *Of the Vanitie and Uncertaintie of Artes and Sciences*, trans. James Sanford (London, 1575), pp. 351–2.

39 Girolamo Cardano, *De rerum varietate*, in *Opera omnia*, 10 vols (Lyon, 1663), vol. iii, pp. 289–93, 317–36.

40 Giambattista Della Porta, *Magiae naturalis, sive de miraculis rerum naturalium* (Naples, 1558), pp. 100–2. See also *idem*, *Natural magick*, trans. anon. (London, 1658), sig. $Cii^r$.

41 Johann Weyer [Johan Wier], *De praestigiis daemonum*, in *Witches, Devils*

*and Doctors in the Renaissance*, ed. George Mora (Binghamton, NY, 1991), pp. 111, 203–7, 259–60, 503–4, 510–11.

42 Reginald Scot, *The Discoverie of Witchcraft* (London, 1584), pp. 16, 35–7, 184–5.

43 John Webster, *The Displaying of Supposed Witchcraft* (London, 1677), p. 23; see also pp. 180–3.

44 *Ibid.*, p. 287; on the limitations of devils, see pp. 215–41.

45 *Ibid.*, pp. 151–63, 267–9 (quotations on pp. 152 and 268).

46 Johannes Trithemius, *Liber octo quaestionum* (Oppenheim, 1515) and *idem*, *Antipalus maleficiorum* (Ingolstadt, 1555), both excerpted in Joseph Hansen, *Quellen und Untersuchungen zur Geschichte des Hexenwahns und der Hexenverfolgung im Mittelalter* (Bonn, 1901), pp. 291–6. See also Zambelli, 'Scholastic and humanist views', pp. 133–7 (quotation on p. 133).

47 Symphorien Champier, *Dyalogus*, in Copenhaver, *Symphorien Champier*, pp. 297–303 (quotation on p. 193).

48 Webster, *Paracelsus to Newton*, pp. 80–3 (quotation on p. 80).

49 Van Helmont, *Oriatrike*, p. 570. See also the comments of Webster, *Displaying*, pp. 259–66.

50 Levinus Lemnius, *The Secret Miracles of Nature*, trans. anon. (London, 1658), pp. 86, 385, 'Preface to the reader'. The important sections are book 2, chaps 1–3, and 'Paraenesis or exhortation', chaps 57–8.

51 H.C. Erik Midelfort, 'Johann Weyer and the transformation of the insanity defense', in R. Po-Chia Hsia (ed.), *The German People and the Reformation* (London, 1988), pp. 237–8.

52 Webster, *Displaying*, pp. 197–215 (corporeality of spirits), 43–53, 66, 73, 147–8 (spiritual 'leagues'), 105, 212–15 (bodies of devils). At pp. 241–2 Webster nevertheless allowed devils to work 'in elemental and corporeal things . . . by natural means, as the applying of fit actives to agreeable passives', thus taking advantage of a commonplace of traditional demonology. Such causation included the bringing of diseases in human bodies and the instigation of the vomitings of the 'bewitched'.

53 *Ibid.*, p. 183, and see pp. 183–97.

54 Thomas, *Religion and the Decline of Magic*, p. 578.

55 R.H. West, *Reginald Scot and Renaissance Writings on Witchcraft* (Boston, 1984). The preface refers correctly to these as Scot's 'fall-back positions'.

Chapter 3

# Demonic affliction or divine chastisement?

## Conceptions of illness and healing among spiritualists and Mennonites in Holland, c.1530–c.1630

*Gary K. Waite*

This essay examines the writings of some sixteenth-century and early seventeenth-century Baptists in the province of Holland on the topics of illness and healing. The Baptists were part of the diverse religious movements of the Protestant Reformation. Appearing first in 1525 in Switzerland and South Germany, the Baptist movement gained tremendous popular support in the Low Countries during the early 1530s, especially under the leadership of the fiery apocalyptical preacher Melchior Hoffman (c.1495/1500–c.1543). Among their unorthodox tenets, Baptists believed that the German reformer Martin Luther and his learned colleagues had not gone far enough, especially on the issue of infant baptism, which they rejected, putting in its place the practice of adult or believer's baptism. Their opponents derisively called them Anabaptists (rebaptizers), a term still used to denote the early, often militant, period of their history. As a result, they were persecuted by both Catholics and Protestants. Dutch Anabaptists had pinned their hopes for a renewal of the world on the return of Christ to the 'New Jerusalem', believed to be the Anabaptist-controlled city of Münster in Westphalia, and when that city fell to its besiegers in late June 1535, many of the disillusioned Anabaptists left the movement entirely. Another grouping was organized by the Frisian former priest Menno Simons (c.1496–1561) into non-violent, separatist church communities that became known as the Mennonites. Some others, such as the Dutch glass painter David Joris (c.1501–56), moved in the direction of spiritualism, which depreciated all external rites in favour of a purely inner or spiritual church.

The question raised by this essay is, given their theological heterodoxy and, for a time, outlaw status, were these Baptists and spiritualists freer to explore unorthodox approaches to medicine than their contemporary Catholic and Calvinist counterparts? How did they relate their religious faith to their medical beliefs and practices? More specifically, did their apparently total rejection of Catholic 'religious magic' predispose them to reject overt acts of supernatural or preternatural healing and to turn to an explicit naturalism?[1]

Sixteenth-century Baptists, like other Europeans, lived in a universe that was personal and organic, in which beneficial and malevolent creatures and forces interfered in human affairs, or could be made to appear to do so by those humans with special knowledge or inbred ability.[2] In this scheme, there was nothing unusual about magic. John Henry, for one, has described it as 'a practical art which used the natural powers of things to achieve certain desired effects'.[3] However, in the sixteenth and seventeenth centuries inquisitors and reformers were on the lookout against diabolical activity in human affairs. The problem came in deciding what was legitimate and supposedly effectual medicine, and what was diabolical and illusory. What learned inquisitors and demonologists sought to suppress was 'popular technique', described by Stuart Clark as 'the enormous repertoire of techniques, recipes and rituals for good health, healing and fertility, for securing good fortune and preventing misfortune'.[4] Most people continued to hold ideas about the origins and cures of illness at odds with those of contemporary clerical reformers and university-trained medical practitioners who sought to change the opinions and practices of their more 'superstitious' flocks.[5] In spite of such attempted suppression, cunning men and women continued in the sixteenth century to provide the bulk of medical services for ordinary people, who themselves possessed a goodly store of basic medical knowledge to cope with daily existence.[6]

As we shall see here, this controversy was also prominent within the Baptist tradition, with one important difference: most Baptist leaders lacked formal education in philosophy or theology. In fact, most were merchants or artisans by trade and by the late sixteenth and seventeenth centuries an increasing number of Mennonite pastors combined their spiritual office (never a full-time occupation) with medical services to their community. Many received formal training as physicians.[7]

As a result of their medical training, a number of Mennonite preachers followed the traditional learned perspective that centred on Galen's theory of the four humours and the notion that an imbalance of one of these caused illness. A course of treatment prescribed by a Galenist usually involved bleeding or purging the patient of the excess humour. This approach filtered down to the populace via contact with professional physicians and surgeons.[8] What caused a specific humoral imbalance was, of course, open to interpretation, though it was agreed that it was internal and usually random. Excesses in diet or astrological conjunctions were often blamed. Some people sought the antecedent in the activity of malevolent witches who worked through diabolical forces, which in turn manipulated the occult powers resident within nature to affect the body of the afflicted person, or to make it appear so. God, of course, was assumed ultimately to be responsible, and some afflictions, such as epidemics, were viewed as divine chastisement for an erring people, calling for processions and public displays of penitence.

Opposing the official Galenic approach were some iconoclastic theorists, the most famous being Paracelsus (1493–1541) who argued that disease was introduced into the human body (the microcosm) from the outer world (the macrocosm) in the form of seeds. Treatment therefore involved the introduction of specially prepared chemicals that corresponded to the macrocosmic affliction. Although spurned by the medical establishment during his lifetime, Paracelsus's approach, based largely on magical techniques,[9] won considerable support throughout Europe after the publication of his controversial writings in the 1570s, leading to a dramatic revival of interest in the alchemical method.[10] As we shall see, the spiritualists and Baptists presented here displayed an acquaintance with a wide range of views, from popular beliefs to both the Galenic and Paracelsian approaches.

## EARLY BAPTISTS AND SPIRITUALISTS

With their divergent views regarding the value of external forms of religion, it would appear that spiritualists (who denigrated the outward manifestations of worship) and Baptists (who emphasized believers' baptism in the hopes of re-establishing the apostolic church) had little in common. Yet, in the Netherlands, a strongly spiritualistic stream flowed within certain segments of the Baptist/Mennonite tradition. The two most important early Dutch Baptist leaders were David Joris and Menno Simons. Although both had been influenced by Hoffman's ideas and were major figures within the early Anabaptist movement in the Low Countries, after the debacle of Münster each took his followers in a different direction to ensure their survival. Joris moved eventually to a fully spiritualistic approach to religion, even allowing outward accommodation to official religion, while Menno insisted on a public display of Baptist faith. By the time of his move to Basel in 1544 Joris was no longer a Baptist, though it seems that many Dutch Baptists continued to read his works (as did many from the other religious camps).

On many questions Joris and Menno were close[11] and both deprecated the power and activity of a corporeal devil, while emphasizing personal, human responsibility for evil. Baptists as a whole rejected the traditional sacramental system, including infant baptism and any rites associated with it, such as the exorcism of infants prior to baptism. Whether or not Menno believed demons could afflict unbelieving humans with bodily torments, his public statements reveal that he saw the root cause of illness among believers as twofold: first, as God's desire to turn them away from concerns of the flesh to higher spiritual goals; and second, as divine chastisement for their residual sinful lusts. There is no expectation of miraculous healing, nor is there even reference to medical intervention, though nowhere does Menno reject this.[12] Resignation to God's will is the central virtue required of all suffering Christians, a not surprising position given the strength of the image of the suffering martyr within the Baptist tradition.

Joris's position on the question of the cause of illness and the believing patient's response is quite similar to Menno's, albeit taken to an extreme. For one thing, Joris denied the independent, corporeal existence of the devil, thus removing his malevolent activity as a cause of illness and, concomitantly, eliminating counter-magic as a potential cure.[13] Joris, moreover, belittled the effectiveness of learned physicians and occult scientists who, in spite of appearances to the contrary, were not able to breathe life into physical matter nor to perceive the true nature of life.[14] When asked if God might allow a sorcerer (*tovenaar*) the ability to debilitate the body of a believer, Joris provided two responses. First, a 'good Lutheran' should give a negative reply, for God would not allow the devil such power. Second, he argues that even the Lutheran position reveals a faith concerned merely with the preservation of the body. What God desires is for the believer to develop a level of distance from physical concerns so that even if a sorcerer or the devil had the power to inflict illness on someone, such an event would be welcomed as a further test of one's faith in God.[15] However, Joris was not one to allow such extreme resignation to lead to a premature demise; in Basel he availed himself of the friendship and medical services of the prominent French doctor, Jean Bauhin.[16]

The most extreme spiritualistic affirmation of resignation in the face of illness is provided by Matthias Wier (1521–60), the younger brother of Johan Wier (chief physician to the court of Cleves and author of the famous *De praestigiis*), and an influential spiritualistic or mystical 'Reformed' thinker.[17] His few writings not only show considerable similarity to those of Joris, but also gained wide support among the Waterlanders, those Mennonites in the region of Holland north of Amsterdam who had come to believe their fellow Mennonites were too strict in their use of the ban and in their doctrinal rigidity.[18] For his part, Matthias regarded illness solely as a chastisement sent from God for the spiritual development of the sufferer. He describes physical suffering 'as a door through which the inner suffering enters', and this inner affliction leads to spiritual purification.[19] Neither the devil nor human, nor even natural agents appear to have been considered as important causes of sickness.[20] Illness, therefore, serves a positive function for the devout believer. One presumes, then, that Matthias discouraged attempts at medical intervention on his behalf. While his more famous brother visited him frequently, judging from Matthias's correspondence it seems their conversations revolved around theological issues, with Matthias warning Johan not to become so proud with his learning that he neglect the wisdom of God. They also discussed the relative merits of the writings of Hendrik Niclaes (the Dutch spiritualist who founded the House of Love) and Dirck Philips (an associate of Menno Simons), and Matthias tried to dissuade his brother from too close an interest in them.[21]

It is not known if Johan attempted to treat his brother. If he did, his ministrations were to little effect, for Matthias died in considerable pain at the age of 39. Surely the physician was frustrated by Matthias's disdain for physical health. In a letter to his brother, Matthias suggests that the best thing that one who is of a pure heart can do for those who are constantly troubled or depressed is to bear with them patiently, for constant physical suffering is a great gift of God.[22] For the righteous sufferer, he concludes, everything comes to good; he ought therefore to 'let the creature fall, and receive everything from the Creator, be it love or affliction'.

## THE WATERLAND MENNONITES: HANS DE RIES AND JAN WILLEMSZ

The general spiritualistic approach to illness, then, was one that viewed all physical affliction as providentially sent for the improvement of the spiritual health of the sufferer. While some, such as Matthias Wier, went to the extreme of neglecting to seek medical attention for their ills, others allowed themselves to be treated. What they all had in common was a rejection of the idea that illness could be caused or cured by diabolical means. This moderate spiritualistic approach was continued within at least one of the Mennonite communities in the Netherlands, the Waterlanders, especially those around Hans de Ries. We will therefore focus on him and on the controversy about his ideas to carry our discussion into the seventeenth century. What we discover are some very interesting developments relating to illness and medicine.

Hans de Ries (1553–1638), merchant and Mennonite preacher in Alkmaar, a town in the northern part of Holland, fled his home in Antwerp where he had practised as a Calvinist. After a period of residency in Holland and Emden, he finally settled down in Alkmaar (temporarily in 1577 and permanently in 1600), where he set up his merchant business and associated himself with the Waterland Mennonites who did not practise what he viewed as the extreme shunning and hairsplitting of many of the Mennonite groups. These ranged in disciplinary strictness from the relatively tolerant Waterlanders to the more conservative and strict Flemish and Frisian branches, though moderates existed in all of these groupings.[23] (Each group's name reflects only its respective region of origin and does not imply that individual members were born there.) De Ries soon became a preacher to the Waterlander community, one who saw his major responsibility as promoting religious unity by emphasizing the inner, spiritual church instead of attempting to recreate the external apostolic church based on a biblical literalism. What is not well known is that De Ries was also a practising alchemist and healer.

According to his anonymous biographer, De Ries's approach as a preacher/healer was one of caring for the health of both the soul and the body. He did not, however, practise what today is described as 'faith healing', but applied his alchemical knowledge to the healing arts, presumably through the treatment of the patient with some alchemically distilled chemical, often called the *Quinta Essentia*. At the same time, he provided good instruction for the 'inner conscience'. Evidently De Ries regarded his alchemical researches as a form of medicine that was both superior to the 'common medicine' practised by the traditional Galenists and more effective in meeting the needs of ordinary people, especially the poor, for whom he waived his small fee.[24] In this posture De Ries was, consciously or unconsciously, reflecting the attitude of Paracelsus who condemned the mainstream medical world that dominated the universities.

De Ries also viewed his medical activity as a corollary to his office of preacher, of caring for both the soul and body, and concluded that this was the only truly effective, or holistic, medicine. In his sermons and writings he frequently used examples from medicine to describe the spiritual world, and characterized Christ as the medicine of the soul and his wounds as true medicine.[25] Faith was required of the patient and played an essential role in the effectiveness of the prescription. It is not known whether De Ries required some act of faith in God on the part of the patient during the healing process itself, or whether the healing of the soul referred to by the biographer was restricted to De Ries's public preaching. Most alchemical theorists regarded the inner purity of the practitioner as an essential requirement for success. Presumably the patient also had to show faith in De Ries's ability as a healer; it may have been the case that the patient's previous frustration with traditionally trained physicians or surgeons made it easier for them to trust this non-traditional healer and presumed 'holy man'.

De Ries's interest in alchemy was not unrelated to his spiritualism. Recent studies suggest that though one need not be a spiritualist to practise alchemy, a spiritualistic approach to religion showed the closest affinity to alchemical methodology and language. The parallels between a spiritualistic conception of Christian progression (such as that of Joris) and the alchemical process of transmutation, are too close to be merely coincidental.[26] According to a number of scholars, the true objective of the sincere alchemist was not the greed for gold, but to discover in the process a means to convert the human 'from a lower to a higher form of existence, from life natural to life spiritual'. The human, not mere metal, was therefore the theme of spiritual alchemy, while Christ's spiritual transformation of the individual corresponded to the action of the alchemist's 'philosopher's stone'.[27] In any event, De Ries's spiritualistic approach and alchemical preoccupations became the subject not only of some interesting stories, but also seem to have initiated a peculiar spirit-inspired approach to medicine and science among a small number of Waterland Mennonites.

The stories are related to us by two Waterlanders who opposed what they viewed as the extreme spiritualistic approach of Hans de Ries and his supporters, favouring instead an emphasis on the written word as sole authority. Actually, the dispute began when De Ries chastened the Amsterdam tailor–preacher Nittert Obbesz (c.1581–c.1636) for teaching rationalistic Socinianism (which among other things disputed the doctrine of the Trinity), to which Obbesz responded by charging De Ries with spiritualistic fanaticism. Those who sided with Obbesz included the physician–preacher Jan Willemsz (1583–1660) and Jan Theunisz (c.1569–c.1637), book printer, innkeeper, brandy distiller and linguist – a controversial figure who acted as the principal propagandist for the Obbesz side.[28] Apart from his support of Obbesz and his acting as a major source for Theunisz's often scandalous reports, Jan Willemsz is important for our study because he left behind a book of sermons in which he describes the relationship between Mennonite religion, popular technique and healing. We will examine this work first and then turn our attention to some of the stories he and Theunisz have preserved.

After completing his medical studies, Jan Willemsz settled in De Rijp where he pursued a long career as both physician and Mennonite preacher.[29] His collection of sermons, completed when he himself lay ill, reveals a perspective similar to the philosophical naturalism of religious reformers and physicians who opposed what they viewed as the superstition and popular magic of ordinary people. Willemsz's disdain for the 'religious magic' of traditional Catholic ritual is very clear, comparing, for example, the Catholics' resort to prayer to saints with pagans who turned to Neptune in times of storm. Christians instead should pray only to God, without any intermediary.[30] Likewise, the devil's work of temptation occurs in the desert of our hearts, and thus he must be opposed there and not with any external or physical means.[31] Like his fellow well-educated contemporaries, Willemsz describes miracles as something above human natural ability and which could be performed only by God's special power. Such miracles are not for us, he continues, just as it is not for us to raise the dead. Satan himself cannot perform miracles, though he can create amazing illusions, with God's permission.[32] Nor can the devil directly bring about illness in humans, for such is caused by humoral imbalance.[33] What the devil specializes in is tempting people so afflicted to misdirect their faith away from God to other supports, such as 'high knowledge', that result in theological dispute or lack of faith altogether.[34] The devil could deceive people either by making them rely upon 'their own wisdom', such as the learned preachers of the mainstream churches, or by deluding them into accepting dreams and visions as valid means of divine communication; surely a reference to some within his own religious community who emphasized the personal inspiration of the Holy Spirit. Some of these make themselves poor (by command of the Holy Spirit), or even go so far as to reject proper medicine when they are ill.

> Some others when in need or sickness use no medicine, needlessly casting into danger their health or sometimes their life, saying who gave it to them, can also take it away. But Syrach expressly states, that the Lord has let the medicine grow out of the earth, and that a wise man should not despise it [Eccles.38:4]. Yes, Christ taught that the sick require the medicine master.[35]

In response to this extremist position – one that, as seen in the case of Matthias Wier, could be a logical extension of spiritualistic principles – Willemsz again and again advises his congregation to 'use all good means of help, which God has ordained to us for the good and the best of the soul and body'. In this way, he suggests, believers can answer the devil, as Christ did, that we must not tempt the Lord our God.[36]

In several sermons concerning Jesus's miracles of healing, Willemsz presents his belief that while the office of pastor, as physician of the soul, was superior to that of a physician of the body, this should not lead any to believe that they could do away with the latter's prescriptions and pretend to rely solely on God's direct mercy. Willemsz believed his combination of the offices of pastor and physician most closely resembled Jesus's own. The procedure for all those suffering any ailment is first to regard the illness as a chastisement of the Lord, intended to lead them to Christ as the true deliverer and receive inner spiritual healing. Second, the patient is to turn to the divinely ordained means of restoring physical health, that is, those who, like Jesus, are 'wise doctors' or 'medicine masters', who will properly analyze the imbalance in the humours and prescribe an appropriate cure. Even the title 'medicine master' implies formal medical education and membership in the guild of physicians as a master.

Faith in God, then, is required for the first, spiritual part of the healing process, while faith in the devout physician is essential for the completion of the physical healing. The patient is strictly forbidden from seeking medical help from any other source, especially from popular magical techniques; furthermore, no mention is made of exorcism.[37] Willemsz warns his congregation against following the example of the 'poor people' who in illness turn to a 'brave and wise' Jew, or to a gipsy soothsayer (*Heydensch Meester*) or to 'any deceitful people, be they liars, sorcerers, fortune tellers (*waerseggers*) and similar ones', instead of trusting in the 'pious and trustworthy medicine masters'.[38]

However, among the over three hundred illnesses chronicled by Willemsz,[39] there were a number that a physician could not heal, such as the leprosy afflicting those who came to Jesus.[40] Often a patient's attempts to be healed were frustrated by other factors. Writing of the woman with the blood flow in Matthew 9:18–27, Willemsz notes that no doctor could heal this woman who was forced to expend her meagre resources to purchase loathsome and useless remedies; she was healed only after turning to Jesus.[41] In other words, the patient's attitude toward God, as well as the healer, was an important factor in the success of the medicine. The art of healing was a gift of the Holy Spirit, bestowed on the properly trained and religiously devout physician. This did not imply, Willemsz argues, that all cures prescribed by that physician would succeed, for often their patients did not follow the doctor's advice or their disposition to God was not a proper one, and without the inner, spiritual healing provided to the penitent patient by the master–physician, Christ, the physical remedies would have little effect.

Willemsz, like De Ries, maintained that religious faith and proper medical care needed to be bound together to be effective. At the same time, attempts at so-called faith healing or other miraculous acts were as ineffectual as the magical techniques of the 'poor people'. Willemsz and his friend Theunisz therefore directed their critical attention towards what they viewed as the strange extremist practices of some of the Waterland Mennonites who followed Hans de Ries and his circle.

## INVENTING AND HEALING BY THE SPIRIT

Although Theunisz was a considerable vexation to his fellow Waterland Mennonites for some time, he clearly had inside information regarding some of the activities of his co-religionists. In several short pamphlets and a booklet, he points out the danger of De Ries's supposed spiritualization of the Word of God. Yet in reality the two sides were not far apart and were eventually reconciled. In brief, Obbesz and Theunisz sought to discredit their opponents by arguing that De Ries was merely following in the footsteps of more notorious spiritualists such as the aforementioned Matthias Wier and David Joris.[42] Furthermore, Theunisz asserts, some of De Ries's people, the 'Peace City Citizens' (*Vredestadsburgers*) – followers of Pieter Pietersz (1574–1651), a builder of windmills and preacher in De Rijp and Zaandam[43] – take the personal communication of the Holy Spirit so far that they claim to be led by the Holy Spirit to create inventions, such as new types of water mill or means to walk under water. Indeed, he continues, De Ries was so inspired, he believed he could transform May dew (which gave butter a reddish colour in spring) into gold![44] These charges naturally lead to the question of Theunisz's reliability, especially of his most scandalous tract, *The Hanssist Mennonite Fanatics History*. Keith L. Sprunger finds the 'startling accusations . . . hardly credible'.[45]

Before accusing Theunisz (and Willemsz, who is apparently his source of information) of creating a polemical work on totally fabricated evidence, it might be well to remember that De Ries was indeed an alchemist. Judging from the work of the Mennonite alchemist and inventor of Alkmaar, Cornelis Drebbel, the alchemical healing elixir or *Quinta Essentia* could be made not only from gold, but also from mineral, vegetable or animal matter.[46] It is not inconceivable, then, that De Ries attempted to produce alchemical gold from May dew. De Ries does not seem to have denied the charge in print, though he certainly did reject Theunisz's charge that he had become for his followers 'Pope Hans'.[47] Likewise, Theunisz's accusation that some of the Waterlanders were relying on the Holy Spirit to inspire them to make unusual inventions had a basis in fact. Drebbel achieved part of his fame for inventing, among other things, a water pump powered by a perpetual motion machine (patented in 1598) and a boat that could travel under water.[48] It therefore does seem true that the spiritualism of some Waterland Mennonites provided an atmosphere conducive to creative thought and innovation, especially when this is linked to their rejection of former traditional authorities (apart from the Scriptures), in particular the Aristotelianism of the universities, as well as their reliance on direct inspiration. Drebbel, trained as he was as an apprentice engraver with no university education, claimed that he had not relied on any of the ancients for his inventions.[49]

It is also clear that one reason why Theunisz found De Ries's emphasis on the direct inspiration of the Holy Spirit so distasteful was that this perspective opened the door of religious leadership not only to gullible fanatics, but also to women. As Joyce Irwin has noted, a spiritualistic approach to religion was much more helpful in raising the status of women than was the biblical literalism of most Baptists and Mennonites.[50] That several of the stories Theunisz relates have women prophets at their centre may not have been mere coincidence. Even if some of the details of the stories have been exaggerated by Theunisz for dramatic effect, there is no reason to doubt their essential veracity. After all, Theunisz presents these accounts as events well known to other Mennonites, and his opponents' criticism about his revelations accused him not so much of telling lies but of telling stories out of school, of presenting them in his pamphlets to a broader audience and hence of bringing discredit to Mennonites as a whole. We can therefore cautiously turn to a few of these stories which relate much more specifically to the subject of this essay.

In his notorious *The Hanssist Mennonite Fanatics History*, Theunisz relates several stories which show how, at least in this circle of Mennonites, popular technique, or at least a more popular understanding of the cosmos, could be combined with radical religion. The sisters Claasdr were the central characters in the first of these. According to Theunisz, these women taught that they could spiritually 'rebirth' adults. They supposedly did so with a fellow Mennonite, Pieter Dircksz, who stood before the bed on which one of the sisters lay. She then began to simulate the contractions of childbirth, calling out to Dircksz, 'Pieter, do you not feel something?'. Finally Dircksz responded, 'I think I feel something', at which the writhing of the woman became more intense and she cried out, 'I bear, I bear', and when she had finished, 'Pieter, I have born you, and you are now a reborn child of God'.[51] Two Mennonite leaders then had an argument about the event, with Lubbert Gerritsz (1534–1612), an Amsterdam preacher and friend of De Ries, describing the event as a result of melancholy (the same diagnosis provided by Johan Wier in his defence of accused witches), and Gerrit Lambertsz, a shoemaker–deacon and another of the *geestverwanten*, defending it as a miracle. (Theunisz's reference to the argument between these two Mennonite leaders adds some credibility to the story itself.) Evidently we have here an event inspired by a popular or magical understanding of the theological concept of rebirth.

If true, the story also reveals that some Mennonite women were seeking to restore their prophetic importance within the Dutch Baptist tradition, one that had been decidedly present in its earliest stages. Melchior Hoffman himself had been inspired by the prophetic utterances of two Anabaptist women prophets in Strasbourg, Barbara Rebstock and Ursula Jost, the latter of whose visions he had published.[52] However, the female prophetic voice had since been suppressed by the resurgence of male dominance over religious leadership, especially after Münster. According to Theunisz, these sisters had also made several prophecies which told their associates to practise community of goods, among other things.[53] Although the story of the rebirthing may have been merely Theunisz's means of discrediting such attempts on the part of women to reassert religious leadership, it is not inconceivable, and is perhaps to be expected, that women would have illustrated the theological concept of rebirth with a physical demonstration of the real thing.

Another event recounted by Theunisz involved a Cornelis Laackhuysen who was staying at the home of a bed-ridden Mennonite sister Judith Lubberts, a stocking darner. Cornelis announced to the three girls also residing there that Judith would undergo a miraculous transformation: in the course of the night she would die and be reborn. The three girls were instructed to keep watch through the night, which they did, noticing that suddenly the patient stopped moving and her eyes became still, as in death. Then Cornelis made his grand entrance, upon which Judith suddenly announced – surely to the fright of the girls – 'oh, there returns the spirit into me, now I am reborn'. When Cornelis interrogated the girls about the miracle they had just witnessed, they were reluctant to view it as such, showing a pronounced scepticism about the supposed death and rebirth. Yet Cornelis and Judith continued to proclaim to others the miracle of the rebirth and of Judith's deliverance from an illness that had brought her close to death.[54]

The final story of a Mennonite visionary experience described by Theunisz to be mentioned here is that of Gerrit Francken, deacon of a Mennonite community in Leiden. He supposedly believed himself to have been led by angels to see visions, one of which occurred during the Christmas season and involved an apparition of a crib in the sky. Apparently his emotional description of this to a mainly Catholic audience had great effect.[55] On a trip from Leiden to Hoorn, to arrange the marriage of his son, Francken seems to have gained the devotion of a dog, which he soon came to regard as an angelic familiar. Because of this he turned down Jan Willemsz's request to be given the animal. When visiting Anthonius Jacobsz in Hoorn, Francken alluded to a special communication with the dog, without further explanation. One morning, however, Jacobsz confronted his visitor with plain evidence that there was nothing unnatural about his pet, saying to Francken,

> 'Gerrit Francken, your dog has shit vilely. Has the hidden meaning of his inspiration thus come to light?' 'What', said Gerrit Francken, 'did you say that it is a dog? It is an angel of God'. 'No', said Anthonius Jacobsz, 'it is a dog, he has shit much too vilely to be an angel'.[56]

Of course, the whole story may simply have been nothing more than Francken pulling his friend's leg. According to Theunisz, however, Francken later revised his belief about the dog when the planned marriage fell through.

Similar stories are described by the storekeeper and pastor of the conservative Old Frisian Mennonite church in Hoorn, Pieter Jans Twisck (1565–1636).[57] For example, he relates the story of Mr Jacob of Hoorn, who believed not only that he no longer had to work with his hands, but also took it upon himself to cast out demons 'by faith' and to heal infirmities (here we do have a Mennonite faith healer). One time a 'rough and rebellious man' came to him with a lame hand and even though Mr Jacob was unable to heal it, the man was so captivated by Mr Jacob's preaching that he refused to criticize the faith healer. Twisck himself disputed with one of Mr Jacob's disciples, who affirmed that his associates could perform the 'true, believing signs, wonders and miracles', even to the point of being able to raise the dead. As further evidence that Mr Jacob was a charlatan, Twisck notes that this supposed holy man bought a lovely house in Hoorn, in which he built many small ovens in order to practice the craft of alchemy.[58] Alchemy (perhaps also Paracelsianism) was evidently repudiated by some Mennonite leaders who linked it with spiritualistic extremism and medical quackery.

What these stories described by Theunisz and Twisck also reveal is that magical notions and popular techniques could be blended in a unique fashion in some Mennonite quarters. In an age when witches were believed to cause illness and exorcists cast out demons by the dozen, these Mennonite stories are not at all surprising, however strange they may seem to a modern reader. But they do reveal a clear difference of approach regarding the level of direct interaction between the divine and human worlds. Many, perhaps most, of the Waterlander leadership evidenced a clear scepticism with respect to visions and miracles, even when attested to by well-regarded associates. Others saw them as a natural outcome of a relationship with the divine. Even those, who sought like Willemsz and Theunisz to discredit the stories, did not, in any direct way, seek to blame the visions and miracles on the immediate work of the devil, though Theunisz believed one could see the 'depths of Satan' in De Ries and his followers.[59] The story of the angel/dog, for example, would have provided Theunisz with an opportunity to accuse his opponents of having demonic familiars. Yet he did not do so. Instead, Theunisz, like Willemsz, resorted to a non-supernatural explanation – the dog was just a dog belonging to a deluded man, visions were caused by praying in dark cellars or by fits of melancholy. For his part, Twisck also turned to a providentialistic explanation when debating the causes of the great plague of mice of 1617. Those witches who confessed to causing the plague were lying, for they could not even make a hair white or black without God's permission. Instead, the plague was ultimately God's chastisement of sinful humanity. Twisck, however, also suggests that there may have been a primarily natural reason for the event, for when God allows a succession of hot summers and dry winters, then one ought not to be surprised that the land was overrun with mice.[60] There was no need, then, to blame the devil or witches when there is clear evidence of natural causation.

The dispute between Hans de Ries and his supporters on the one side and Jan Willemsz and Jan Theunisz on the other, may have had as much to do with their different approaches to healing as to the precise theological differences that received the greatest publicity. The Galenist Willemsz was a strong supporter of traditional university medicine and of the professionalization of the physician's craft.

De Ries, on the other hand, appears to have been something of a Paracelsian, identifying with the Swiss theorist's rejection of the stranglehold that the university elite had over the medical profession. While both Willemsz and De Ries combined the healing arts with their preaching office, their combinations were quite distinct. De Ries's approach, with its emphasis on Paracelsian or alchemical methodology and the direct inspiration of the Holy Spirit was more open to innovation and helpful popular techniques, perhaps even faith healing. De Ries's attitude seems to have encouraged an atmosphere of inventiveness within the spiritualistic Mennonite communities of Northern Holland that perhaps helped inspire one of the most famous inventors of his day, Cornelis Drebbel. Given the examples presented here, it may also have fostered an environment receptive to alchemical pursuits. For example, not only did the Flemish Mennonite preacher and university-trained physician Galenus Abrahamsz (1622–1706) take De Ries's spiritualism to its ultimate conclusion of advocating a purely invisible church, but he too attempted, at least once, to create gold by means of alchemy.[61]

Willemsz's approach strikes the modern reader as being the more rational one, combining a biblical literalism with the naturalism of the university-trained physician. At the same time, both sides depreciated the role of the devil in causing illness, seeking its cause instead in divine activity or natural developments. As a result of recent studies by Marijke Gijswijt-Hofstra and Hans de Waardt, we now know that later Mennonite writers, such as Jan Jansz Deutel (d.1657), Abraham Palingh (1588/89–1682), and Antonius van Dale (1638–1708), among others, came out strongly against the prosecution of so-called witches and for a naturalistic interpretation of their supposed acts.[62] This examination of the views of some earlier spiritualists and Mennonites has illustrated that the works of Palingh and Van Dale were the climax of a century-long tradition within the Dutch Baptist reformation that depreciated diabolical interference in human affairs, usually offering in its place a 'common sense' explanation of supposed magical events. Such an approach is revealed in Theunisz's account of the supposed 'Mennonite miracles' and in the sceptical reaction of many of his co-religionists. That most Mennonite leaders came from the artisanal and merchant strata of society, or practised medicine, generally kept them away from much of the theological speculation of the universities and mainstream churches. Their spiritualistic inheritance from the sixteenth century also played a role in this development.

In any event, the Waterland Mennonites regarded illness as a divine and natural event, lacking any significant diabolical interference; an interesting position during the age of heightened fears of demonic activity and witch hunts.

## ACKNOWLEDGEMENTS

Funding for this research was graciously provided by the Social Sciences and Humanities Research Council of Canada and the University of New Brunswick. All translations are my own.

## NOTES

1 Sjouke Voolstra, ' "The colony of heaven": the Anabaptist aspiration to be a church without spot or wrinkle in the sixteenth and seventeenth centuries', in Alastair Hamilton, Sjouke Voolstra and Piet Visser (eds), *From Martyr to Muppy: A Historical Introduction to Cultural Assimilation Processes of a Religious Minority in the Netherlands: The Mennonites* (Amsterdam, 1994), pp. 15–29, esp. pp. 16, 20.
2 Keith Thomas, *Religion and the Decline of Magic* (New York, 1971), pp. 631–68.
3 John Henry, 'Doctors and healers: popular culture and the medical profession', in Stephen Pumfrey, Paolo L. Rossi and Maurice Slawinski (eds), *Science, Culture and Popular Belief in Renaissance Europe* (Manchester and New York, 1991), pp. 191–221, esp. p. 217.
4 Stuart Clark, 'The rational witchfinder: conscience, demonological naturalism and popular superstitions', in Pumfrey, Rossi and Slawinski (eds), *Science, Culture and Popular Belief*, pp. 222–48, esp. pp. 226–7. See also Stuart Clark, 'Inversion, misrule and the meaning of witchcraft', *Past and Present*, 87 (1980): 98–127, esp. pp. 99–100; and *idem*, 'The scientific status of demonology', in Brian Vickers (ed.), *Occult and Scientific Mentalities in the Renaissance* (Cambridge, 1984), pp. 351–74.
5 Bengt Ankarloo and Gustav Henningsen (eds), *Early Modern European Witchcraft: Centres and Peripheries* (Oxford 1990), p. 13.
6 Henry, 'Doctors and healers', p. 199.
7 Voolstra, ' "The colony of heaven" ', p. 25; Piet Visser, *Broeders in de Geest*, 2 vols (Deventer, 1988), vol. I, p. 111.
8 Henry, 'Doctors and healers', pp. 197–205.
9 *Ibid.*, p. 213.
10 Walter Pagel, *Paracelsus: An Introduction to Philosophical Medicine in the Era of the Renaissance*, 2nd edn (Basel, 1982); Allen G. Debus, *The Chemical Philosophy: Paracelsian Science and Medicine in the Sixteenth and Seventeenth Centuries*, 2 vols (New York, 1977).
11 Samme Zijlstra, 'Menno Simons en David Joris', *Doopsgezinde Bijdragen*, nieuwe reeks 12–13 (1986–87): 71–80.

12 For example, see Menno Simons, 'Letter of consolation to a sick saint (1557)', in J.C. Wenger (ed.), *The Complete Writings of Menno Simons* (Scottdale, PA, 1956), pp. 1052–4.

13 Gary K. Waite, 'David Joris en de opkomst van de sceptische traditie jegens de duivel in de vroeg-moderne Nederlanden', in Gerard Rooijakkers, Lène Dresen-Coenders and Margreet Geerdes (eds), *Duivelsbeelden in de Nederlanden* (Baarn, 1994), pp. 216–31; *idem*, ' "Man is a Devil to himself": David Joris and the rise of a sceptical tradition towards the Devil in the Early Modern Netherlands, 1540–1600', *Nederlands Archief voor Kerkgeschiedenis*, 75 (1995): 1–30.

14 David Joris, *Twonder-boeck: waer in dat van der werldt aen versloten gheopenbaert is*, 2nd edn (1551) ([Vianen, 1584]), part II, $9^{v}$–$10^{r}$.

15 In a bound volume, with 42 MS tracts, University of Amsterdam, MS 65–82, $68^{r}$–$71^{v}$.

16 Gary K. Waite, *David Joris and Dutch Anabaptism, 1524–1543* (Waterloo, 1990), pp. 181–2, 189.

17 E. Simons, 'Matthes Weyer, ein Mysticker aus der Reformationszeit', *Theologische Arbeiten aus der rhein. wissenschaftliche Predigerverein*, new series, 9 (1907): 30–49.

18 Sjouke Voolstra, 'The path to conversion: the controversy between Hans de Ries and Nittert Obbes', in Walter Klaassen (ed.), *Anabaptism Revisited* (Scottdale, PA, and Waterloo, Ontario, 1992), 98–114, esp. pp. 103–4.

19 Matthias Wier, *Dat Boeck der Sproecken Inhoudende veel schone onderwijsingen/ hoe een yegelijck tot reynighinghe synder sonden ende om tot die wedergheboorte te comen hem schicken sal* ([Vianen?], n.d.), p. 74.

20 *Idem*, *Grondelijcke Onderrichtinghe/ van veelen Hoochwichtighen Articulen/ eenen yeghelijcken die tot reyniginghe zijnre Sonden/ ende in die wedergheboorte begheert te comen/ seer dienstelijck. Door den hooch-van-Godt-verlichten M.W. met synen vrienden/ bekenden ende bywoonderen tot verscheyden tijden so Schriftelijck als mondelijck gehandelt ende wtghesproocken* ([Vianen?], 1584), pp. 9–14.

21 *Ibid.*, pp. 34–5, 41–5.

22 *Ibid.*, pp. 51–2.

23 Visser, *Broeders*, vol. I, pp. 82–133; Cornelius J. Dyck, 'Hans de Ries and the legacy of Menno', *Mennonite Quarterly Review*, 62 (1988): 401–16.

24 Anonymous, *Kort-Verhael Van het Leven ende Daden van Hans de Ries Outste/ ende Leeraer der Waterlantsche-Gemeenten* (De Rijp, 1644), pp. 56–8.

25 Hans de Ries, *Ontdeckinghe der dwalingen/ misduydinghen der H. Schrift ende verscheyden mis-slagen/ begrepen in seecker Boeck/ ghenaemt RAECH-BESEM* (Hoorn, 1627), pp. 61–2.

26 Gary K. Waite, 'Talking animals, preserved corpses and Venusberg: the sixteenth-century worldview and popular conceptions of the spiritualist David Joris (1501–1556)', *Social History*, 20 (1995): 137–56, esp. pp. 153–6.

27 James R. Keller, 'The science of salvation: spiritual alchemy in

Donne's final sermon', *Sixteenth Century Journal*, 23 (1992): 486–93, esp. p. 487.

28 Keith L. Sprunger, 'Jan Theunisz of Amsterdam (1569–1638): Mennonite printer, pamphleteer, renaissance man', *Mennonite Quarterly Review*, 68 (1994): 437–60. Further on Theunisz, see Voolstra, ' "The colony of heaven" ', pp. 101–04; Piet Visser, 'Aspects of social criticism and cultural assimilation: the Mennonite image in literature and self-criticism of literary Mennonites', in Hamilton, Voolstra and Visser (eds), *From Martyr to Muppy*, pp. 67–82, esp. p. 77; and Visser, *Broeders*, vol. I, pp. 37–40, 68–78.

29 Piet Visser, *Dat Rijp is moet eens door eygen Rijpheydt vallen: Doopsgezinden en de Gouden Eeuw van De Rijp* (Wormerveer, 1992), pp. 36–8; Visser, *Broeders*, vol. I, p. 72.

30 Jan Willemsz, *Postilla, Dat is Wtlegginge der Sondachs en Hoge feestdachs Euangelien door het gantsche Iaer* (De Rijp, 1647), p. 252.

31 *Ibid.*, pp. 335–54.

32 *Ibid.*, p. 1154.

33 *Ibid.*, pp. 926–7, 1021–36.

34 *Ibid.*, p. 342.

35 *Ibid.*, p. 345.

36 *Ibid.*, p. 353. Willemsz's argument on this and many other points is reminiscent of other Protestant providentialists, such as the English Calvinists examined in David Harley, 'Spiritual physic, Providence and English medicine, 1560–1640', in Ole Peter Grell and Andrew Cunningham (eds), *Medicine and the Reformation* (London and New York, 1993), pp. 101–17.

37 For Catholic resort to exorcism, see Charles Caspers, 'Duivelbannen of genezen op "natuurlijke" wijze. De Mechelse aartsbisschoppen en hun medewerkers over exorcismen en geneeskunde, ca. 1575–ca. 1800', in Willem de Blécourt, Willem Frijhoff and Marijke Gijswijt-Hofstra (eds), *Grenzen van genezing: Gezondheid, ziekte en genezen in Nederland, zestiende tot begin twintigste eeuw* (Hilversum, 1993), pp. 46–66, esp. pp. 52–3. For the medical debate over exorcism in sixteenth- and seventeenth-century Holland, see Hans de Waardt, 'Van exorcisten tot doctores medicinae: geestelijken als gidsen naar genezing in de Republiek, met name in Holland, in de zestiende en de zeventiende eeuw', in *ibid.*, pp. 88–113; and *idem*, 'Chasing demons and curing mortals: the medical practice of clerics in the Netherlands', in Hilary Marland and Margaret Pelling (eds), *The Task of Healing. Medicine, Religion and Gender in England and the Netherlands 1450–1800* (Rotterdam, 1996), pp. 171–203.

38 Willemsz, *Postilla*, p. 1035.

39 *Ibid.*, p. 1127.

40 *Ibid.*, pp. 935, 1121.

41 *Ibid.*, pp. 1127–8.

42 [Nittert Obbesz], *Raegh-besem. Seer bequaem Om sommige Mennonijtsche Schuren te reynigen vande onnutte Spinnewebbens, sotte grollen, en ydelheden eeniger Geest-drijveren, Swinckveldianen ende des selfs voorstanderen, die op hun bysondere drijvingen ende inspraken steunen tot verminderingh van't*

*beschreven woordt Godts* (Amsterdam, 1625), pp. A4$^r$, E1$^r$, E3$^v$–F4$^v$; Jan Theunisz, *Jan Willemsz. Raegh-stock, Voor Nittert Obbesz. Raegh-beesem. Ofte eenighe Spreucken oft redenen ghetoghen uyt het Boeck van Jan W. Medecijn ende Bisschop over de Komen-lannen op de Rijp teghens den Gheestdrift ofte Geestdriverye, van Pieter Pietersz. ende Claes Jacobsz. mede-vermaanders, ende teghen andere Geestdryveren met hun* (Amsterdam, 1627), p. 6.

43 Visser, *Broeders*, vol. I, pp. 37–43; Visser, *Dat Rijp*, pp. 41–5.

44 Theunisz, *Jan Willemsz*, p. 3.

45 Sprunger, 'Jan Theunisz', p. 454.

46 Cornelis Drebbel, *Grondige oplossinge van de Natuur en Eygenschappen der Elementen . . . Als mede Een klare beschrijving van de Quinta Essentia* (Amsterdam, 1688), p. 567.

47 Sprunger, 'Jan Theunisz', pp. 452–4.

48 For more on Drebbel and his alchemy and inventions, see F.M. Jaeger, *Cornelis Drebbel en zijne Tijdgenooten* (Groningen, 1922), pp. 9–10; Gerrit Tierie, *Cornelis Drebbel (1572–1633)* (Amsterdam, 1932), pp. 18–25; also anon. 'Kort verhaal van het leeven des beroemde natuurkenner Cornelis Drebbel', in Cornelis Drebbel, *Kort begrip der Hoofdstoffelycke Natuurkunde of Inleiding tot de Kennis der Eigenschappen van de vier Elementen* (Amsterdam, c.1800).

49 Cornelis Drebbel, *Een Kort Tractaet van de Natvere der Elementen, ende hoe sy veroorsaecken, den wint, reghen, blixem, donder, ende waeromme dienstich zijn* (Haarlem, 1621), pp. 8–9.

50 Joyce L. Irwin, *Womanhood in Radical Protestantism 1525–1675* (Lewiston, 1979), p. xxix.

51 [Jan Theunisz], *Der Hansijtsche Menniste Gheest-drijveren Historie, Ofte kort Verhael van de ghepretendeerde Ghesichten/ Inspraken/ Openbaringen/ende haer Acten/ by onse tijden. Voort-komende uyt de leeringe ende drijven van een invvendigh, ofte onbeschreven Woordt, van Hans de Rys* ([Amsterdam], 1627), p. 30.

52 Klaus Deppermann, *Melchior Hoffman: Social Unrest and Apocalyptic Visions in the Age of Reformation*, trans. Malcolm Wren, ed. Benjamin Drewery (Edinburgh, 1987), pp. 203–13.

53 Within the Baptist tradition, the practice of community of goods was not restricted to Münster or the Hutterites: see James M. Stayer, *The German Peasants' War and Anabaptist Community of Goods* (Montreal and Kingston, 1991).

54 [Theunisz], *Der Hansijtsche Menniste*, pp. 31–2.

55 *Ibid.*, p. 35.

56 *Ibid.*, p. 36.

57 Marijke Gijswijt-Hofstra, 'Doperse geluiden over magie en toverij: Twisck, Deutel, Palingh en Van Dale', in A. Lambo (ed.), *Oecumennisme: Opstellen aangeboden aan Henk B. Kossen ter gelegenheid van zijn afscheid als kerkelijk hoogleraar* (Amsterdam, 1989), pp. 69–83.

58 Pieter Twisck, *Chronijck vanden onderganc der tijrannen ofte Jaerlycklche Geschiedenissen in Werltlycke ende Kercklijke saecken*, 2 vols (Hoorn, 1620), vol. II, pp. 1441–2.

59 Jan Theunisz, *Brief Aen de Broederen van Komen-Jans-volck in Waterlant, ende op de Rijp* (Amsterdam, 1627), single-page broadsheet.
60 Twisck, *Chronijck*, vol. II, p. 1737.
61 H.W. Meihuizen, *Galenus Abrahamsz, 1622–1706* (Haarlem, 1954), pp. 148–50.
62 Gijswijt-Hofstra, 'Doperse geluiden'; Hans de Waardt, 'Abraham Palingh en het demasqué van de duivel', *Doopsgezinde Bijdragen*, 17 (1991): 75–100; *idem*, 'Abraham Palingh. Ein holländischer Baptist und die Macht des Teufels', in Hartmut Lehmann and Otto Ulbricht (eds), *Vom Unfug des Hexen-Processes: Gegner der Hexenverfolgungen von Johann Weyer bis Friedrich Spee* (Wiesbaden, 1991), pp. 247–68.

Chapter 4

# A false living saint in Cologne in the 1620s

## The case of Sophia Agnes von Langenberg

*Albrecht Burkardt*

Shortly after St Catherine's Day in 1621 Gertrud Foer, a nun of St Vincent's convent in Cologne, was suffering from a painful fracture of her knee which made walking impossible for her without the aid of a crutch. Consulting a physician brought no relief, nor did her subsequent recourse to the hangman (*Scharffrichter*) with his reputed healing powers.[1] After these failures, Gertrud turned to other, 'alternative', means of healing. As we should expect of a good nun, this decision, encouraged by her family, did not appear to lead to any kind of 'superstitious' practices. In recommending herself to the prayers of another pious nun in the nearby monastery of St Clara, Gertrud appeared rather to avail herself of one of the most conventional 'spiritual' means towards health offered by the church: the intercessory prayer.[2]

This minor incident would not attract the reader's attention if Gertrud had contented herself with such pious practice. But prayer was not enough for Gertrud and her hope for recovery was based above all on the person she chose to pray for her. So great was her confidence in the nun of St Clara's that, not satisfied with recommending herself to the nun's prayers, Gertrud insisted on meeting her, as she was convinced that by talking personally with the nun and by complaining of her misery and pain, she would recover her health.

Gertrud's hopes were not wasted. With the permission of her superiors, on St Blasius's Day 1622, more than two months after her accident, she visited St Clara's where she talked to the nun. On the way home she was suddenly delivered from her suffering. A document now preserved in the Vatican Archives bears witness to this grace and its author, the abbess of St Vincent's, left no doubt as to whose merits had brought about this incident: 'that this grace was given to us through the prayers of Sophia of Langenberg, professed nun in St Clara's, that is what I wanted to stress . . . with my own hands'.[3] Obviously the document reveals more than a simple recourse to a traditional church ritual. Between the world of learned or popular magic and the established cult of saints, their relics and miraculous images, it indicates the existence of a form of curing which, though widespread in other Catholic areas, has not yet been observed for the Cologne medical market: the recourse to a 'living saint'[4] whose reputation of sanctity led to a genuine, though unofficial and more or less discrete, cultural exercise of charismatic gifts.[5]

For the Catholic authorities, dealing with such a phenomenon was a difficult matter precisely because this practice could not be seen as an officially established cult. Indeed, it was during this very period that the papacy, confronted with the enormous wave of sanctity it had itself encouraged within the Counter-Reformation movement, tightened the rules concerning canonization procedures. These measures imposed by the Holy Office concerned people who had died with a reputation of sanctity; the concern for orthodoxy and for avoiding scandals was all the greater when living saints were involved.[6]

There was no need for papal wisdom to make it clear to the local authorities that a charismatic mediator of the supernatural must be treated with suspicion. At a time when witch hunting in Germany was about to reach its peak in a tremendous wave of persecution, it was obvious to any observer that such a person could as easily have been inspired by the devil as by God. For one of the masters of northern witchcraft theory, Jean Bodin, the question of how to make the distinction between the two was at the heart of the whole enterprise of demonology.[7] But even if one descends from Bodin's somewhat Manichaean viewpoint – and his crucial statement on devilish inspiration under a pious or even holy appearance – to a mere day-to-day level of confrontation with the supernatural, members of the secular or regular clergy played an important part in the mediation of magical practices, at least as far as Cologne was concerned.[8] This was especially true of men, and the case of Cologne seems to be quite similar to that of Naples where men, and in particular monks or clerics, were the practitioners of 'learned magic', based on the study of books. Meanwhile, the world of 'popular magic', based on oral traditions, was largely dominated by poor lay women.[9]

The Naples example also shows, as does our own case, that nuns, though better protected inside the walls of convents, could be no less active mediators of the supernatural. It is difficult to establish a distinction between nuns practising with the reputation of living saints and women practising in the surrounding world, just as it is difficult to draw clear distinctions between magical practices and legitimate church rituals.[10] As to Gertrud Foer, the source is silent about what happened during our nun's visit to St Clara's, but even supposing that a completely 'legitimate' form of action had ended in a clearly miraculous event, it was a commonplace among theologians that such a fact, while justified by its edification of the faithful, did not necessarily prove the reliability of the intercessor.[11]

While Gertrud Foer may not have had to worry about the character of her grace, provided that its effects lasted, her intercessor's reliability was far from being taken for granted. Indeed, Sophia Agnes von Langenberg was not destined to become a venerated saint. It is true that in exceptional cases during the same period some future saints succeeded in overcoming the substantial difficulties they encountered with their spiritual authorities before finally becoming venerated. Sophia was to experience the opposite. Having taken her vows in 1614, she acquired her reputation of sanctity during a long illness in 1621–22. But, in April 1622, as soon as her *fama* became publicly known, serious doubts started to arise about its consistency. It is true that this questioning did not initially have very dramatic consequences. However, in 1626, the convent of St Clara was the setting of an important series of demonic possessions and it was during this period that the nun's reputation was definitely transformed into that of a person inspired by the devil. Sophia was executed within months.

It is in this guise, with the reputation of a 'witch', a 'foolish' or 'possessed' person, that Sophia Agnes von Langenberg has found a modest place in Cologne's local history. This place in history is an uncomfortable one because, in 1626, Sophia's name was linked above all with the well-known affair of Catharina Henot, an aristocrat whose condemnation as a witch was mainly due to the denunciations of the nun of St Clara's. Subsequently, Catharina's execution, in May 1627, triggered the only major wave of witchcraft persecution in Cologne – a period which lasted until 1630 and resulted in almost 30 victims being burnt at the stake.[12]

The moving case of Catharina Henot who was condemned to death in a trial which far exceeded the common procedures applied to the *crimen exceptum* puzzles contemporary scholars as much as it scandalized its first historians, including Friedrich Spee.[13] However, in light of what happened to Sophia, it seems clear that the demonic possession invoked in the case of Catharina Henot has been consistently underestimated by historians of this witch hunt, who have treated the only 'visible' origins of the accusation against Catharina, including the denunciation by Sophia Agnes von Langenberg, as trivial.[14] For other witch-hunting regions in Germany demonic possessions have been recognized as typical starting points of persecution waves.[15] Is not such a mechanism even more convincing against the emotional background of the fall from grace of a so-called saint in one of the most distinguished monasteries of Cologne?

However, Sophia's progress – from a reputation for sanctity to its 'falsification' and translation into a case of demonic possession and finally into the beginnings of a witch hunt – was not one approved by all parties. The case of Sophia Agnes von Langenberg gave rise to different appreciations of its 'nature' – over the course of time, but also in the eyes of the different authorities involved. The subsequent changes of perspective were accompanied each time by the takeover of the case, or at least an attempt to do so, by another institution interfering in the business, procedures which involved a great deal of conflict between these different authorities which were continuously overshadowed by questions concerning the distribution, loss or gain, of institutional power.[16]

The background to these conflicts between various church institutions can readily be understood. It is true that the highest spiritual power of the region was Cologne's Archbishop, who was also the temporal ruler of the surrounding Electorate (*Kurköln*). The regular clergy, however, were largely exempt from his prerogatives and directly subject to the Holy See and thus, in Cologne, to the papal *Nunzio* residing there.[17] These exempted institutions would appeal to that functionary whenever they saw their rights encroached upon by the Archbishop, and the *Nunzio*, moreover, was also responsible for their spiritual supervision. That is why we owe most of the information concerning our case to the investigations of Pier Francesco Montoro, *Nunzio* from 1621–24, and in particular to his correspondence with the secretary of state in Rome.[18]

## SOPHIA'S 'CALLING'

The primary spiritual authority of St Clara's was confided to its confessors, the Franciscans of Cologne. It was under their guidance that Sophia's particular vocation had developed and it is among them that we find the immediate supporters of her sanctity – in particular her personal confessor who, as Montoro put it, 'demonstrates much esteem for her, writing her biography, conserving her belongings as relics, and not content with relating her visions, in her own presence he calls her the "Chosen of the Lord", the "Bride of God" '.[19]

It is not possible here to go into a detailed analysis of the different traits which compose the nun's reputation of sanctity, but if one considers Montoro's few indications against the background of the Franciscan spiritual traditions, it is not difficult to imagine that the nun's life was modelled on the traditional image of female sanctity spread by the mendicant orders in the later Middle Ages: one of a woman who 'not particularly well educated, tended to a strongly emotional expression of religious sentiment, formed strong ties with a spiritual director', and was 'inclined to mystical experiences', centred on a particular 'eucharistic devotion' and on the Passion of Christ.[20] This model was perhaps slightly modified at the beginning of the seventeenth century by the influence of the Counter-Reformation Spanish mystics, and in particular by the example of St Teresa, whose *Vita*, by F. de Ribera, had been published for the first time in the German vernacular in Cologne in 1621.[21]

I would like to pay more attention, however, to the question of how Sophia actually acquired the reputation of a charismatic healer. We may begin with Montoro's statements about the case, mentioning that Sophia's supporters not only glorified her victorious fight against the devil's temptations, but also her own miraculous recovery, 'relating as a marvel that having died she had then been resuscitated'.[22] The two elements are revealing. Both might be interpreted as tests in an act of initiation confronting the future saint with the most difficult trials on the road to sainthood: the 'incarnation' of evil – and death. And while the first may give proof of the saint's reliability, the second will establish, in particular, her thaumaturgical capacities. In that latter respect, recent research has pointed to the parallels between the Christian saint and the phenomenon of shamanism where the acquisition of charisma often follows the successful mastery of the crisis of a dangerous illness.[23] Indeed it may seem evident how these mechanisms of vocation work in Christian notions and traditions. The saint acquires his charismatic, thaumaturgical gifts by the radical imitation of Christ's Passion. Taking upon himself, as did Christ, the suffering and evil of the world, he becomes for his devoted patients a reliable agent of salvation.[24] And from that point of view the pious parallels, so strongly criticized as idolatry by the Protestant movement, between Christ and the life of certain saints, in particular that of St Francis, appear comprehensible.[25]

Thus, it is not very surprising that Sophia's *fama* was based on a long-lasting agony and its extraordinary outcome. On the threshold of death, in a series of visionary journeys to the gates of heaven, Christ himself finally called her to her spiritual functions and sent her back into her corpse on earth.[26] Consequently the very proof of this vocation was her miraculous recovery itself. And against the background of the aforementioned spiritual traditions it seems natural that the initial act of that recovery was performed by her (completely shattered) confessor himself when marking Sophia's languishing body with a crucifix and with the sign of the cross on the very sites of Christ's stigmata. This was just the starting point for a whole chain of events alternating between visionary contacts with the divine on the one hand, and miraculous signs on the other.

The first proof of Sophia's sanctity had been given on her own behalf; now her gifts could be used for other people. Given the particularly explicit nature of what was literally a calling, it is clear that Sophia herself knew her status full well, and indeed she did not hesitate to emphasize this vocation whenever she felt any resistance against her. If such behaviour might appear somewhat smug as opposed to a good saint's humility, Sophia's methods as a practitioner do not appear to have transgressed the limits of prudent spiritual assistance by means of prayer and confidential, semi-confessional conversation. That is what is illustrated by Gertrud Foer's visit to the nun, for which we fortunately have a more direct account in the testimony of Sophia's confessor. Having listened to Gertrud's motivation for coming to see her, Sophia tried to determine the possible 'spiritual' causes of Gertrud's illness – some particular sin, perhaps, an insufficient exercise of her duties as a nun, or God's will to prove her patience and humility. Of course this examination did not lead to a veritable confession of Gertrud's sins, but nevertheless it seemed to provoke some repentance ('so that the poor maid was crying bitterly'), to which Sophia Agnes replied with a friendly exhortation to spiritual improvement and confidence in God.[27] It was this kind of 'purification' which enabled Sophia to pray for Gertrud, which she did immediately after the nun's departure. The rest of the story we know.

Instead of searching for the origins of Gertrud's illness in external 'supernatural' causes – a spell for instance – or having recourse to some kind of 'automatic' (sacramental or magical) ritual, Sophia thus stressed her 'patient's' own faults as the origin of her suffering. The repentance of these faults became the condition of her intercession for a recovery which mirrored the patient's unburdened conscience.[28]

## SOPHIA'S CASE IN ROMAN PERSPECTIVE: THE DOUBTS OF *NUNZIO* MONTORO

Whereas the events described so far had been handled in a more or less confidential sphere, in April 1622 – more than a year after the curing of Gertrud Foer – they were suddenly brought to public notice by one of the most emphatic miraculous signs. On Easter Sunday a crucifix hanging in the nun's *cella* started to bleed. For the monastery's confessors this event must have constituted the zenith of a whole series of signs confirming Sophia's sanctity. However, the papal *Nunzio* who was immediately called to the scene offers us, with his critical distance, a completely different way of appreciating this affair. It is not even the miracle itself which made Montoro abandon his rather lenient passivity toward the case. What counted was the way in which the event had been treated and which transformed the whole into a definitely public affair. Immediately after the event, the confessors exhibited the crucifix to a mass of people gathered that Sunday in the church of St Clara, and without the *Nunzio*'s intervention 'they would have already decided to carry it in procession through the whole town'.[29]

It is obvious that the confessors' actions were not at all in accordance with the procedures required in such a case; the Council of Trent called for a strict verification of a possible miracle before allowing publicity of any kind.[30] As the opposite had happened, Montoro's situation was embarrassing. It was no longer possible to hide the traces of the event; on the day of the miracle Montoro did not even dare to remove the blood from the crucifix, since the nuns' agitation in that case would incur the risk of uproar, 'there being an infinity of people in the church and the square'.[31] However, it was impossible to let matters ride. This might have been conceivable if the event had taken place in public, but having happened in the *cella* of a nun whose reputation – given the demonic temptations Montoro had been told of – could be suspect, the risk of a later discovery of fraud and the scandals this might provoke was too high. This danger was even more devastating in its possible effects as the 'heretics' in the city were ready to seize such opportunities to ridicule the Catholic faith.[32]

Montoro's provisional solution was a complex one. After locking the crucifix up in a room of the convent and sealing off the door, he convened a committee of churchmen to investigate the miracle. At the same time, he seemed to want to let the affair cool off a bit, 'all the more so since if the miracle is proved we can always publish it, whereas in the opposite case, with time passing, the curiosity of the people will have been greatly dissipated'.[33]

Accustomed to such supernatural cases – many of which did not end well – the *Nunzio* was above all concerned about the public effects of such an affair and to avoid scandals. Preserving a positive public image was what really served the glory of God, much more than the truth of a particular miracle, and all the more so since it was clear to him that such a 'truth' was far from being proved by just the material solidity of the given fact. Thus, the first step in the miracle's verification – the certificate of no less than ten physicians that the liquid on the crucifix was real blood – led only to the exclusion of a first possible doubt: the suspicion of 'imposture or human art'.[34]

And yet, an even more disquieting doubt persisted. Although it was clear to everyone that a real miracle exceeding the limits of nature could only be performed by God, the devil was constantly expected to be the author of 'illusions' that were hard to distinguish, for human beings, from signs of divine origin. And since Sophia was well known for her demonic temptations, Montoro's commission had good reasons to suspect some deception. However, as divine intervention was not yet excluded, the commission turned to a golden rule of the authoritative administration of the supernatural. It is not the miracles which determine the legitimacy of a *causa*, but precisely the opposite: 'it seems to these Fathers that in order to find out whether there is a miracle or some fraud, one should examine her [Sophia's] life and virtues'.[35]

In that respect, Montoro had more than one reason to have

doubts about Sophia's case: 'the root is infected'! Her father was, though a Catholic, the counsellor of a Protestant prince. Her mother was said to have been involved in witchcraft affairs, and Sophia herself did not even seem to have an honest vocation as a nun: 'they say that she became a nun because of the despair she felt not to have been married to a young man she was in love with'.[36] And in fact that is what seemed to have been the original reason for her temptations, the devil having tried to seduce her by his promise to make her regain her beloved. Those promiscuous temptations actually seemed to have been prolonged in the life of the monastery itself: 'there are interests of nuns with friars' – favoured by a too liberal handling of the nuns' enclosure, 'a failing of almost every monastery in this town'.[37] In Sophia's case the suspicion even fell upon her confessor himself: 'a very young confessor for that kind of business, good looking and rather robust, who enters the enclosure whenever he likes'.[38]

Thus Montoro's doubts were based in a sense on the almost classic images of the enemy in the age of confessions. If the possibility for the transmission of witchcraft from a mother to her daughter was widely accepted among the partisans of persecution, the father's contacts with heresy were no less harmful to Sophia's reputation. And both roots of corruption, coming from outside the monastery, led consequently to the again significant triad on the inside, to a suspect religious vocation, an inclination towards demonic seduction and, finally, 'carnal vices'.

It is interesting to note in this context, that Sophia's confessor had also linked some first doubts about the consistency of the nun's visions announcing her forthcoming recovery to the influence of her parents. But he had done so in a benevolent sense. During her state of incurable suffering and terrible anxiety without the release of death, Sophia's visions had seemed to be the expression of some forces preventing her from finding eternal peace; a phenomenon typically produced by parents who, either by not fulfilling a pious vow or by loving their children too much in the hour of death, prevented them from dying.[39] It was only after a longer conversation with Sophia's father, and after his tearful acceptance of the confessor's exhortation 'that he should sacrifice her to God', that these reservations about Sophia's continuing visions ceased.[40] This was the second time that the nun had needed to be 'liberated' from her parents' will, for her entry into the monastery had already been retarded by her father's long resistance.

Thus, Montoro's and the confessor's point of view concerning Sophia's background were as contradictory as they were analogous. Whereas, for the latter, the nun's trajectory to holiness was closely linked to the preceding renunciation of and liberation from the world, and in particular from her family, Montoro seemed to be convinced that Sophia could not escape from these origins – and that her ecstatic crisis was the outcome of this. Nevertheless, and in spite of these serious doubts about Sophia's reliability, Montoro's conclusions about the whole affair were astonishingly pragmatic. Since the confessor's presence happened to be linked just as closely to the miraculous aura of the nun as to the dangers of promiscuity, the most evident and incisive measure to take was to separate him from Sophia, replacing him with a zealous, prudent and aged person 'who will teach her the exercise of humility, patience and the other virtues, and will make her return to an ordinary life'. So time would decide 'whether there is in her the true spirit of God'.[41]

And indeed, as far as the *Nunzio*'s involvement was concerned, the measures taken in this affair did not go further. Some weeks after Montoro's first letter they were approved in their entirety by Rome.[42] Although this relative leniency must also be seen in the local context of a considerable spreading of the vices of the flesh amongst Cologne's clergy,[43] one might nonetheless speak here of a specifically Roman position dominating this second phase of Sophia's destiny. In Italy too 'false' female saints were persecuted attentively by the Inquisition,[44] but to prevent the feared public scandals resulting from such affairs, the sanctions considered appropriate against such nuns came down, more or less, to reinforced enclosure.[45] Of course such a destiny was hard enough to bear for the women concerned, since they saw themselves confronted with the most dishonourable accusations, including the traditional couple of heresy and sexual perversion. But at least the alternative between demonic and divine inspiration does not appear to have been as frightening in the Italian perception as it was in the northern witch-hunting countries.[46] It is therefore not by chance that Montoro's conclusions on Sophia's case are not only contemporaneous with the aforementioned reforms concerning canonization procedures, but also with the famous *Instructio*, worked out by the Inquisition, in which Rome expressed a remarkably sceptical view of the persecution of witchcraft – a position very similar, by the way, to that of Spee's *Cautio criminalis*.[47]

But above all, coming back to the case of Sophia, the danger of demonic agencies does not seem to have been sufficiently pressing for Montoro to let it take precedence over political considerations. According to the *Nunzio*, the change of confessor had to be carried out 'in some way which does not raise the slightest suspicion'.[48] This was not only designed to avoid Sophia's suspicion, but also, once more, to prevent the probable scandals which might arise from further publicity about the affair: an argument which counted even more strongly for the method of dealing with the carnal vices suspected in the monastery. This overwhelming fear of scandals was not only based on the hay which the 'heretics' could possibly make of them. There were at least two other distinct elements. The convent of St Clara's was one of the most distinguished monasteries in Cologne and any effort at reform had to avoid questioning the honour of Cologne's and the Electorate's most distinguished families whose unmarried daughters were often destined to religious life there.[49] In addition the *Nunzio* and the Holy See had some interest in not dramatizing these affairs. Since they were directly responsible for the supervision of the regular clergy, these scandals could too easily lead to a questioning of the papal prerogatives by the alternative spiritual power in Cologne, the Archbishop.

Thus, the desire to prevent public scandal – the same motive which was at the origins of Montoro's involvement in the case – also set its limits and made him search for a benevolent solution.

## FROM 'FALSE SANCTITY' TO WITCHCRAFT: THE 'NORTHERN' PERSPECTIVE

Due to an outbreak of the plague, Montoro left Cologne some months after the miracle and went no further in the investigation of the event. Having been finally convinced that the miracle was 'a mere imposture', his last act in the case, again some months later, was the removal of the crucifix from the monastery – once more 'to prevent the opportunity for new scandals'.[50] But in St Clara things did not cool down. Most likely due to the disillusionment surrounding Sophia's case, and perhaps in part due to the plague, the monastery for a long time became the theatre of demonic possession and the Franciscans themselves turned to exorcism. As the situation did not improve, Cologne's Vicar-General, Johann Gelenius, decided, in 1626, to intervene himself in the affair.[51]

This intervention undoubtedly provoked an unpleasant feeling of *déjà vu* for Montoro's successor, Pier Luigi Carafa, for Montoro had already been confronted with exactly the same problem. Independently of Montoro the Vicar-General then in office had started to investigate the miracle, thus violating, in the *Nunzio*'s view, the papal prerogative. The Vicar-General had argued for the application of the decrees of the Council of Trent, which required every miracle to be verified by the Bishop. To the *Nunzio*, this reasoning – easily to contradict – hid more fundamental motives: the Archbishop and his collaborators' tendency tendency wherever and whenever possible to restrict papal rights in favour of their own, primarily economic, concerns. A watchful defence was thus necessary 'regarding everything concerning the Holy See whose authority is so weak in these regions that, if one cedes in one point, one loses everything'.[52]

One can imagine that Gelenius's intervention in the case must have raised the same preoccupations for Carafa, who took a clear position in favour of the Franciscans who had been accused of not working vigorously enough against the ongoing possessions.[53] Montoro's commission had in fact included the Archbishop's representative, a measure which had been, at the time, an effective diplomatic move to maintain the papal juridical primacy in the case while avoiding any more serious conflict with the Archbishop. The outbreak of possessions, however, seemed to Gelenius to justify a much more uncompromising handling of the affair. While Montoro had hesitated to intervene too rigorously in the case – partly to avoid compromising the honour of certain distinguished families – the desire to preserve that honour was now used to favour the opposite line of action. Gelenius's central argument for his exorcisms in the monastery was that the Archbishop had been asked by the relatives of certain nuns to conduct them[54] and it is obvious that this argument was not only used for strategic reasons.

Apart from the power struggle between the *Nunzio* and the Archbishop, and notwithstanding the latter's reinforced attempts to take over the spiritual authority in the convents under papal prerogatives,[55] the Archbishop, and even more so his Vicar-General, had a serious personal interest in the case. Gelenius did not even shrink from a measure which clearly showed that Sophia was still at the centre of the whole affair. Not only did he demand a solid re-examination of the miracle which thus – four years after the event – still seemed to be the decisive enigma, but he went so far as to remove Sophia from the monastery and put her into confinement.[56] Even here he acted with some justification. To get around the lengthy and persistent legal conflict with the Franciscans concerning the monastery's spiritual supervision in general, the Archbishop had called, in the case of Sophia, upon an institution which had thus far not been directly concerned with the affair: the Roman Inquisition itself.[57] It was from this institution that he not only obtained permission to investigate the miracle,[58] but even 'to torture, and also to come to a definitive judgement' against the nun, henceforth 'under investigation . . . for magic, idolatry, and other very serious excesses'.[59]

With the results of this investigation, we enter the last phase of the evolution described above: the beginnings of a wave of witchcraft persecution in Cologne. However much the Holy Office recommended to the Archbishop, in the same authorization, to keep in mind 'the clemency of Rome', it nonetheless gave way to the assertion, in Sophia's case, of a typically 'northern' perspective toward demonic affairs. Whereas Gelenius's predecessor had been among Sophia's supporters, whose enthusiasm had to be restrained by the *Nunzio*,[60] the new Vicar-General's revision of the case made her the first victim of the persecution wave in Cologne. Her execution on 31 January 1627 was thus the last step in the steady decline in the reputation of this nun once venerated as a living saint.[61]

Nevertheless, the affair of the miracle remained constantly in the background of the witch hunt. Catharina Henot was questioned on the subject of the crucifix and was even accused of having bewitched and murdered the churchman to whom Montoro had entrusted the crucifix when he was forced to leave Cologne. Moreover the very last victim of the persecution, Christina Plum, was condemned to death, partly because of her connections with 'the false miracle of the cross in St Clara's'.[62]

It would be worth reanalysing the whole persecution wave against this background; in the meantime at least the fate of the crucifix can be traced. This object – 'which they say spreads blood . . . by the work of the Devil' – seems to have worried the Holy Office so much that it could not be left in the hands of the Archbishop's representatives. 'To restrain the diversity of opinions formed by the common people' the Inquisition preferred another solution – to take the crucifix directly to Rome.[63]

## ACKNOWLEDGEMENTS

This article is a first overview of the subject. A more detailed study is in preparation, in which I will publish archival material on the case. Quotations and notes have therefore been limited. I would like to thank Marc Naimark and Patricia Simonson for assistance with the English.

## NOTES

1 On the healing activities of the hangman in Cologne, see R. Jütte, *Ärzte, Heiler und Patienten: Medizinischer Alltag in der frühen Neuzeit* (Munich, 1991), pp. 27, 108.
2 E. Lengeling, 'Fürbitten', in *Lexikon für Theologie und Kirche*, (Freiburg, 1960), vol. 4, col. 461–2. For Cologne, see Jütte, *Ärzte, Heiler und Patienten*, pp. 157–158.
3 Archivio Segreto Vaticano (ASV), Archivio Nunziatura Colonia (ANC) box 83, fo. $307^r$.
4 On the Cologne medical market, see Jütte, *Ärzte, Heiler und Patienten*; On 'alternative means' of curing, see *ibid.*, pp. 131–62.
5 J.-M. Sallmann, *Naples et ses saints à l'âge baroque (1540–1750)* (Paris, 1994); G. Zarri, 'Le Sante vive. Per una tipologia della santità femminile nel primo Cinquecento', *Annali dell'Istituto Italo–Germanico di Trento*, 6 (1980): 371–445.
6 On the measures decreed by the Holy Office in 1625, see the comments of Sallmann, *Naples et ses saints*, pp. 111–13. On the suspicion against living saints, see notes 10 and 44 below.
7 Jean Bodin, *De la démonomanie des sorciers* (Paris, 1587), p. 15.
8 G. Schwerhoff, *Köln im Kreuzverhör. Kriminalität, Herrschaft und Gesellschaft in einer frühneuzeitlichen Stadt* (Bonn, 1991), pp. 429–30, 440–1.
9 J.-M. Sallmann, *Chercheurs de trésors et jeteuses de sort. La quête du surnaturel à Naples au XVIe siècle* (Paris, 1986), pp. 141–91.
10 For the different uses of magic and its constant fusion with rituals or traditional motifs of the church in Cologne, see Jütte, *Ärzte, Heiler und Patienten*, pp. 149–57; Schwerhoff, *Köln im Kreuzverhör*, pp. 428–36. For Naples, see Sallmann, *Chercheurs de trésors*, 145; *idem*, 'La Sainteté mystique féminine à Naples au tournant des XVI^e^ et XVII^e^ siècles', in S. Boesch-Gajano and L. Sebastiani (eds), *Culto dei santi, istituzioni e classi sociali in età preindustriale* (Rome, 1984), pp. 681–702, esp. pp. 690–2.
11 Angelo Rocca, *De Canonizatione sanctorum commentarius* (Rome, 1601), p. 65.
12 Schwerhoff, *Köln im Kreuzverhör*, p. 427; F. Siebel, *Die Hexenverfolgung in Köln* (Bonn, 1959). On Catharina Henot, including a few remarks on Sophia Agnes von Langenberg, see *ibid.*, pp. 52–62; and L. Ennen, *Geschichte der Stadt Köln*, (Düsseldorf, 1880), vol. 5, pp. 773–83.
13 G. Schormann, *Der Krieg gegen die Hexen. Das Ausrottungsprogramm des*

*Kurfürsten von Köln* (Göttingen, 1991), pp. 52–6; F. Spee, *Cautio criminalis oder Rechtliches Bedenken wegen der Hexenprozesse*, ed. J.-F. Ritter (Munich, 1982), p. 190.

14 Schormann, *Der Krieg gegen die Hexen*, p. 54; Siebel, *Die Hexenverfolgung*, p. 60.

15 W. Behringer, *Hexenverfolgung in Bayern. Volksmagie, Glaubenseifer und Staatsraison in der Frühen Neuzeit* (Munich, 1987), p. 177; C. Ernst, *Teufelaustreibungen. Die Praxis der katholischen Kirche im 16. und 17. Jahrhundert* (Bern, 1972), pp. 23–6.

16 For a classical study of a similar affair, see M. de Certeau, *La Possession de Loudun* (Paris, 1990). For another important case of possession in the archdiocese of Cologne, some decades after Sophia's case, see R. Decker, *Die Hexen und ihre Henker: Ein Fallbericht* (Freiburg, 1994).

17 A. Franzen, *Der Wiederaufbau des kirchlichen Lebens im Erzbistum Köln unter Ferdinand von Bayern, Erzbischof von Köln 1612–1650* (Münster, 1941), pp. 244–6, 255–65. On the *Nunzio*, *ibid.*, pp. 36–50, and M.F. Feldkamp, *Studien und Texte zur Geschichte der Kölner Nuntiatur*, 2 vols, Collectanea Archivi Vaticani, 30–1 (Vatican City, 1993).

18 *Nuntiaturberichte aus Deutschland nebst ergänzenden Aktenstücken. Die Kölner Nuntiatur*, im Auftrage der Görresgesellschaft hrsg. v. Erwin Iserloh, vol. 6, bound in 2 vols: *Nuntius Pietro Francesco Montoro 1621–1624*, bearb. v. K. Jaitner (Munich, 1976) (hereafter NBK VI, 1/2). There is a short description of the case in G. Chaix, *De la cité chrétienne à la métropole catholique: Vie religieuse et conscience civique à Cologne au XVI*[e] *siècle*, thesis for State doctorate (Strasbourg, 1994), pp. 995–8.

19 NBK VI, 1, p. 240, no. 221, Montoro to Ludovisi, Cologne, 17 April 1622.

20 R. Kieckhefer, *Unquiet Souls: Fourteenth-Century Saints and their Religious Milieu* (Chicago, IL and London, 1984), p. 32. On the devotion of the Passion, *ibid.*, pp. 89–121.

21 G. von Gemert, 'Theresa de Avila und Juan de la Cruz im deutschen Sprachraum. Zur Verbreitung ihrer Schriften im 17. und 18. Jahrhundert', in D. Breuer (ed.), *Frömmigkeit in der frühen Neuzeit*, Chloe, Beihefte zum Daphnis, 2 (Amsterdam, 1984), pp. 77–107, esp. pp. 88–99.

22 NBK VI, 1, p. 252, no. 231, Montoro to Ludovisi, Cologne, 24 April 1622.

23 Sallmann, *Chercheurs de trésors*, p. 152; *idem*, *Naples et ses saints*, pp. 243–51; G. Klaniczay, *The Uses of Supernatural Power* (London, 1990), pp. 95–110, 129–50.

24 A. Burkardt, 'Reconnaissance et dévotion: les Vie des saints et leurs lectures au début du XVIIe siècle à travers les procès de canonisation', *Revue d'histoire moderne et contemporaine* 43: 2 (1996): 214–33..

25 Bartholomeo de Ridoncio, *De confirmitate vitae beati Francisci ad vitam Domini Jesu (1380–1390)* (Milan, 1510). On the Protestant polemics against these traditions, see R. Schenda, 'Die protestantisch–katholische Legendenpolemik im 16. Jahrhundert', *Archiv für Kulturgeschichte*, 52 (1970): 28–48.

26 This mechanism of vocation also forms part of the medieval traditions of female sanctity. See P. Dinzelbacher, *Vision und Visionsliteratur im Mittelalter* (Stuttgart, 1981), pp. 39, 51; *idem*, 'Körperliche und seelische Vorbedingungen religiöser Träume und Visionen', in T. Gregory (ed.), *I sogni nel medioevo* (Rome, 1986), pp. 57–86. In spite of the geographic and temporal proximity and other astonishing analogies, the case of Sophia Agnes von Langenberg differs considerably from that of Evert Willemsz described by Willem Frijhoff in this volume. It is true that the two protagonists found their charismatic vocation in a sort of juvenile conversion crisis triggered by a dangerous illness. But the types of vocation are different. Whereas Sophia incorporates traditional traits of female sanctity centred on mystical experience and a thaumaturgical practice, Evert appears more in the guise of popular prophet. In the two conversion crises themselves this difference finds its expression, beyond the same experience of illness, in differing ways of communication with the divine. Evert owes his godly messages to apparitions. The Holy Ghost descends upon him, just as the Spirit descended upon the disciples. Sanctioned by this biblical tradition, such a 'calling' was appropriate of course for prophetic vocations, but it is not surprising that Evert was not by any means a charismatic healer. The healer's calling finds its expression in a very different way of communicating with the sacred. Sophia 'leaves the earth' by means of her visionary journeys, and it is this transgression of the border between life and death which founded her thaumaturgical capacities. For the traditional distinction between apparitions and visions, see Dinzelbacher, *Vision*; for several examples of such ecstatic healers, see W. Behringer, *Conrad Stoeckhlin und die Nachtschar. Eine Geschichte aus der frühen Neuzeit* (Munich, 1994).

27 ASV, ANC box 83, fo. 257r.

28 On these different explanations of the supernatural origins of illness and the rareness of a position like Sophia's in Cologne, see Jütte, *Ärzte, Heiler und Patienten*, pp. 46–54.

29 NBK VI, 1, p. 242, no. 222, Montoro to Ludovisi, Cologne, 17 April 1622.

30 A. Michel, *Les Décrets du Concile de Trente* (Paris, 1938), p. 596 (XXVth session).

31 NBK VI, 1, p. 239, no. 221.

32 *Ibid.*, p. 252, no. 231.

33 *Ibid.*

34 *Ibid.*, p. 240, no. 221.

35 *Ibid.* On the criteria of the *discretio spiritum*, see J.-M. Sallmann, 'Théories et pratiques du discernement des esprits', in *idem* (ed.), *Visions indiennes, visions baroques: les métissages de l'inconscient* (Paris, 1992), pp. 91–116.

36 NBK VI, 1, p. 252, no. 231. Apart from these indications by Montoro, we have no further information on Sophia's biographical background.

37 *Ibid.*, and also p. 240, no. 221.

38 *Ibid.*, p. 240, no. 221.
39 ASV, ANC box 83, fo. 310[r].
40 *Ibid.*, fo. 310[v].
41 NBK VI, 1, p. 240, no. 221.
42 Ibid., p. 263, no. 245, Agucchia to Montoro, Rome, 7 May 1622.
43 Ibid., pp. 268–9, no. 252, Montoro to Ludovisi, Cologne, 8 May 1622. For a broader characterization of this 'moral status', see Franzen, *Der Wiederaufbau*, pp. 167–75, 246–54.
44 G. Zarri (ed.), *Finzione e santità tra medioevo ed età moderna* (Turin, 1991); *idem* and L. Scaraffia (eds), *Donne e fede. Santità e vita religiosa in Italia* (Rome and Bari, 1994).
45 Sallmann, 'La sainteté mystique féminine', pp. 697–701; *idem*, *Naples et ses saints*, pp. 177–210.
46 J. Tedeschi, 'Inquisitorial law and the witch', in B. Ankarloo and G. Henningsen (eds), *Early Modern European Witchcraft. Centers and Peripheries* (Oxford, 1990), pp. 83–118.
47 *Idem*, 'The Roman Inquisition and witchcraft: an early seventeenth century "Instruction" on correct trial procedure', *Revue de l'histoire des religions*, 200 (1983): 163–88. For a famous example of an application of this *Instructio*, see C. Ginzburg, *I Benandanti* (Turin, 1966), pp. 176–81. See also Decker, *Die Hexen und ihre Henker*, pp. 279–312.
48 NBK VI, 1, p. 240, no. 221.
49 *Ibid.*, p. 240, no. 221, 252–3, no. 231, 268, no. 252.
50 NBK VI, 2, p. 852, no. 1123, final relation of Montoro to his successor Carafa.
51 *Nuntiaturberichte aus Deutschland* [as note 18], vol. 7/1: *Nuntius Pier Luigi Carafa 1624–1627*, bearb. von Josef Wijnhoven (Munich, 1980) (hereafter NBK VII/1), p. 549, no. 812, Carafa to Barberini, Liège, 20 Nov. 1626.
52 NBK VI, 1, p. 251, no. 231.
53 NBK VII/1, p. 549, no. 812.
54 Historisches Archiv des Erzbistums Köln, E–Bc 5, fo. 161[r].
55 Franzen, *Der Wiederaufbau*, p. 246.
56 *Ibid.*, n. 66; Th.P. Becker, 'Hexenverfolgung in Kurköln: Kritische Anmerkungen zu Gerhard Schormanns "Krieg gegen die Hexen" ', *Annalen des Historischen Vereins für den Niederrhein*, 195 (1992): 204–14, esp. p. 213.
57 The Holy Office had been informed several times about the affair, but until then it had not taken a stand. See, for instance, NBK VII/1, p. 68, no. 2.
58 *Nuntiaturberichte aus Deutschland* [as note 18], vol. 7/2: *Nuntius Pier Luigi Carafa 1627–1630*, bearb. von Josef Wijnhofen (Munich, 1980), 39, no. 1110, Millino to Carafa, Rome, 23 Oct. 1627.
59 Biblioteca Apostolica Vaticana, Barb. lat. 6334, fo. 314[v], Rome, 1 Nov. 1626.
60 NBK VI, 1, p. 252, no. 231.
61 Hauptstaatsarchiv Düsseldorf, Kurköln, box 23, fo. 247[r]; I am very grateful to Dr Thomas Becker who told me of this archival evidence, discovered by Hanna Stommel. See also Thomas Becker, 'Hexen-

verfolgung im Erzstift Köln', in *Bensberger Protokolle*; H. Stommel, *Quellen zur Geschichte der Stadt Erftstadt*, vol. 4 (both forthcoming). It is difficult to explain the obvious contradiction between the sceptical attitude of the Holy Office towards witchcraft affairs and its blessing of the Archbishop's takeover of Sophia's case. However, beyond the fact that the Inquisition could not foresee the outcome of the affair (the persecution wave in the Electorate was only about to start), one cannot exclude the possibility that the decision was motivated above all by political considerations. Given Gelenius's excellent reasons for taking over the spiritual authority at St Clara's, the Holy Office might have found it wise to invert Montoro's reasoning (cited above) and thus to concede Sophia's case to the Archbishop; it 'cedes in one point' in order not to 'lose everything' – that is, the papal prerogatives.

62 The text of this condemnation has been edited by Siebel, *Die Hexenverfolgung*, pp. 150–1 (quotation p. 150); for C. Henot, see the indications given in her famous letter, *ibid.*, pp. 147–50, written in prison to her brother Hartger, 147, 149. See also NBK VI, 2, p. 852, no. 1123.

63 NBK VII/1, p. 690, no. 1045, Millino to Carafa, Rome, 28 Aug. 1627.

Chapter 5

# Popular Pietism and the language of sickness

## Evert Willemsz's conversion, 1622–23

*Willem Frijhoff*

### AN UNCOMMON ORPHAN

During the summer of 1622 and the following winter, the town of Woerden in the province of Holland was a hive of rumours. A sudden sickness, physical troubles and a spiritual experience had stricken a 15-year-old tailor's apprentice, named Evert Willemsz, a native of the town.[1] He claimed to be in communication through an angel with his heavenly Father. The boy lived at the local orphanage together with his elder brother Pieter and two younger half brothers. Evert's family name appears to have been Bogaert, but he never used it other than in its Latin form Bogardus; which is how he was known at Leiden University where he matriculated in 1627, and also after 1633 as a minister of the Dutch Reformed Church on the island of Manhattan in New Netherland (the present-day State of New York).[2]

We know nothing for certain about his parents. Evert lost his natural father, Willem Bogaert, when he was very young. He was educated by his stepfather, Muysevoet, who must have died, like Evert's mother, some years before the boy's spiritual experience, perhaps in the plague year 1617–18.[3] The four brothers were then placed in the town orphanage of Woerden. Members of Evert's stepfather's family are known to have been small artisans, mostly shoemakers, but as no account of any property appears in the administration records of the orphanage, the family was without means. Without parents, without the help of a local family network, without money or property and having an uneducated (though not necessarily illiterate) background, Evert had virtually no opportunities to rise in society. But he had got something else: intelligence and faith.

What happened to Evert Willemsz in 1622–23 is known to us from two contemporary pamphlets which confirm each other and partly repeat the same information.[4] Their editor was Lucas Zas, headmaster of the small local grammar school and an eye witness to the events. However, the pamphlets' true author was Evert himself, for the text of the pamphlets consists for the most part of the messages which he wrote down during his spiritual experience when he was temporarily deaf and dumb. During this time, he communicated through written notes, referred to as 'copies' in the pamphlets. Each slip of paper contained both the questions and the answers in a dialogue with one person who had come to confer with Evert. Other notes contained his spiritual messages, written under the impulsion of an angel's apparition or after his ecstatic experiences. His own version of the summer experience of 1622, written down some weeks afterwards in a long hymn, was also added.

It was not Evert himself but Master Zas who made a coherent story out of the notes, but without any rewriting of Evert's own words and without literary pretensions. The pamphlets were printed immediately. The manuscript of the first pamphlet was hurriedly carried by Master Zas to Utrecht on Friday, 20 January 1623, during Evert's second spiritual experience, when he was still waiting for his redemption. The second manuscript was first checked against Evert's own handwritten notes by the Woerden town council and the church consistory, and then ordered by them to be brought to a zealous Calvinist bookseller in Amsterdam, Marten Jansz Brandt, who published them immediately. Both pamphlets were reprinted at least once, an indication of the public attention which the boy enjoyed for a time.

The decisions taken by the Woerden town council on Evert's behalf demonstrate that we are not dealing with a religious hoax.[5] In fact, the council never ceased to favour him above other pupils. In particular, the orphanage master and school inspector Gerrit Gijsbertsz Vergeer, a wealthy cloth merchant who from the very beginning was one of the leaders of Calvinist orthodoxy in Woerden, appears to have been Evert's mainstay on the council. In 1622 Evert was admitted to the Latin school, four years later the new town organist was instructed to teach him music; in 1627 he was authorized to leave for Leiden University and in 1629 the Woerden scholarship at the theological college at Leiden was granted to him.

Apparently, the events of 1622–23 are strewn with the classical commonplaces of adolescent conversion; the most direct course to achieving a successful identity, to use Erik Erikson's terms.[6] Evert follows the psychosomatic patterns of what Freudian psychiatrists call a conversion hysteria. However, in reducing his experience to the stereotyped outlines of a psychiatric model, we would lose our hold on the multiple meanings of the event: personal, social, religious and cultural. Besides, the pamphlets were not presented as the exemplary story of a youthful hero who remains above the event and his calling, as we see in the accounts of many other young Protestant religious enthusiasts, some of which date back to before Evert's time.[7] The boy's reluctance to endorse the interpretation of his experience by the authorities, either religious or political, may also be the reason why the story of Evert Willemsz was not later used in edifying literature. It has remained the life story of a real young man, its impact limited to the time period in which it happened.

## PHYSICAL DISABILITIES AND HEAVENLY MESSAGES

In the spring of 1622 Evert finished his elementary education and, while living in the orphanage, almost completed his two-year apprenticeship with master tailor Gijsbert Aelbertsz, whom he loved very much for his piety and for their discussions about God's word. This very companionship may well have opened his eyes to his true vocation – not as a tailor, but as a minister.

According to the story in the pamphlet, Evert had been seriously ill for some time. He had barely recovered when other physical phenomena manifested themselves. From 21 to 30 June 1622, he neither ate nor drank (see Appendix). By isolating himself from the community he caused a sensation among the thirty-odd children of this densely populated orphanage, in which all deviations from the everyday routine were welcome. Evert's refusal of the daily aggregation ritual of meals taken in common was the most efficient way to bring him to the attention of both the orphans and the trustees. The pamphlets show clearly how concerned the matron of the orphanage was about his well-being, not to mention her embarrassment about the disorders in the group caused by Evert's dealings with heaven.

This first phase of physical isolation was followed by a second which lasted throughout the summer, from 30 June to 8 September. Evert was stricken deaf and dumb. He could neither speak nor hear and occasionally he lost his sight, 'as also for a long time the proper use of his reason' (B6).[8] This phase of physical paralysis, with the privation of almost all use of the senses, served as a climax. It suggests a slowly intensifying struggle which led naturally to a new, crucial moment of transition. It prepared Evert for a third, ecstatic phase, which again lasted for nine days, from 8 to 17 September 1622. Evert returned to fasting and still could neither hear nor speak, but this last phase was circumscribed by the double apparition of an angel of the Lord. This points to the true meaning of Evert's experience: communication with heaven. The angel delivered to him a message from the Father (*his* Father): he had to convert people and admonish them to repent, to deliver themselves from their sins. The heavenly origin of the message and the veracity of Evert's encounter with the angel would be proven and legitimated by his deliverance from the physical disabilities with which God had stricken him, and a return to his previous state of health. The angel brought a second message of social conversion for himself, to which we will return later.

After the angel's first appearance, Evert went into a trance-like state and a long period of ecstatic writing. For entire days he wrote his heavenly messages on little slips of paper, mostly simple messages of a repetitious nature:

> Spread the word, spread the word, for God is sore displeased that word of his wondrous works is not spread. Oh spread the word, oh my dear friends, I beg you, spread the word, for God is displeased that his godly things are not communicated throughout the whole world. Spread the word, then, oh spread the word.
>
> (A3)

The message was just as simple as the knowledge of the world which the young tailor's apprentice had acquired. He repeated it throughout the pamphlets: there are good men and bad; God wants the good to repent, so his word must be spread and the signs must be read. As the background to this message, we can detect a very simplified form of belief in double predestination as defended by orthodox Calvinism and confirmed in 1618–19 by the Synod of Dordrecht. It was quite similar to the grassroots form of everyday theological discussion at Woerden which appears in the documents around the denominational struggles of the 1610s and 1620s: the bad are damned and the good are elected. But God will punish even the good if they do not publicly behave as his perfect faithful.[9]

The signs of God's wrath were easy to detect – the repeated plagues, dearth (implying famine) and war (A2–4, B24–6). This traditional liturgical triad (*a peste, fame et bello libera nos, Domine*) was preceded by the 1618 comet ('the rod', A3) as their portent.[10] But the most important sign of all was God's wondrous work in his faithful child Evert Willemsz. Having first stricken him with sickness and deprived him of the use of his bodily functions, He will sovereignly deliver him at the moment chosen by Himself and announced through the angel's intervention. To believe in the truth of Evert's spiritual experience was therefore to believe in God's work with all his elected people. Evert had no doubt whatsoever about his own election. The affliction which God had put upon him was the very proof of his election. God visits the one He loves. Evert felt like Christ; he suffered for his Father, but finally reconciled his will with God's will (Luke 22:42; B7, B10). Evert knew for sure that he was one of the 144,000 elected who would sing the hymn of the Lamb (Apoc. 14:1–5, 15:3; B17–18). But he did not take Christ's place; though he may have been tempted by the role of a godly mediator, he finally remained at his human place, as a messenger and a minister of God.

Evert's texts certainly reveal a form of youthful radicalism that linked up well with the firm positions of the predestinarians and which was more easily satisfied by the pious and straightforward intolerance of orthodox Calvinism than by the political accommodations of Arminian latitudinarianism and humanistic toleration. He did not worry about subtleties such as the why, the when or the how. In his perception, there was no clear distinction between heaven and earth, nor between time and eternity. The present day and the Last Judgment overlapped; the sins were great and punishment was near. However, Evert was not naïve. He followed the apocalyptic mainstream of orthodox Protestantism but kept his eyes fixed upon his own destiny. He willingly used church and civil authority for his divine goal, but refused to become a 'will-less' victim of these powers, as we shall see later. In a rhymed message Evert resumed his position telling us which were the evil ones' sins:

O woe that ever we were born,
So angry is the Lord,
That people will not live
According to God's word . . .
For people now are very full

Of excess and of pride
They give themselves to drunkenness
And adultery besides.
People commit so many sins
That God cannot abide . . .
The Lord will soon come down to us
To punish all the bad.
That is the meaning of the rod [the comet]
So frightfully sad.

(A3)

## PERSONAL ACHIEVEMENT

During Evert's first spiritual experience everything remained enclosed within the boundaries of the orphanage. In time, however, his activities drew attention in Woerden, all the more so when the young man found his impresario in Master Zas. Lucas Zas (c.1591–1636), the son of a Gouda schoolmaster, had worked prior to his appointment as a headmaster and precentor at Woerden as a teacher of Latin and French at Utrecht and nearby Montfoort. In addition to the two pamphlets, in 1628 he published a play on parents' responsibility for their children's education and the choice of a profession (*Borgerliicke Huyshoudingh*). The pious play includes a panegyric of the sacred ministry, from which young Evert may have borrowed some traits of his ecclesiastical calling. In 1631, Zas edited a rhymed translation of Juan Luis Vives's life rules, the *Introductio ad veram sapientiam*. In the introductory poems to this edition, he overtly criticized the hypocrisy of the new Calvinist elites. In Zas, Stoa and Bible met each other; humanistic concern went together with orthodox belief and he was Woerden's independent intellectual, the ideal partner for an independent believer.

Zas came running as soon as Evert had him called, collected the messages and had them printed. He understood what happened. Evert had good reason to choose Master Zas. Besides his call to repentance which was meant for outsiders, he had a personal message to share with the headmaster. So, on 17 September, just before his first deliverance:

> I hope that God will release me this night so that I may again hear and again speak: I do not know this by myself, but through the Spirit of God, which will enlighten me . . . If He has the

> power to inflict things upon me, He also has the power to deliver me again: for do we not read in God's word that He made the deaf hear, the blind see, the crippled walk, the dumb speak [Matthew 11:5; 15:30] . . . Does He not then have the power to give back two of my five senses? Oh yes, I have had that trust and I still have it. But when I have recovered my speech and my hearing, it pleases God and the Spirit of God that I go to school until the time has come for me to do the work by which I shall be blessed. I intend then to become a minister and nothing else. Then you shall see what the Spirit of God shall work through me. I must no longer sew, when I have finished my clothes; for it pleases God Almighty and the Spirit of God that such shall no longer be my work. I must fear the Lord, as the angel of the Lord has commanded me, and that I must do.
>
> (B11)

Evert's corporal and spiritual experiences, his sickness and his ecstasy, made him aware of his real vocation, the sacred ministry. He used the impact which the event made on the local community to achieve this calling and to turn his life in another direction. But to be credible, it had to be legitimized by higher authority. This legitimation, announced by an angel of the Lord, was to occur by a ritual of deliverance. Since it adopted the symbolic language of the community, it would not only point to heaven, but restore the boy to his social group. Sickness and health were therefore not only metaphors of a spiritual destiny, but also instruments of social approval. For Evert, the process of healing was his supernatural calling made visible to man. Healing was not simply a personal benefit, but could be a sign of heaven meant to change the course of individual and social life.

Evert's first deliverance took place nine days after the beginning of his ecstatic experience. Was this a spiritual metaphor for the nine months of pregnancy, previous to his rebirth as a converted Christian in the Pietistic and Puritan spiritual tradition?[11] Evert himself spoke of his 'laying down the old Adam, in order to begin a new life, in all virtue and godliness' (B8). Since he adopts here the very terms of the Pietistic idiom, we may certainly conclude that he was also acquainted with the central themes of its spirituality and in particular with the spiritual symbolism of illness and recovery; illness was closely linked to sin, recovery to conversion from a sinful life to the regeneration of the old Adam as a true Christian, under the exclusive impulsion of the Holy Ghost. No magic, no demonology. Evert's devil was no more than God's biblical opponent in hell.

Evert was then spiritually reborn in an accelerated process, just as he had been physically born 15 years earlier. In the Almighty God, who caused him to be reborn, he recognized his new father. The place of his rebirth was the orphanage, where the orphans, rector and matron – who was addressed by Evert affectionately as 'my mummy' and indeed seems to have been a new mother to him – were standing around him and praying. They sustained his spiritual birth pains in singing together Psalm 100, as he had predicted in one of his notes some days before. Carried away by the dynamics of the ritual, all of a sudden Evert was singing with them. He had recovered his ability to hear and speak and was now completely his old self, but reborn as a new Adam. Three days later, the magistracy of Woerden, convinced by God's own support of Evert's words, authorized him to leave the tailor's shop and, without having to earn his own living, to attend the Latin school, following his self-chosen adviser Zas.

Thus, while his messages had from the very first moment a universal goal, Evert's first deliverance chiefly served his own, personal achievement. It was God's legitimation of a career turn which would otherwise have been virtually unthinkable for a poor orphan without any fortune or family. Evert needed protection at the right point. His heavenly recovery from a godly affliction procured him two powerful friends: headmaster Zas, who from that moment acted as his spiritual mentor; and councillor Vergeer, who as orphanage master and school inspector was in charge of the orphan's material well-being and education. Both men gave him their firm support over the years.

## THE WOERDEN COMMUNITY

In itself, Evert's message was of course not sufficient to win the unconditional trust of all the people around him, especially since, three years after the National Synod of Dordrecht had established Calvinist orthodoxy, few cities in Holland were torn apart by religious conflict as much as Woerden. As a matter of fact, Evert's spiritual dealings provoked scepticism and resistance in the town. As the boy himself reminds us, critics grumbled that they would beat the deaf and dumbness out of him:

They have called out with pride,
And still cry noisily
That they might punish me,
And beat me terribly
So that to me again
Speech and hearing be given.
Oh woe, oh woe such people,
For God knows up in heaven!

(B34)

Woerden was not in all respects an average Dutch town. Its position on the Rhine made it a strategic place, provided with a garrison. Apart from its market function, Woerden possessed many tile and brick yards along its two rivers, which employed most of the town's population of about 3,500. But Woerden was an utterly divided town, torn apart by three competing confessions: Lutheranism, liberal Arminianism and orthodox Calvinism. Lutheranism had invaded Woerden almost by accident, and when in 1572 the town joined the rebels under the prince of Orange, it was on the express condition that the free exercise of the Confession of Augsburg be guaranteed. However, the rebellious States-General started an active policy of Calvinization, and by 1602 Calvinism had become the only official religion in a still mainly Lutheran town. Soon Calvinism itself was torn in two bitterly opposing factions. From 1617 the Arminians, who by then dominated the town council (and had sole use of the church) had to face public opposition from a dissenting orthodox consistory supported by a steadily increasing number of town councillors and by one of the two burgemeesters. By the end of September 1618, the *stadhouder*, Prince Maurits, dismissed the Arminian members of the magistracy and replaced them with orthodox Calvinists. They took over the church as well. The following year, the Synod of Dordrecht formally condemned the Arminians and cut short the languishing dialogue with the Lutherans.

The Arminians offered active resistance. They were particularly numerous among the labourers in the brick and tile yards, rough customers who inspired the magistracy with terror. The fear of a popular insurrection brought the town council to impose radical repression, with the active help of the States of Holland. By 1622–23 the Lutherans still formed about a third of the population and the Arminians accounted for more than 40 per cent, though they were the poorest. The Calvinists, meanwhile, made up approximately a quarter of the population, but they were in a leading position in the town and countryside, many of them being social climbers. At this time, the opposition between the three factions was sharper than ever before. The Arminians were heavily fined for their conventicles and the Lutherans for keeping up their own rituals: christening and marrying at home, and preaching at funeral services. The two Arminian ministers were forced to leave the town, while one of the new Calvinist ministers, Henricus Alutarius, assaulted the Lutherans in 1623 with a theological treatise proving that Luther had been a true Calvinist and that his successors had perverted the true (Calvinist) meaning of the Confession of Augsburg. Two years earlier, he published a small Reformed catechism for the orthodox education of the local youth. Confronted with the two oppositional groups, who both claimed their seniority and their good faith, the Calvinists badly needed a justification of their rights.

In this religious landscape Evert's spiritual experience naturally acquired special meaning. In fact, the question is twofold. Where did he stand himself, and which religious party took him as an emblem? The two questions are, of course, interrelated, but there was room for manoeuvre and Evert did not hesitate to seize this opportunity. We do not know for sure if his parents were orthodox Calvinists, but the Woerden orphanage, founded just after the beginnings of Calvinist penetration, functioned as one of the main agencies of Calvinization in the town. Evert's elder brother Cornelis Bogaert married the sister of a radical young Calvinist, Cornelis Paludanus, who after actively combating Arminianism at Woerden, taught himself theology. He was admitted as a candidate for the ministry in the very months of Evert's ecstasy, and in 1625 acquired a parish near Woerden. The two ministers, Everhardus Bogardus (as a student and a preacher Evert Willemsz used this Latinized name) and Cornelis Paludanus were made guardians to the children of Cornelis Bogaert in 1636. Paludanus's fervour may have inspired young Evert, who was clever enough to reject the difficult way of a self-taught theologian and therefore claim his access to the Latin school. Evert's half brother Pieter Muysevoet became an orthodox schoolmaster at the nearby village of Linschoten, and Evert himself obtained his ministry at New Amsterdam as a favourite of the orthodox party within the Amsterdam consistory, which in those years decided on appointments to the overseas churches.

In fact, the three brothers must have been closely akin to the zealous Calvinist minister, Vincent Muysevoet or – Dutchified – Meusevoet (1560–1624). This minister was the son of a Flemish shoemaker who, as a convinced Calvinist, had fled into exile in Norwich, England in 1568. Vincent went back to Holland in 1586 with the new Calvinist governor, the Earl of Leicester. He served first as a minister at Zevenhoven near Woerden, then at Schagen near Alkmaar where he terrorized the Arminians. He has some fame in the history of Dutch Calvinism because of his work as a cultural broker. Between 1598 and his death in 1624 he translated more than 30 Puritan and Pietistic treatises from English into Dutch, including virtually all the works of the famous Puritan divine William Perkins (1558–1602) and some of King James I.[12] He was largely responsible for the introduction of Puritan Pietism into the Netherlands.

The second marriage of Evert's mother with a Muysevoet must have made Vincent Evert's uncle, hence Evert's acquaintance with the Pietistic idiom and the Puritan doctrine of regeneration. It was probably no accident that Meusevoet's second English translation, in 1599, was that of Perkins's treatise on sickness and death.[13]

## PUBLIC LEGITIMATION

With this spiritual genealogy in mind, Evert's second ecstasy may receive a new interpretation. Spiritual experience is, of course, embedded in social traditions of bodily control and physical constraint. Prayer, fasting, visions, celestial messages and miraculous healing adopt traditional forms of communication between heaven and man.[14] Such forms, stored in what we may call the 'social memory' are prerequisites for the production of spiritual experience by the subject. But they also make it recognizable for the target group which shares with the subject a network of traditions and meanings, and form with him or her what Fish has called an 'interpretive community'.[15] In accentuating the basic features of such traditions, the theatrical expression of spiritual experience is a guarantee for its appropriate transmission, not only to the target group, but also to others who may recognize the traditional forms without immediately giving them the same meaning as the target group.

In the second phase of his spiritual experience, Evert tended to overaccentuate its theatrical expressions because his aim was no longer his self-promotion as an agent of God, but the adhesion of as many social groups as possible to his message. Of course, his target group was the elected (his own religious entourage), but he also wished to draw the other religious groups in the town. Whereas the spiritual traditions were from the very beginning easily recognized by all, Evert's major concern was now the transmission of their true meaning. Even apart from God's commission, there was also a good personal reason for his obstinacy. The passing from youth into adulthood involves entrance into public life, with an individual life project that must be acknowledged by the community (see Luke 2:46–7). Since many in Woerden still remained rather sceptical, it was vital, not only for the victory of orthodox Calvinism but also for Evert's achievement of his own personal identity, to make his experience credible to the unbelievers. Hence its second stage.

Four months after his spiritual regeneration, on a Wednesday morning, 18 January 1623, Evert got up with a severe headache. Again, he isolated himself in the particular way permitted by the close community of the orphanage. He refused to eat or drink and predicted that he would again lose the ability to hear or speak and indeed that happened about noon. This time it lasted only three days. Perhaps Evert's experience was now more intense and more exhausting (as minister Alutarius suggested), perhaps passing on his message did not need more time. Anyway, Evert now behaved in a completely different way. He was still surrounded by the group of orphans, who found this break in the daily routine extremely interesting and who perhaps shared collectively or intensified his spiritual excitement. Instead of a target group as in the first phase, the orphans were now made Evert's assistants, the new target group being the unbelievers outside. With their help providing testimonies, Evert now orchestrated public recognition of the turn in his career and in his mission. One by one he called the representatives of the various institutions which made up his social horizon into the room which had been put at his disposal. Together, they legitimized his actions for the whole town.

First came the matron as representative of the household sphere; then Evert's eldest brother as a representative of his family; the rector of the Latin school as the main agent of literate culture in the town; Evert's former employer, master tailor Gijsbert Aelbertsz; the ruling mayor, contractor Jan Florisz van Wijngaarden; and finally the minister, Domine Henricus Alutarius, in the name of the church council. The whole community, as far as it was significant for a young man's world picture – lay and clerical, public and private – paraded symbolically past the chair from which Evert sent his messages out into the world. In the process, each was assigned a task related to his mission.

The church was never absent in those days, and certainly not at Woerden where confession was a major element of group identity. The social recognition of Evert's experience needed the approval of the ecclesiastical leaders of his group, the two orthodox Reformed ministers. Both came to see him, but only one of them was expressly summoned by Evert as his judge. This was Domine Henricus Alutarius (c. 1592–1633), a strong character, orthodox without being sectarian (as was indeed his colleague Jacobus Cralingius), an excellent theologian, popular preacher and also a practising physician.[16] We do not know for certain what he thought initially of Evert's spiritual experience, but there is no evidence of any medical treatment by the minister. In this case Alutarius's concerns were not medical but ecclesiastical. He doubted the truth of Evert's religious experience, even though – or perhaps especially because – both lived in the same sphere of orthodoxy. Would Evert's experience conform to the Calvinist canon of scriptural exegesis and could it support the interests of the orthodox party at Woerden, or was it to be combated as detrimental to the purity of faith and the cohesion of the church? And how to measure the dangers?

Domine Alutarius therefore looked for instruments, signs which could incorporate what was happening to Evert into the discourse of dogmatics and the logic of the church order. Hence his questions:

DS ALUTARIUS: Did the Lord make any special promise to you or any other disclosures that he will keep you alive without the usual means of eating and drinking which he wants us to use for our preservation?

EVERT: Yes, he certainly did; for that is my promise from the voice that said to me that God would keep me healthy and powerful in this world; for that is spoken by the mouth of the angel who said it to me.

DS ALUTARIUS: In the New Testament the Lord does not speak to his people through visions and divine revelations like in the Old Testament. And the Holy Ghost warns us that we must not lightly depend on such things since there have been many who have believed them and have been deceived. Therefore, I beseech you that you ponder deeply whether you are doing these things on a firm foundation. Especially since much will depend on it and it will be everywhere publicized; for that reason, we must act very carefully and be assured of everything before we reveal it to others. Will you repeat to me here once again what kind of outcome you think there will be for you? But take care not to strain your heart too much; better keep it for tomorrow and write it out in detail.

EVERT: What I have written is truthful, for the spirit of God is indeed in me. But I have not much read the Old and New Testaments. But what God is doing, He is doing through a punishment as an example for all people so that people will repent; for God is very angered, and that because people do not live according to his word; for God lets many miracles take place, but we cast them to the wind. So take this to heart. (B26)

Evert here puts himself emphatically in the realm of the deed. God speaks to and through him by way of reality. His miracles and the apparitions of the angel precede His words, which are nothing but explanations of what anybody is capable of seeing through his own eyes. The proof of Evert's legitimacy lies therefore in what happens to him, not in the text of the Bible, which he has hardly read. At least, so he said. And perhaps it was true in so far as his familiarity with the word of God seems more connected to oral transmission, hearing or discussion in particular situations (the tailor's workshop, the orphans' recreations, church going and catechism), than systematic.

But Evert did not avoid discussion. On the contrary, the way in which he constructed his public mission was totally directed towards a discursive, public proclamation. He had, however, learned a lesson from the first phase of his spiritual experience: the discourse could no longer come from himself, as if he were an untouchable and irrational child prodigy. On the contrary, as a candidate to adulthood he had to submit himself to the public, reasoned acknowledgement of his fellow adults. Hence the importance of the discussion about the legitimacy of his claims. Evert's second deliverance was therefore of a public nature. It still took place in the orphanage, but Evert announced it well in advance. When at a given moment he saw the other orphans gathered around the hearth fire, writing and talking, his consciousness was reactivated. He wrote on a slip of paper that the rector and the ministers should be brought, and then he asked them all to sing together a most appropriate psalm, apparently found by opening the Bible at random: 'Out of babes and sucklings hast thou ordained strength' (Psalms 8:2). During the singing, Evert regained successively the use of his senses until he left the condition of babe mentioned in the psalm and sang along with the rector and the ministers as an adult.

This was sufficient proof for both ministers. On the next day, a Sunday, Evert was allowed to read in church before the whole congregation the responses of the Heidelberg catechism to the 35th question, 14th Sunday. Again a very appropriate text: 'What do we call what is received from the Holy Ghost?', for had Evert not repeatedly emphasized that the Holy Ghost was working through him? We may consider this reading as the last rite of passage which achieved Evert's official entrance into public life. From this point on, he was empowered to speak in public with adults, though this very confirmation of the change in his life's direction provoked new harsh criticism in the town.

Evert then played his last trump. Two nights later all the orphans were awakened, including Evert's two little brothers who slept in the same bed with him. Evert was talking aloud in his sleep. The matron was fetched from downstairs. Troubled, she woke him and asked whether something was wrong. Evert calmed everyone down and persuaded them to go back to bed. He had hardly gone back to sleep himself when he started speaking aloud again, as if in a dream. Pieter, five years older than he, obviously knew his younger brother's tricks. He had pen, paper and candle ready, and wrote Evert's long rhymed message down for us. The beginning and end again set the tone:

> O woe, o woe, people with pride and excess,
> Oh ye people mean and heartless,
> Your lives today are so godless . . .
> All that is spoken here
> Will help you ward off sin.
> Stop speaking blasphemous words;
> Think before you begin.
> Then God his blessing to you will give,
> And I will depart eternal life to live.
>
> (B34–5)

This dictated dream – the most classical form of a message from the hereafter, a judgment of God – brought the last Calvinist critics over into Evert's camp. God himself had legitimized Evert's spiritual experiences and his public mission while he was unconscious. The next day the magistrate called the witnesses, including Evert's brothers, to appear before him, authenticated the whole story and gave the church council orders to have it published as quickly as possible in Amsterdam. And so it happened.

## EPILOGUE

Although Evert's gradual legitimation among the dominant Calvinist party at Woerden is well documented, we know very little about his acceptance by other local confessional groups. Six years later, the Amsterdam chronicler Claes van Wassenaer (1571/2–1629), a former Calvinist preacher and also a university trained physician, argued that the whole story was a fraud and that the fasting orphan had been a simulator.[17] However, the publication of this popular chronicle did not prevent the Woerden magistracy from providing Evert Willemsz with the town scholarship at Leiden six months later, nor the Amsterdam consistory from having a very positive opinion of his abilities and sending him successively as a comforter of the sick to the Coast of Guinea in 1630 and as an ordained minister to New Netherland in 1632. The unfavourable sentence of the critical chronicler remains in a sense a mystery and we may well wonder whether this sceptic deserves more credit than the believers.

Yet, there is no trace of any sickness whatsoever in Evert's later life. On the contrary, his transitional experience made him exceptionally fit for the spiritual function of a comforter of the sick in reputedly the most murderous of all Dutch possessions, the Coast of Guinea (present-day Ghana), where he worked and studied in 1631–32. Evert's very survival of the Guinea experience suggests that he was far from having a sickly constitution. He was a strong man with a fierce temper, who in New Netherland got himself the reputation of a heavy drinker and died accidentally in a shipwreck at the age of 40. His sickness and healing in 1622–23 had been a transitory phenomenon; instruments of his maturation as an individual, images of God's intervention in human matters and metaphors of Evert's own spiritual development. His sickness in youth had been primarily a matter of his soul and a language of his mind.

It is precisely on this point that a comparison with the case of Sophia Agnes von Langenberg of Cologne is illuminating (see

Albrecht Burkardt, writing in Chapter 4 of this volume). Analysis reveals notable differences in gender, age, confession and social status between the nun of noble extraction and the tailor's apprentice living at an orphanage. But structural similarities prevail. For the awakening of their calling, the spiritual procedures corresponded in both cases with pre-established models of sanctity involving familiar metaphors and religious idioms, easy to interpret by the local community. The sense of being reborn, the conversion to a new life, was the cultural form in which this shared conviction was moulded. In both cases a two-stage model appears. First, personal holiness was achieved through a near-death experience (agony, sickness and the loss of the senses followed by ecstasy), whereas the proof of the authenticity of the subject's experience was provided by his or her miraculous healing, attributed to God's intervention. The differences are related to the idioms of holiness characteristic for each particular confession and are hence essentially accidental: for the Catholic woman redemption was achieved through the traditional devotion to Christ's Passion, and perhaps the Eucharist, while for the Protestant boy it came through the new key ritual of singing psalms.

In the second stage, after an interval which served as a time of maturation, public recognition was sought, with the help of spectacular public signs taken from the social memory that were able to suggest meaning. For the Catholic nun this was the miracle of the bleeding cross, while the Calvinist orphan – educated in a spirit of individual sanctification – returned to a more theatrical and discursive presentation of his own experience. In both cases, this second stage did not aim at the self-fashioning of the subject as a saint, but at the adhesion of the masses to the message. It turned out differently for each once they had been verified publicly (in one case by the *Nunzio*'s committee, in the other by the ministers and the town magistrate). The nun was rejected and sent back to her origins, while the boy was allowed to grow socially and spiritually. In both cases an epilogue to the second stage intended the final legitimation of the experience, at the intersection with the supernatural: demonic possession in the convent, a heavenly dream in the orphanage.

To conclude, three aspects merit particular attention in relation to gender. First, the impact of gender seems evident in the way personal 'vocation' was achieved. While young Evert constructed his own career, was authorized to express himself autonomously and was credible in himself, Sophia Agnes remained largely a victim of male ecclesiastical (and perhaps medical) authority. Second, in the stage of public recognition the nun appeared from the outset as a suspected fraud, whereas the boy was treated as a performer, working hard at getting a legitimation which seemed, after all, probable from the very beginning. Third, these two godly persons might well pertain to two different gender-related traditions of holiness, the nun a representative of a tradition of female sanctity, embedded in practices of suffering, self-chastising and healing, whereas the boy appeared both at Woerden and in his later American life as an active community builder of a charismatic nature. In both cases, it took the common language of sickness to reveal them to themselves and to be instrumental in the disclosure of their social calling.


## ACKNOWLEDGEMENTS

For the translation of Evert's own texts in this essay I am indebted to James F. Cool of Wilmington, Ohio.

## APPENDIX

Times, rhythms and modalities of Evert's spiritual experience

| *Day* | *Date* | *Fasting* | *Deaf and dumb* | *Blind* | *Loses his senses* | *Sees an angel* | *Writes messages* |
|---|---|---|---|---|---|---|---|
| | **1622** | after recovery from illness | | | | | |
| Tuesday | 21 June | nine days | | | | | |
| Thursday | 30 June | | | | | | |
| | | | 70 days | intermittently | | | |
| Thursday | 8 September | | | | | ■ | |
| | | nine days | | | | | nine days |
| Saturday | 17 September | | | | | ■ | |
| | | | | first deliverance | | | |
| | four months (123 days) | | | | | | goes to school |
| | **1623** | | | | | | |
| Tuesday | 17 January | | | | | | |
| Wednesday | 18 January | headache | | | | | |
| | *morning* *afternoon* | | predicts | | | ■ | |
| Thursday | 19 January *evening* | | | | | | |
| Friday | 20 January | | | | | | |
| | | three days | | | | | |
| | *afternoon* | | | | | | says 'yes' |
| Saturday | 21 January *3.00/4.00 pm* | | | | regains consciousness | | |
| | *6.00 pm* | | sings | | | | |
| | | drinks | | | | | |
| | | | | | second deliverance | | |
| | *8.00 pm* | eats | | | | | |
| Sunday | 22 January *afternoon* | | | | | speaks in church | |
| Monday | 23 January | | | | | goes to school | |
| Tuesday | 24 January *6.00 am* | | | | | speaks in his sleep, dreams aloud | |
| Thursday | 26 January | | | public recognition | | | |

## NOTES

1 This essay is based on the material collected for my book *Wegen van Evert Willemsz: Een Hollands weeskind op zoek naar zichzelf (1607–1647)* [Pathways of Evert Willemsz: A Dutch orphan child in search of himself, 1607–1647] (Nijmegen, 1995), where full references to all sources are given. I shall quote here only the most essential evidence.

2 Evert Willemsz's life story from the Leiden matriculation in 1627 is well known under his Latinized name Everhardus Bogardus. He died in 1647 at the age of 40 in a shipwreck off the coast of Wales, near Swansea, leaving a widow (Annetgen or Anneke Jans, a Norwegian woman) with nine children. As a central figure in the 1643–45 Indian wars, violently opposed to the disastrous policy of West India Company governor, Willem Kieft, he is one of the main characters of early New York historiography. However, the appreciation of his ministry and personality differs greatly among authors. These different images are discussed in my book. The most reliable English version of his life is in Q. Breen, 'Domine Everhardus Bogardus', *Church History*, 2 (1933): 78–90. On his New Netherland family, see G.O. Zabriskie, 'Anneke Jans in fact and fiction', *New York Genealogical and Biographical Record*, 104 (1973): 65–72, 157–64. As his family name never occurs in the Woerden sources, the story of his youth has only recently been recognized as pertaining to the same person.

3 The family relations appear in Evert's brother Cornelis Bogaert's second will, 12 Sept. 1636: Gemeentearchief Leiden, Notarieel archief, inv. no. 265, akte no. 63 [Municipal Archives of Leiden, notarial records 265, deed 63].

4 Lucas Zas [Zasch, Zasius] (ed.), *Waerachtighe ende seeckere gheschiedenisse/ dewelcke is gheschiedt binnen de Stadt Woerden/ hoe dat Godt almachtich zijn Wonder-werck heeft betoont aen een seecker Wees-kindt genaemt Evert Willemsz* (Utrecht, 1623) and *Waerachtige Geschiedenisse/ Hoe dat Seker Wees-Kindt binnen Woerden/ out ontrent xv. jaren/ tot tweemalen toe vanden Heere met stommigheyd/ doofheyd/ somtijts oock met blintheyt besocht/ ende van het gebruyck syns verstants berooft zijnde* (Amsterdam, 1623) [Den Haag, Koninklijke Bibliotheek, Pfl. Knuttel 3500–3501]. Both pamphlets have been reprinted at least once. On the pamphlet genre, see C.E. Harline, *Pamphlets, Printing and Political Culture in the Early Dutch Republic* (Dordrecht, 1987).

5 On this problem, see W. Christian Jr, *Apparitions in Late Medieval and Renaissance Spain* (Princeton, NJ, 1981), pp. 188–203; G. Zarri (ed.), *Finzione e santità tra medioevo ed età moderna* (Turin, 1991); M. Cuénin, 'Fausse et vraie mystique: signes de reconnaissance, d'après la *Correspondance* de Jeanne de Chantal', in J.-P. Massaut (ed.), *Les Signes de Dieu aux XVIe et XVIIe siècles* (Clermont-Ferrand, 1993), pp. 177–87.

6 See W. Frijhoff, 'Enfants saints, enfants prodiges: l'expérience religieuse au passage de l'enfance à l'âge adulte', *Paedagogica historica*, 29: 1 (1993): 53–76. For the vast literature on conversion models in

English and American Puritanism, the counterpart of Evert's adolescent conversion, see the surveys by L. Bergamasco, 'Hagiographie et sainteté en Angleterre', *Annales ESC*, 48: 4 (1993): 312–42; P. Caldwell, *The Puritan Conversion Narrative: The Beginnings of American Expression* (Cambridge, 1983); K. von Greyerz, *Vorsehungsglaube und Kosmologie: Studien zu englischen Selbstzeugnissen des 17. Jahrhunderts* (Göttingen and Zürich, 1990).

7 See L.F. Groenendijk and F.A. van Lieburg, *Voor edeler staat geschapen: Levens – en sterfbedbeschrijvingen van gereformeerde kinderen en jeugdigen uit de 17e en 18e eeuw* (Leiden, 1991); F.A. van Lieburg, *Levens van vromen: Gereformeerd piëtisme in de achttiende eeuw* (Kampen, 1991); L.F. Groenendijk, 'De spirituele (auto)biografie als bron voor onze kennis van de religieuze opvoeding en ontwikkeling van Nederlandse piëtisten', in L.F. Groenendijk and J.C. Sturm (eds), *Leren geloven in de Lage Landen: Facetten van de geschiedenis van de religieuze opvoeding* (Amsterdam, 1993), pp. 57–90.

8 The letters A and B after quotations in this essay refer to the pamphlets described in note 4. A refers to the Utrecht edition, B to the Amsterdam edition. They are followed by the number of the page.

9 See the depositions on Petrus Cupus and Petrus de Bricquigny, Reformed (Arminian) ministers at Woerden, in Algemeen Rijksarchief, Oud Synodaal Archief, inv. no. 157 [General State Archives at The Hague, Old Synodal Archive, 157].

10 On the 1618 comet and its meaning, see S. Drake and C.D. Malley (eds), *The Controversy on the Comets of 1618* (Philadelphia, 1960); J. Cats, *Aenmerckinghe op de tegenwoordige staert-sterre, en drie lofdichten op Philips Lansbergen*, introduced by G.J. Johannes (Utrecht, 1986); E. Jorink, 'Hemelse tekenen: Nederlandse opvattingen over de kometen van 1618', unpub. Master's thesis, University of Groningen, 1993.

11 See on the relationship between illness, healing and orthodox spirituality, A. Wear, 'Puritan perceptions of illness in seventeenth-century England', in R. Porter (ed.), *Patients and Practitioners. Lay Perceptions of Medicine in Pre-Industrial Society* (Cambridge, 1985), pp. 55–99; D. Harley, 'Spiritual physic, Providence and English medicine 1560–1640', in O.P. Grell and A. Cunningham (eds), *Medicine and the Reformation* (London and New York, 1993), pp. 101–17; M.J. van Lieburg, 'Zeeuwse piëtisten en de geneeskunde in de eerste helft van de 17e eeuw: Een verkenning van het werk van W. Teellinck en G.C. Udemans', in H.J. Zuidervaart (ed.), *Worstelende wetenschap: Aspecten van de wetenschapsbeoefening in Zeeland van de zestiende tot in de negentiende eeuw* ([Middelburg], n.d. [1987]), pp. 63–86.

12 C.W. Schoneveld, *Intertraffic of the Mind: Studies in Seventeenth-Century Anglo–Dutch Translation, with a Checklist of Books Translated from English into Dutch 1600–1700* (Leiden, 1983); W.J. op 't Hof, *Engelse piëtistische geschriften in het Nederlands, 1598–1622* (Rotterdam, 1987), 441–55.

13 W. Perkins, *Salve voor een sieck mensche, ofte een tractaet vervatende de*

*natuere, onderscheydentheden ende soorten des doots*, trans. V. Meusevoet (Amsterdam, 1599, reprinted 1604, 1620).

14 These traditions and the way Evert Willemsz uses them are analyzed in chapters 8–11 of my book.

15 S. Fish, *Is There a Text in This Class? The Authority of Interpretive Communities* (Cambridge, Mass., and London, 1980).

16 We know from another source that, at the same time, Alutarius was medically treating a peasant from the neighbourhood stricken with 'salvation panic'. Just like Francesco Spiera 70 years before, the peasant was convinced of being eternally damned by God and let himself die. Alutarius took him into his house, in order to observe him and to treat what he considered to be a psychic disorder. See W. Frijhoff, 'Medical education and early modern Dutch medical practitioners: towards a critical approach', in H. Marland and M. Pelling (eds), *The Task of Healing: Medicine, Religion and Gender in England and the Netherlands 1450–1800* (Rotterdam, 1996), pp. 208–10. On Spiera, see M. MacDonald, ' "The fearfull Estate of Francis Spira". Narrative, identity and emotion in early modern England', *Journal of British Studies*, 31: 1 (1992): 32–61.

17 C. van Wassenaer, *Historisch verhael alder ghedenck-weerdichste geschiedenissen, die van den beginne des jaeres 1621 . . . tot 1632 voorgevallen sijn*, 21 vols (Amsterdam, 1622–35), vol. XV (1629), fo. 64$^{ro}$. Following Wassenaer, A.Th. van Deursen calls Evert 'a notorious faker', *Plain Lives in a Golden Age: Popular Culture, Religion and Society in Seventeenth-Century Holland*, trans. M. Ultee (Cambridge, 1991), pp. 257–8.

Chapter 6

# Charcot's demons

## Retrospective medicine and historical diagnosis in the writings of the Salpêtrière school

*Sarah Ferber*

For more than 20 years, between 1874 and 1897, several members of the so-called Salpêtrière school in Paris, under the inspiration of the energetic and innovative neurologist Jean-Martin Charcot, published a body of historical and clinical works which compared historical accounts and illustrations of witchcraft, demonic possession and ecstatic spirituality with contemporary cases of diagnosed hysteria. Historical texts were republished and given clinical annotations, and in clinical texts these doctors described the behaviour of patients they had diagnosed as hysterical by reference to behavioural analogies found in early modern texts. This historiographical and clinical practice was referred to as 'retrospective medicine'.[1] The project had its apogee in the production of the *Bibliothèque Diabolique Bourneville*, a well-known series of eight works published between 1882 and 1897 under the direction of Charcot's younger colleague, Désiré-Magloire Bourneville.[2] Members of the group also wrote commentaries which explicitly refuted supposed miracles and cases of possession of the nineteenth century.[3]

The assiduity with which Charcot and his colleagues – most conspicuously Bourneville, but also Gilles de la Tourette, Gabriel Legué, Paul Richer, Charles Richet, Paul Regnard and others – applied themselves to this historical research was remarkable.[4] Jan Goldstein has proposed that an anticlerical impulse was at the heart of their rediagnosis of supernatural explanations as hysteria, and has remarked that this project was 'not just a jeu d'esprit of the Salpêtrière school but one of its constant preoccupations and an integral part of its public image'.[5] Representing their clinical work and their secularizing philosophy within a historical sweep, Charcot and his colleagues inscribed themselves in the story of progress, for, as Charcot's close colleague Paul Richer wrote, without its historical dimension the study of hysteria would be 'incomplete'.[6]

In a feminist reading of the use of historical material by the Salpêtrians, Michèle Ouerd has argued that the historical comparisons made by Charcot and his colleagues demonstrate that the avowedly humane practices of the Salpêtrière clinicians were the manifestations of a persistent misogynistic ideology. She argues that a pathologization of all femininity was at the heart of the hysterical diagnosis and suggests that there might have been more in common between Charcot and his colleagues and witch hunters than there was difference. The practice of each, Ouerd suggests, was primarily informed by the desire to colonize the 'dark continent' of femininity.[7]

This chapter provides an account of the historical readings of hysteria, given by Charcot and his colleagues, in relation to early modern demonic possession and witch hunting. Following on from the observations of Goldstein, my aims are to present a historiographical reflection which will show in detail the ways in which the group's use of historical analogy lent a moral depth to their clinical and scientific enterprise, and to consider the possibilities and limitations of such a reading of the past. This will be followed by a discussion of Ouerd's comparative treatment of early modern texts and nineteenth-century authors, and finally by a brief consideration of some of the perceived parallels between possession and hysteria, and early modern exorcists and witch hunters and nineteenth-century doctors.[8]

## THE POLITICS OF DISEASE

Charcot and his colleagues used historical literature at the time of an unprecedented rise in the diagnosis of hysteria at the Salpêtrière hospital – the major asylum for women in Paris.[9] Charcot's incumbency as head physician began in 1862 and was distinguished by his campaign for a redefinition of hysteria as an organic ailment originating in the nervous system.[10] This campaign was a conspicuous feature of the 'medical materialism' of the late nineteenth century and Charcot was one of its chief proponents.[11] Goldstein has argued that the increase in the proportion of inmates diagnosed as hysterical at the Salpêtrière can be associated with the republican anticlericalism of Charcot and his colleagues. She depicts 'a tight network of republican politicians and scientist politicians' who promoted anti-Catholic views and Comtean historical positivism in the 1870s and 1880s. Furthermore, Goldstein argues that the way in which the group (and particularly Bourneville) built their public and professional identities around the new and, it was stressed, definitive hysteria diagnosis can be seen as an important affirmation of positivism.[12] The group's promotion of a new and avowedly more scientific diagnosis of hysteria, she argues, formed a neat 'fit' with the anticlericalism of republican leaders such as Gambetta.[13] She also suggests that by fixing on a disease which had historically competed with supernatural explanations to account for the behaviour of witches and demoniacs, Charcot may have seen that the promotion of the hysteria diagnosis could be an effective means to make an oblique attack on the Catholic church.[14]

Early modern cases of demonic possession and the question of witch hunting had already surfaced many times during the nineteenth century, most notably in the works of Michelet, Calmeil and Briquet.[15] However, the direct precursor of the Salpêtrière school's interest appears to have been Alexandre Axenfeld, who delivered a series of public lectures at the Paris Faculty of Medicine in 1865 on the Dutch physician Johan Wier. In these lectures, Axenfeld celebrated Wier's claim that accused witches should be treated humanely in the courts on the grounds that they were ill.[16] Axenfeld extended this to argue for the notion that criminality was involuntary and the result of individual pathology, a position which militated directly against the idea of free will and thereby provoked the ire of the pro-Catholic Paris medical faculty.[17]

For the Salpêtrière school, the reading of historical texts involved not only the recategorizing of possession, spiritual ecstasy and the behaviour of accused witches according to new clinical descriptions of hysteria, it embodied the moral project of exposing the 'barbarity' of religious interpretations for their failure to allow that accused witches were merely ill.[18] The doctor Charles Richet wrote: 'Among the *aliénées* at the Salpêtrière, there are sick women who would have been burnt in another time and whose sickness three centuries ago would have been seen as a crime.'[19]

In the process of reinscribing demonic possession as hysteria, the group proclaimed their own technical prowess against clerical interventions in (usually) female displays of hysteria. Bourneville and Regnard wrote:

> To calm hysterics down, priests in former times employed exorcisms, and still recommend them today; . . . [but] we doctors, we have more active agents: not counting the compression of the ovarian region . . . we make use of . . . chloroform, ether, amyl nitrite, valerianates of amyl and ethyl, ethyl bromide, Leyden jar [an electrical device], the compressor, electric current, and so on.[20]

Elsewhere, however, Gabriel Legué acknowledged the capacity of church ritual to have real effects, and Charcot himself, in his late essay on faith healing appeared to be leaning towards a greater acceptance of the power of the imagination, while still opposing the possibility of supernatural intervention.[21]

## THE USES OF HISTORY

By locating examples of hysteria in history, Charcot added weight to the claim that he had identified a perennial phenomenon, misunderstood until his own time, when a restitutive order could be imposed on its manifestations. The discovery of hysteria in the past lent credence to the idea that there was a natural law governing the varied manifestations of the affliction. The observation of nature, Charcot and Richer wrote, would lead to a conclusion of the 'indisputable marks of a pre-established order' and to knowledge of 'a scientific law' about hysteria.[22] They wrote: 'We have demonstrated the existence of a fixed and immutable law, in the place where up until now authors have only seen disorder and confusion.'[23] Elsewhere, historical accounts are referred to as showing a 'complete similitude' between past and present occurrences,[24] and Charcot and Richer invoked the rhetoric of revelation to describe the persistence of identical symptoms across time, speaking of a 'hidden reason' under apparent disorder.[25]

Historical cases were also invoked to insist that the symptoms of hysteria were not chaotic and changeable, but were immutable 'across the ages'.[26] Possibly as a response to accusations of over-diagnosis of hysteria at the Salpêtrière, Charcot and Richer argued that hysteria should not 'be considered . . . as the special malady of our age'[27] and stated that the newly refined claims about the nature of hysteria were 'valid for all countries, all times, all races'.[28]

The definition of hysteria as a nervous disorder also shifted the meaning of hysteria away from its previous clinical and etymological association with the womb, thereby aligning it to neither male nor female physiology exclusively. In the words of Charcot and Richer, 'the exact meaning [of hysteria] no longer has anything to do with its etymology'.[29] However, as Ruth Harris has observed, Charcot 'did little to sever the link between the disease and a vision of female sexual lubricity and indelicacy'.[30]

Charcot's claim to have found natural laws which governed hysteria derived not so much from a discovery of its physical causes, which was never made, as it did from a systematic taxonomization of the stages of the hysterical fit – a description which was Charcot's chief contribution to theorization about hysteria and which served, among other things, to set the boundaries between hysteria and epilepsy.[31] The hysteria of Charcot's conception was referred to as *la grande hystérie* or *hystéro–épilepsie*.[32]

The stages of the hysterical fit were grouped into four periods which were said to be clearly discernible. First was the *période épileptoïde*, characterized by flailing of the limbs and unconsciousness. This was followed by the *période des contorsions et des grands mouvements* or *période de clownisme*, characterized by spasmodic movements. The third phase, the *période des attitudes passionelles*, involved predominantly verbal and hallucinatory displays, while the *période terminale* saw the attack resolved in displays of pain and anguish.[33] The whole attack was said to take place, as a rule, within the space of around 15 minutes, though it could go on for hours or even a whole day.[34] Each stage was said to contain a number of identifiable phases, the second phase incorporating the so-called *variété démoniaque*, named for its resemblance to accounts of demonic possession.

Having established these symptoms of hysteria, the task remained to seek them out in historical accounts of possession, witchcraft and ecstasy, to 'translate' early modern texts into modern clinical categories for modern readers. For example, in the heavily annotated autobiography of Jeanne des Anges – the possessed superior of the Ursulines at Loudun in the 1630s – Legué and Tourette wrote:

> The hysteria of Sister Jeanne is very complete from a symptomatic point of view . . . The phenomena of the attack here are very varied. It is a question here of the 'variety by immixture of lethargic phenomena' described by M.P. Richer in his chapter VII.[35]

And in a description of the paroxysms depicted in a medieval picture of possession, Charcot and Richer noted: 'The attitude of the young possessed boy given here by the artist is noteworthy. This curving over backwards must be seen as the *arc de cercle*, so common in hysteria.'[36] The method was procrustean: if a historic representation of a phase of the attack did not correspond to the clinical picture devised by Charcot, it was judged to be incorrect, misperceived. For example, in describing a fifteenth-century picture of a person having a convulsion – which Charcot and Richer considered likely to be an attack of hysteria or of epilepsy – they wrote: 'Whatever kind of convulsion it is, the flaccid appearance of the open hands does not appear to have any reason to be there.'[37]

It is worth noting that, while the ostensible purpose of these comparisons was to etch a clear clinical image of hysteria, the language of the demonic and of witchcraft served equally the rhetorical purpose of arresting the readers' attention and signalling that the terrain of religious and psycho–sexual disorder was being entered. For example, the title of Charles Richet's article 'Les Démoniaques d'aujourd'hui' invited readers to see hysterics as demoniacs and, in its text, he referred without qualification to a hysterical patient as a 'demoniac'.[38] Furthermore, in the *Iconographie photographique de la Salpêtrière* published by Bourneville and Regnard, a young woman named Geneviève, one of the 'famous' hysterics of the Salpêtrière, was described as being a 'succubus', because of her erotic hallucinations of a nocturnal lover at the hospital. The authors affirmed 'Geneviève is a succubus', yet a footnote intended to show the historical sense of this reference only mentions 'incubi' (male demons) and suggests a confusion, intended or not, between the identity of the woman and her imagined 'diabolic' lover.[39] A chapter in the second volume of the *Iconographie*, headed 'Succube', which describes the progress of the same case, is illustrated by a photograph of a placid-looking woman, head downcast and her hands in her lap, the photograph bearing the caption '*Hystéro–épilepsie: Succube*'.[40]

## PERFECT KNOWLEDGE, PRAISE AND BLAME

Most of the texts produced by these clinicians either traced or implied a historical narrative which culminated with their own discovery of the true causes of hysteria, or which – in the absence of a strong aetiology – enunciated a theoretical position from which the truth could be revealed 'as science progresses'.[41] Underpinning their readings of past events was the aim of achieving perfect knowledge. The use of historical texts, which supplied at once abundant 'clinical' evidence and flawed interpretations, lent credence to these writers' own claims of having arrived at a state of perfect knowledge about hysteria. Concerning the possessions at Loudun in the 1630s, Gabriel Legué wrote: 'These miracles, about which such a fuss was made, were but the strange phenomena of a malady today perfectly understood: hysteria', while Bourneville, in a deft move, wrote that although the known scientific laws were 'less perfect today than they will be in the future, they are quite enough to explain everything which is reputed to be miraculous'.[42] Charcot, in his preface to the autobiography of Jeanne des Anges, wrote by way of complement of the 'incontestably imperfect' knowledge of the seventeenth century.[43]

Yet to the extent that the project of these authors was also a moral one – an observation made in a different context by Georges Didi-Huberman – these avowedly scientific readings were apt to apportion blame.[44] For example the belief that hysterical women, both in the past and in modern cases, were seen to have an affinity with religiosity could align them with the wilful ignorance of the clergy, and punitive or sarcastic comments encouraged an identification of the innocent sick woman with the culpable church, regardless of the woman's illness. The supposed tendency of hysterics to hold grudges and to exaggerate ills done to them was conflated with the role of the possessed in the prosecution for witchcraft of the priest Urbain Grandier at Loudun in 1634, and Bourneville referred to Jeanne des Anges as the 'principale actrice' in the affair.[45]

For the purposes of science, however, it was necessary to subsume this apparent responsibility to the illness of hysteria, to diminish the play of will within hysteria itself and keep it securely within the parameters of a psycho–physiological pathology. The incapacity of hysterics (or the possessed) to act of their own accord was underlined. Legué wrote of the nuns at Loudun: 'the tendency to simulation being nothing but a consequence of the malady, the moral responsibility must disappear completely',[46] and he wrote elsewhere that the nuns at Loudun were 'absolutely not responsible' for what happened there.[47] Charles Richet nimbly surmounted the dilemma posed by this construction of the responsibility of the possessed when he wrote of Louise Capeau, a possessed nun at Aix in

1610–11, that she was 'more mad than wicked, but wicked in her madness'.[48]

Bridging the historical distance between the new truth of hysteria, its *sens exact*, and its historical 'misinterpretations' also entailed a moral evaluation of the responses of past historical figures who had encountered hysterical phenomena. Historical actors, notably artists and doctors, were seen either as heroes, prisoners of their time (possibly both at once) or, usually in the case of priests, as perpetrators of untruth, attached to the dead historical weight of supernatural explanations.

Several of the works produced by the group mention the role of doctors in early modern cases of possession. Marc Duncan, Pierre Yvelin and Claude Quillet, who actively opposed the exorcisms in the famous cases at Loudun, Louviers and Chinon, are cited for their 'wise and humane' opposition to claims of demonic possession.[49] Reginald Scot, Cornelius Agrippa, Paracelsus and, of course, Wier are also mentioned. Yet while the conclusions of doctors in early modern cases of possession often drew upon the explanation of possession as *mal de mère*, surprisingly little attention is paid to the scientific endeavour of any authors other than Wier; they are judged almost solely on their intentions. Their erroneous science was exonerated by the fact that they were, in effect, trapped in time. In the case of Wier, his 'eminent services to humanity' are saluted, for as Alexandre Axenfeld expressed it, while Wier's 'head' was mired in the credulity of the sixteenth century his 'heart' had belonged to progress.[50]

Towards artists from earlier centuries who were believed to have inaccurately represented the visible realities of a hysterical attack, however, Charcot and Richer were less indulgent. When the 'evidence' was clearly before them, they argued, artists had no excuse to go beyond 'the exact observation of nature'. 'It is not enough,' he wrote, 'to deform at one's pleasure and make things strange at will.'[51] Thus representations of demonic possession and ecstasy in art were assessed for their approximation to modern hysteria and the artist's inclination to depict or ignore the evidence was evaluated accordingly.

Charcot and Richer expressed disappointment at a picture by Raphael which gave an 'inaccurate' representation of possession, notwithstanding Raphael's artistic abilities. They wrote: 'It was, then, intentionally, that such a master falsified and modified nature.' They concluded tartly that they would 'not formulate here a judgment on this system of attenuation of the truth'.[52] Conversely, when referring to an image which shows a possessed woman holding up her thumb and two forefingers in what was normally a priestly gesture, they asked: 'By what contradiction did the artist give this gesture to the hand of a slave of the demon? We think that it is necessary to see this as a proof of the sincerity of the painter', who had followed what he had seen in nature.[53]

In accounts of their own perceptions, the Salpêtrière group depict themselves as having achieved a state of moral transparency, which saw them as mere conduits of truth, their identities and perceptions precisely parallel with their place in historical time. Their passivity is stressed. Gabriel Legué wrote: 'Everywhere the sickness is the same, everywhere the same symptoms. . . . The great analogy of all these ailments struck us.'[54] And responding to the accusation that he diagnosed hysteria everywhere, Charcot stated: 'To those who would reproach me for always talking of hysteria . . . I respond with this "mot" from Molière: "I say the same thing, because it always is the same thing." I confirm, and nothing more.'[55] These readings suggest an association of a particular time period with a particular morality, a move which conflates the 'we' and the 'now', and endows the late nineteenth-century writers with a guarantee of their own scientific rightness and moral authority. At the same time, it renders them innocent of personal motivations, enabled by their time to 'objectify' themselves as part of a greater process.

## THE USES OF ANALOGY

I want to turn now to the comparison offered of nineteenth-century medical works with early modern texts by Michèle Ouerd and to discuss the historiographical questions that her analysis raises. In her account of nineteenth-century medical writers' work on witch hunting and possession, Ouerd traces a series of parallels between their accounts of their own clinical practice and the practices of witch hunters, noting the Salpêtrière group's enthusiasm for making favourable comparisons of their own work with that of exorcists and witch hunters. Some of Ouerd's observations of parallels between nineteenth-century medical attitudes and those of witch hunters are quite striking. For example, the article contains a chart across two pages which parallels extracts from the *Malleus maleficarum* and a selection of texts of nineteenth-century medical authors on hysteria. The selected texts indicate direct parallels between concerns about the hereditary nature of witchcraft and hysteria, suicidal tendencies of both witches and hysterics, and their shared tendencies to fickleness, wilfulness and suggestibility.[56]

More noteworthy still is Ouerd's observation concerning the introduction by Bourneville to an account of the seventeenth-century case of Barbe Buvée, a nun accused by her possessed sisters of causing their possession through witchcraft. Here, Bourneville cites the practice of exorcists pricking the possessed or burning them to test for insensitivity (*anasthésie*, or *hemianasthésie*, in the language of new hysterical diagnosis). Defending the modern practice of pricking hysterics, Bourneville notes that 'inexperienced' observers might see the use of pricking as 'a little inhumane', but that it is not. Burning, on the other hand, he rejects as barbaric, saying he has never seen it done. However, at the very end of the same text to which Bourneville had written the introduction, the author, Samuel Garnier, describes the use not only of pricking on hysterics by modern doctors, but also of fire to detect their insensibility.[57]

Ouerd's comparison of these texts is the product of a stream of feminist scholarship which has been essentially concerned with establishing a filiation of immutable patriarchal behaviours and may be seen as similar, ironically, to Charcot's and his colleagues' own reading of history.[58] In the case of the Salpêtrière school, analogy was used to affirm discontinuity between the medical and clerical professions by reference to a perceived continuity in their patients. Ouerd, in an ironic move, observes analogies in order to express an absence of discontinuity. In each case, the moral imperative is palpable and the historical distance between the two periods collapsed – and in each case, little room is left for suggesting ambiguities in the interpretation of the historical material. Thus, while Ouerd's analysis certainly revealed the misogyny which underpinned the work of the Salpêtrière school, her selection of historical material also had the effect of obscuring the fact that women in many cases of possession, though often manipulated by exorcists, occupied an ambivalent position in relation to authority. For example, they were heavily implicated in the prosecution of several priests for witchcraft, and several possessed women also occupied prominent places in public religious life in the seventeenth century.

Yet it would seem cavalier to ignore the parallels which might be drawn between the work of Charcot and his colleagues and the history of cases of demonic possession and witch hunting, particularly when the nineteenth-century readings actively invited such a comparison. These readings presented apparently striking analogies, both in the behaviour of the women – which the clinicians and early modern authors described – and in their own behaviour, to which we are witness through their texts and to which Ouerd has drawn our attention. By indicating what Charcot and his colleagues saw as the relationship between the behaviour of the possessed and of accused witches, and that of hysterics, and in their use of these texts to heighten the contrast between their own diagnoses and those of the clergy, they left a space for later readers to compare their own behaviours with those of the exorcists and the witch hunters against whom they defined themselves.

Analogies other than those elicited by Ouerd and the Charcot group may be found in the literature of Charcot and his colleagues and of the sixteenth and seventeenth centuries, and these may be relevant to the writing of other histories about the relationship between the two periods, particularly regarding the professions of medicine and the priesthood in relation to women. It may be possible to see that these professions were neither necessarily antagonistic opposites in regard to their humanity, nor exclusively twin pillars of oppression.

## The analogy of free will

Attention might be usefully drawn to the question of the will in both these historical contexts. As we have seen, the case promoted by Axenfeld's arguments for the 'illness' of accused witches had had important implications for the status of the doctrine of free will.[59] In the work of Charcot and his colleagues this was extended to include the historical 'exoneration' of possessed women who, as we have noted, had contributed evidence to secure the prosecution of several priests for witchcraft. For Charcot, the possibility that his patients were actually using their will and 'faking' their hysterical symptoms was, however, always present and became, in the opinion of one commentator at least, a major sticking point against the claim that hysteria had a physiological base.[60] But Charcot remained committed to the demonstration that the will was absent in the performances of hysterics and that they were primarily suffering from a disease. The entire interpretive edifice of the performances of hysterics was reliant on the idea that their behaviour was proceeding according to laws which existed outside both their control and that of the clinician. Fraud or any degree of intention among the hysterical women called into question the integrity of both the laws and the clinicians. Here continuity can also be seen with Charcot's own emphasis upon the undesirability of the exercise of the will in the perception by doctors and artists faced with potentially hysterical phenomena.[61]

Similarly, in cases of demonic possession in the early modern period, a concern prevailed with demonstrating the absence of the will of the possessed. This occurred in a historical period where the renunciation of the will in the quest for spiritual perfection was a critical aspect of religious life. It was also a time when the consignment of the will to the devil by witches – through the donation of a hair, for example, or through seduction – became a key element in witch prosecutions. Thus all the tests which were performed upon the possessed, from tests in foreign languages to trials of extraordinary physical strength, were carried out in order to ensure that the devil and not the woman was totally in control of the woman's actions. If the woman's own volition were detected, or any degree of collusion with an exorcist exposed, the claim of possession was instantly debunked and the woman risked prosecution for witchcraft, her exorcists risking public ridicule.[62]

For exorcists in early modern France, the body of the possessed was the index of the will, presumed to be 'legible' independently of the sufferer's conscious control. Successful exorcism was a way of gaining access to religious truth: it showed the power of the clergy to intercede at a level where no other profession could, and demonstrated the ability of exorcists to make the possessed speak as demonic oracles, as sources of truth unmediated by the sufferers' will. In the context of exorcism, the 'somatic conversion' of cognitive phenomena into bodily signs was understood to take place within the sphere of the numinous, and to be controlled by church magic. If the body failed to display its lack of will, the possessed or ecstatic was deemed fraudulent or merely sick.[63] Similarly, in the case of the Charcot school, the body of the hysteric was presumed to be able to demonstrate the power of the psychophysiological illness of hysteria to swamp or pre-figure the will, and thereby to demonstrate the truth of Charcot's scientistic proposition about the true nature of hysteria.

## The analogy of the female body

In the literature of both the early modern period and in the nineteenth century, an appeal is present to a literate public with titillating descriptions of female bodies and behaviours, which also traded on the *frisson* of the demonic. In both instances, the literate were flattered at being permitted to handle topics such as demonic power and lurid sexuality by the presentation of these subjects as learned discourse. In the case of the Charcot school, this was achieved by the use of a heavy overlay of taxonomic phraseology and critical references to the superstitions of the church. In the early modern period, authors on both sides in contentious cases of possession affirmed the scholarly nature of their own undertakings and the danger of permitting 'the vulgar' to discern the presence of demons.[64]

Charcot and his colleagues, early modern exorcists and witch hunters – and also, importantly, early modern opponents of exorcism and witch hunting – were trying to diminish the power of the devil or of belief in it, and to protect from superstition those less well equipped intellectually and emotionally than they.[65] There was in each period a paternalistic reliance on defining the social world in terms of an imagined audience which required the protection of a learned, but not necessarily sceptical elite. This link is largely obscured by the Salpêtrians because of their desire to emphasize the rupture brought about by the rise of science and the French Revolution.[66]

## Political analogy

Cases of possession in early modern France, like the hysteria diagnoses of the late nineteenth century, are also episodes in history when 'female disinhibition' had a major role in what were questions of public political consequence. Part of the reason why a vast quantity of polemical literature was produced around cases of possession in the early modern period in France was the relationship of the cases to major political and jurisdictional issues, concurrent with and related in a number of ways to anxieties about the power of the devil. In the sixteenth and seventeenth centuries, the possession of Nicole Obry, which occurred at the height of the Wars of Religion, and that of Marthe Brossier at the time of the implementation of the Edict of Nantes, are prime examples, as is the Richelieu-sponsored execution of Urbain Grandier at Loudun in 1634, following accusations by possessed nuns.[67] For the nineteenth century, Goldstein's analysis has shown the importance of the Salpêtrière school's analysis of hysteria to its members public and 'mainstream' political life.

In this context, it may be possible to see hysteria and possession each in a metaphorical light; to see, for example, nineteenth-century hysteria as the embodiment of the disordered knowledge and haphazard religious manifestations over which scientific knowledge sought to establish itself, but which it also required in order to be reflected in a positive light. Similarly, demonic possession in the early modern period, as Stuart Clark has argued, might be seen as a metaphor for the state of the world, which exorcists portrayed as requiring the miracle of exorcism to forestall apocalypse.[68] At the heart of each was the use of the body, usually a female body, which was at once a representation of disorder, a means of understanding disorder and a means of overcoming it. Here, Ouerd's evocation of the 'dark continent' of femininity as the preoccupying subject of witch hunters, exorcists and nineteenth-century doctors rings especially true – with the added possibility that it was not only femininity which was at issue, but a relationship between femininity, or at least physicality, and the pressing metaphysical and political issues of the day.

## Analogy concluded

This 'use' of the possessed and of hysterics was, as we have seen, partly made for political reasons. On the purely pragmatic front, it enabled powerful men to criticize and attack other political opponents obliquely, by mediating their polemic through the bodies of the possessed or hysterics. But it is also important to assert that neither the behaviour of exorcists in the sixteenth and seventeenth centuries, nor that of the Charcot group, need be seen as necessarily or exclusively cynical, if indeed it was cynical at all. As Ouerd's demonstration of the 'blindness' of the Charcot group members to their own actions has shown us, the inconsistency between their claims of humanity and their own actions were clearly overwhelmed by their sense of place in history. And it should not be forgotten that they were part of a tradition of opposition to the inhumanity of witch hunting – a tradition to which our own liberal era is heir, if in more nuanced forms.

By sketching some additional fields of comparison, I have sought to demonstrate that there may be uses for the device of analogy which can incorporate the history of ideas within considerations of institutional and professional practice, and public performance. Taking the structural similarity between Ouerd and the Charcot school as a point of departure, I have pointed to the possibility of expanding the terrain of reflection on the two historical periods by exploiting the relationship between these periods which these two sets of readings have established. I am suggesting, in other words, that there may be ways in which analogy can be used in order to trace correspondences which would be made irrelevant or obscured by traditional synchronic or diachronic analyses.

However, in admitting a sense of provisionality in the task of addressing why Charcot and his school were so deeply engaged in establishing relations with the historical past, I want to suggest that their use of early modern texts might be seen in part as a means not only of establishing a distance between themselves and the clergy, but also a way of establishing a kind of heredity and a lineage. Certainly, this involved their assumption of the mantle of a kind of hieratic authority.[69] It might also not be too far-fetched to suggest that, in establishing a kind of inverted professional genealogy, they gave expression to an ambivalence about their own rapid and wholesale distancing not only from the historical past but also from many of their 'backward' contemporaries in the course of making their own, not insubstantial, contribution to the 'civilizing process'.

## ACKNOWLEDGEMENTS

I gratefully acknowledge the assistance of the Ian Potter and George Alexander Foundation and the University of Melbourne History Department Research Fund, each of which aided in the preparation of this paper. My thanks are also due to Denise Meredyth and Charles Zika for their valuable comments, and to Jenny Ferber for her support.

## NOTES

1 J.-M. Charcot and Paul Richer, *Les Démoniaques dans l'art* (Amsterdam, 1972), p. vi. The phrase 'retrospective medicine' was coined in 1869 by Emile Littré, a doctor and republican politician: Jan Goldstein, *Console and Classify: The French Psychiatric Profession in the Nineteenth Century* (Cambridge, 1987), pp. 369–70.

2 The titles in the *Bibliothèque Diabolique* were: D.-M. Bourneville and

E. Teinturier, *Le Sabbat des sorciers* (Paris, 1882 and 1890); A. Benet, *Procès verbal fait pour délivrer une fille possédée par le malin esprit à Louviers (1591)*, introduction by Vicomte B. de Moray (Paris, 1883); Jean Wier, *Histoires, disputes et discours* [*De praestigiis daemonum*, 1563] [as n. 17] and Thomas Erastus, *Deux dialogues*, preface by D.-M. Bourneville and a biographical essay on Wier by A. Axenfeld (Paris, 1885); D.-M. Bourneville, *La Possession de Jeanne Fery (1584)* (reprint of *Histoire admirable et véritable des choses advenues à l'endroict d'une religieuse professe du couvent des Soeurs noires de la ville de Mons en Hainaut*) (Paris, 1886); Jeanne des Anges, *Soeur Jeanne des Anges, Supérieure des Ursulines de Loudun: Autobiographie d'une hystérique possédée*, ed. and annotated by Gabriel Legué and Gilles de la Tourette, preface by J.-M. Charcot (Paris, 1886) (the edition of this work, published with Michel de Certeau, 'Jeanne des Anges' and Ferdinand Cavallera, 'L'Autobiographie de Jeanne des Anges d'après des documents inédits' (Grenoble, 1990), will be used for citation in this chapter); P. Ladame, *Procès criminel de la dernière sorcière brûlée à Genève le 6 avril 1652* (Paris, 1888); Samuel Garnier, *Barbe Buvée, en religion Soeur Sainte-Colombe, et la prétendue possession des Ursulines d'Auxonne (1658–1663)*, preface by D.-M. Bourneville (Paris, 1895); J.-M. Charcot, *La Foi qui guérit*, preface by D.-M. Bourneville (Paris, 1897). All titles were published at the offices of the journal *Progrès médical*. See also two editions of the historical piece by Paul Regnard, 'Les Sorcières', in *La Revue scientifique de la France et de l'étranger: revue des cours scientifiques* (3rd series), 1 April 1882, pp. 385–97, and in *Les Maladies épidémiques de l'esprit: sorcellerie, magnétisme, morphinisme, délires de grandeurs* (Paris 1887), pp. 1–98, and Paul Richer, *Etudes cliniques sur l'hystéro-épilepsie ou grande hystérie* (Paris, 1881), pp. 615–726 ('Notes historiques').

3 See D.-M. Bourneville, *Science et miracle* (Paris, 1875), a clinical interpretation of the reputed stigmata of a Belgian woman, Louise Lateau; Richer, *Etudes cliniques*, pp. 670–6, 701–15, 718–26.

4 As Ruth Harris noted, Charcot 'proposed a picture of feminine disinhibition which . . . was overtly and unceasingly compared to convulsive religious episodes': J.-M. Charcot, *Clinical Lectures on Diseases of the Nervous System*, ed. and introduced by Ruth Harris (London, 1991), p. xix.

5 Goldstein, *Console and Classify*, p. 372. See also an earlier version of Goldstein's chapter on Charcot: 'The hysteria diagnosis and the politics of anticlericalism in late nineteenth-century France', *Journal of Modern History*, 54 (1982): 209–39. See also Mary James, 'Hysteria and demonic possession', in Basiro Davey, Alastair Gray and Clive Seale (eds), *Health and Disease: A Reader*, 2nd edn. (Buckingham, 1995), pp. 55–61.

6 Richer, *Etudes cliniques*, p. 615. The historical study of hysteria no longer need risk being incomplete, following the invaluable publications of Mark S. Micale, 'Hysteria and its historiography: a review of past and present writings', *History of Science*, 27 (1989): 223–61, 319–51; *idem*, 'Hysteria and its historiography: the future perspective',

*History of Psychiatry*, 1 (1990): 33–124. See also the major survey by G.S. Rousseau, 'A strange pathology: hysteria in the early modern world', in Sander Gilman *et al.*, *Hysteria Beyond Freud* (Berkeley, CA, 1993), pp. 91–221.

7 Michèle Ouerd, 'Dans la forge à cauchemars mythologiques: sorcières, praticiennes et hystériques', *La Sorcellerie* (1978), Les Cahiers de Fontenay, nos 11–12 (Paris, 1992), pp. 103–58, esp. p. 124. See also Elaine Showalter, *The Female Malady: Women, Madness and English Culture, 1830–1980* (New York, 1985), pp. 145–54.

8 Here I am considering some of the implications of Lyndal Roper's trenchant question, posed in the introduction to *Oedipus and the Devil* (London, 1994), p. 2, where she asks how we might conceive of 'the historical'. While Roper's argument is primarily informed by a concern to see human subjectivity and individual experience addressed in historical writing, my own intention is a more limited attempt to retain on the historiographical landscape 'outmoded' forms of historical writing as an acknowledgment of the continuity in the discipline and of the possibilities of revisionism in history writing.

9 Goldstein, *Console and Classify*, p. 322.

10 Ruth Harris, introduction to Charcot, *Clinical Lectures on Diseases of the Nervous System*, p. xv; Goldstein, *Console and Classify*, chap. 9; Ouerd, 'Dans la forge', p. 116; Roy Porter, 'The body and the mind, the doctor and the patient: negotiating hysteria', in Gilman *et al.*, *Hysteria Beyond Freud*, pp. 225–85, esp. pp. 255–60.

11 Porter, 'The body and the mind', p. 238. Patrick Vandermeersch has argued that the notion that demonological explanations were replaced with physical explanations of psychic phenomena, was a myth perpetrated by mid- to late nineteenth-century writers. Echoing Goldstein, he proposes that the myth arose from an anticlerical impulse and allowed these writers to bypass the incongruous fact of Pinel's 'moral treatment' of hysteria. Vandermeersch argues for a more rigorous exploration of the processes of 'secularization' in nineteenth-century France: 'The victory of psychiatry over demonology: the origin of the nineteenth-century myth', *History of Psychiatry*, 2 (1991): 351–63. See also Goldstein, *Console and Classify*, p. 5 and *passim*.

12 Goldstein, *Console and Classify*, p. 361.

13 Bourneville, for example, was both a member of the *Conseil Municipal* of Paris and a member of the Chamber of Deputies. Other significant aspects of the relationship between the later Third Republic and medical culture were the laicization of the public hospital system and the creation of a Chair in Diseases of the Nervous System in the Paris Faculty of Medicine in 1882, destined from its creation to be filled by Charcot: Goldstein, *Console and Classify*, pp. 361–77.

14 *Ibid.*, p. 373.

15 Jules Michelet, *La Sorcière* (Paris, 1862); L.-F. Calmeil, *De la folie considérée sous le point de vue patholigique, philosophique, historique et judiciaire* (Paris, 1845); Pierre Briquet, *Traité clinique et thérapeutique de l'hystérie* (Paris, 1859).

16 Goldstein, *Console and Classify*, pp. 355–6.

17 In 1885, the third publication in the *Bibliothèque Diabolique* was Wier's *De praestigiis daemonum*, published as *Histoires, disputes et discours*, and preceded by an abbreviated version of Axenfeld's work on Wier.

18 Bourneville wrote of 'the great battles of the scientific spirit against barbarity' in his preface to Wier, *Histoires, disputes et discours*, p. vi. (All translations are mine.)

19 Charles Richet, 'Les Démoniaques d'aujourd'hui', *Revue des Deux Mondes*, 37 (1880): 340–72, at p. 340.

20 D.-M. Bourneville and P. Regnard, *Iconographie photographique de la Salpêtrière*, 3 vols (Paris, 1876–80), vol. II, pp. 173–4.

21 Gabriel Legué, *Documents pour servir à l'histoire médicale des possédées de Loudun* (Paris, 1874), p. 4; Charcot, *La Foi qui guérit*. Patrick Vandermeersch has noted that Pinel too acknowledged the capacity of exorcists to effect 'real' changes in the possessed: 'The victory of psychiatry over demonology', p. 357. Pierre Janet spoke of the psychological treatment that he employed as a form of exorcism: 'Un cas de possession et l'exorcisme moderne', in *Névroses et idées fixes* (Paris, 1898), p. 402. It was also argued, however, that the church provoked the hysteria of the possessed, see De Moray's introduction to Benet, *Procès verbal fait pour délivrer une fille possédée*, p. xviii.

22 Charcot and Richer, *Les Démoniaques dans l'art*, p. 109.

23 *Ibid.*, p. 91.

24 Bourneville, in Wier, *Histoires, disputes et discours*, Preface, p. ii.

25 Charcot and Richer, *Les Démoniaques dans l'art*, p. 109.

26 Preface to Jeanne des Anges, *Autobiographie*, p. 8.

27 Charcot and Richer, *Les Démoniaques dans l'art*, p. v.

28 Goldstein, *Console and Classify*, p. 327 (citing Charcot, 'Leçon d'ouverture', *Progrès médical*, 100 (1882): 336); see *ibid.*, pp. 330–1 and Etienne Trillat, *Histoire de l'hystérie* (Paris, 1986), p. 50.

29 Charcot and Richer, *Les Démoniaques dans l'art*, p. vi.

30 Introduction to Charcot, *Clinical Lectures on Diseases of the Nervous System*, p. xi. Notwithstanding both the Salpêtrière group's insistence on the phenomenon of hysteria in men and the fact that there were numerous cases of possession (and indeed witch trials) in the early modern period which involved men or children, the majority of the literature upon which Charcot and his colleagues drew concerned cases of possession in women, just as the majority of their own hysteria patients were female. Their choice of literature reflects, however, the intense literary and polemic preoccupation in early modern France with possession among women. See Robert Mandrou, *Magistrats et sorciers en France au XVII^e^ siècle: une analyse de psychologie historique* (Paris, 1968); Michel de Certeau, *La Possession de Loudun* (Paris, 1970); H.C. Erik Midelfort, 'The devil and the German people: reflections on the popularity of demon possession in sixteenth-century Germany', in Steven Ozment (ed.), *Religion and Culture in the Renaissance and Reformation* (Kirksville, MO, 1989), pp. 98–119; D.P. Walker, *Unclean Spirits: Possession and Exorcism in*

*France and England in the Late Sixteenth and Early Seventeenth Centuries* (London, 1981); Sarah Ferber, 'Mixed blessings: possession and exorcism in France, 1598–1654', unpub. PhD thesis, University of Melbourne, 1994. On Charcot's work on hysteria in men, see Mark S. Micale, 'Charcot and the idea of hysteria in the male: gender, mental science and medical diagnosis in late nineteenth-century France', *Medical History*, 34, (1990): 363–411; Jan Goldstein, 'The uses of male hysteria: medical and literary discourse in nineteenth-century France', *Representations*, 34 (1991): 134–65.

31 Richer, *Etudes cliniques*, p. 615.

32 Charcot and Richer noted, however, that not all types of supposed demonic possession could be reclassified as hysteria. They added that mental alienation, epilepsy and hypochondria and other ailments might also be present: Charcot and Richer, *Les Démoniaques dans l'art*, p. 91.

33 *Ibid.*, pp. 92–106.

34 *Ibid.*, p. 102. Charles Richet noted the possibility of a 'demoniacal' attack lasting for several days: 'Les Démoniaques d'aujourd'hui', p. 359.

35 Jeanne des Anges, *Autobiographie*, p. 99.

36 Charcot and Richer, *Les Démoniaques dans l'art*, p. 8.

37 *Ibid.*, p. 22.

38 Richet, 'Les Démoniaques d'aujourd'hui', pp. 341, 355. Richet's emphasis on the denial of supernatural intervention and on the cruelty of the church also led him to confuse at times the categories of demoniacs and witches, and to imply that demoniacs were burned as witches, which rarely occurred.

39 Bourneville and Regnard, *Iconographie*, vol. I, pp. 103–4.

40 *Ibid.*, vol. II, pp. 202, 206, plate 39.

41 Legué, *Documents pour servir à l'histoire médicale*, p. 83. Charles Richet spoke of 'une maladie incomplètement connue, dont la science n'a pas encore pu approfondir la nature bizarre et complexe': 'Les Démoniaques d'aujourd'hui', p. 351.

42 Gabriel Legué, *Urbain Grandier et les possédées de Loudun* (Paris, 1880), p. 307; Bourneville, *Science et miracle* (Paris, 1875), p. 1.

43 Jeanne des Anges, *Autobiographie*, Preface, p. 7.

44 See the edn of G. Didi-Huberman of *Les Démoniaques dans l'art* (Paris, 1984), p. 174.

45 Bourneville and Regnard, *Iconographie*, vol. I, pp. 100–03; Preface to Garnier, *Barbe Buvée*, p. i.

46 Legué, *Urbain Grandier* , p. 313.

47 Legué, *Documents pour servir à l'histoire médicale*, p. 82.

48 Charles Richet, *L'Homme et l'intelligence* (Paris, 1884), p. 367. Louise Capeau's 'demons' had testified against Louis Gaufridy, a priest accused of causing Capeau's possession.

49 Bourneville, preface to Garnier, *Barbe Buvée*, p. xviii.

50 Wier, *Histoires, disputes et discours*, Preface by Bourneville, p. vii; *ibid.*, Axenfeld, biographical note on Wier, p. xvi.

51 Charcot and Richer, *Les Démoniaques dans l'art*, p. 109.

52 *Ibid.*, p. 31.
53 *Ibid.*, p. 21.
54 Legué, *Documents pour servir à l'histoire médicale*, p. 5.
55 Charcot, *La Foi qui guérit*, p. 22.
56 Ouerd, 'Dans la forge à cauchemars mythologiques', pp. 118–19. Ouerd here uses texts from a range of nineteenth-century writers, including Taguet, Huchard, Falret, Richet, Esquirol and Raviart.
57 *Ibid.*, pp. 120–1; Garnier, *Barbe Buvée*, pp. xi, 91. Similarly, Pierre Janet noted in an 'ironic' aside that he and other doctors might be seen as similar to witch prickers because of their tests on hysterics: A.R.G. Owen, *Hysteria, Hypnosis and Healing in the Work of Jean-Martin Charcot* (New York, 1971), p. 74.
58 For a quite different feminist reading of the behaviour of hysterics, see Jacqueline Carroy-Thirard, 'Figures de femmes hystériques dans la psychiatrie française au 19e siècle', *Psychanalyse à l'Université*, 4 (1974): 313–24. In stressing the agency of the highly-publicized hysterical women at the Salpêtrière, the author suggests that they may have had a degree of complicity in regard to their treatment by doctors, suggesting a kind of 'reciprocal seduction' in which the women took initiatives to achieve their own desire within the context of the medical discourse: *ibid.*, p. 323.
59 Goldstein, *Console and Classify*, pp. 355–6.
60 Trillat, *Histoire de l'hystérie*, pp. 163–6.
61 Goldstein has noted, importantly, that the notion of the 'diseased will' also had implications for Catholic practice at the level of paraliturgy, negating prayer, confession and the possibility of divine intervention: *Console and Classify*, p. 270.
62 See, for example, the debunking of a famous case of possession promoted by militant Catholics following the Wars of Religion, by a doctor, Michel Marescot, *Discours véritable sur le faict de Marthe Brossier de Romorantin prétendue demoniaque* (Paris, 1599). See also the contribution of Albrecht Burkardt in this volume (Chapter 4).
63 For example, Elisabeth de Ranfaing, a possessed woman who lived in the first half of the seventeenth century, was warned that if she was found to have made a pact with the devil which gave her the powers of a possessed person, she would be punished: Rémy Pichard, *Admirable vertu des saints exorcismes sur les princes d'enfer possédant réellement vertueuse Demoiselle Elisabeth de Ranfaing* (Nancy, 1622), p. 85.
64 See Sanson Birette, *Refutation de l'erreur du vulgaire, touchant les responses des diables exorcisez* (Rouen, 1618); Léon d'Alexis [Pierre de Bérulle], *Traicté des energumènes, suivy d'un discours sur la possession de Marthe Brossier* (Troyes, 1599).
65 See Ruth Harris, introduction to Charcot, *Clinical Lectures on Diseases of the Nervous System*, p. xxxiv, on Charcot's and Tourette's anxieties about the effects of spiritualist practices on susceptible minds.
66 Bourneville, *Science et miracle*, p. 1; Goldstein, *Console and Classify*, p. 371.
67 See Walker, *Unclean Spirits*, pp. 19–42; Mandrou, *Magistrats et sorciers en France*, pp. 163–73.

68 Stuart Clark, ' "The Demoniacke World": possession, exorcism and eschatology in early modern Europe', *The Society for the Social History of Medicine Bulletin*, 41 (1987): 12–15.
69 Goldstein speaks of the 'imperfectly severed religious roots of the early psychiatric practitioner': *Console and Classify*, p. 5.

Chapter 7

# Breaking the boundaries

## Irregular healers in eighteenth-century Holland

*Hans de Waardt*

In the eighteenth century, in almost all the towns of densely urbanized Holland, the political authority that was personified by the college of *burgemeesters* had a thorough grip on medical activities within their jurisdictions. Normally, the *Collegium medicum* was the highest level in the structure that was thus created. It supervised the work of the physicians, the local surgeons, the apothecaries and the midwives. The surgeons and the apothecaries had been allowed to organize themselves in guilds; a privilege that was ordinarily denied to the midwives. In theory all irregular healers were obliged to ask the local magistrates for permission to practise in their district. The *burgemeesters* then asked the advice of the *Collegium medicum* and, if the petitioner wanted to operate on patients, that of the surgeons' guild as well. The boundaries that separated the towns from the outside world protected the inhabitants against unlicensed medical practitioners.

In practice, however, just as in France or England, great numbers of itinerant mountebanks and charlatans offered their panaceas on every market square.[1] Sedentary empirics could be found in the centre of most towns, and though belief in witchcraft had lost much of its vigour in eighteenth-century Holland, professional cunning men were still available to assist the bewitched.[2] Some of these irregular healers were perhaps nothing but ordinary swindlers, but others were well-trained specialists who could offer their patients genuine help.[3]

This chapter deals with the careers of three irregular healers who all tried to cross the boundaries that separated them from the medical market in the Dutch towns. Many irregular healers tried to bypass the official procedure or to influence its outcome by manipulating the physicians' and surgeons' organizations, the magistrates or the patients themselves. The careers of these three healers are exemplary for the different ways in which this was attempted. The patients often played a vital role in these encounters. Ever since Roy Porter's appeal to incorporate the patient's view into medical history, a growing number of historians have devoted at least part of their energy to this aspect,[4] but until now very little has been said about the position of the patients of irregular healers. In particular, the position of members of the lower social strata has remained outside the scope of most studies. This has largely resulted from a restricted choice of sources, and so the sources used in this chapter include many patient testimonies, often in their own handwriting.

The framework of this chapter owes much to Lucinda Beier's study of the casebook of the London surgeon Joseph Binns.[5] Binns, however, was a regular healer, whereas the healers on whom this contribution focuses were at best admitted for only a brief period as members of a recognized organization of medical practitioners.

Porter has argued that the communication between irregular healers and their patients normally took the form of a one-way speech. Such healers flooded their potential customers with publicity to catch their attention, whereas the clients were an audience of 'relatively silent and passive' spectators.[6] It will be argued here that the relationship between irregular healers and their patients was not necessarily one sided. Many irregular healers, both itinerant and sedentary, only managed to gain admission to a town because they were supported by a number of its inhabitants. On the other hand, there were also healers who showed no interest at all in their patients. The German Johan Christoph Ludeman belonged to this second category.

## JOHAN CHRISTOPH LUDEMAN

In the eighteenth century the astrologist and uroscopist Johan Christoph Ludeman was without any doubt the most renowned irregular healer in the Netherlands. Apart from a few lacunae, the course of his life is fairly well known. He related much about it himself[7] and his mistress added a few odd details,[8] as did several contemporaries.[9] A recent biographical sketch sums up many of the known details.[10] Ludeman was born in 1683 in the small North German town of Harburg. When he was 30 years old the local, very orthodox Lutheran clergy, who strongly disapproved of his sympathies for the ideas of Paracelsus and Jacob Böhme, forced him to leave his home town.[11] In the sixteenth century the German physician Paracelsus had argued that every physician should be familiar with astrology and should have a perfect knowledge of minerals and metals,[12] and from the works of the mystic Jacob Böhme, Ludeman learned how to become a reborn Christian. These convictions brought with them great problems in his Lutheran home town, and in any case his neighbours disdained him because he habitually abused his wife Dorothea. In 1711 Ludeman went bankrupt, which further exacerbated his situation. Two years later he arrived in Amsterdam.

Shortly after his arrival in Amsterdam Ludeman started to practise as a uroscopist and astrologist, without asking the *Collegium medicum* or the *burgemeesters* for permission. Around the same time he met Brita Beyer, a Swedish woman who shared his admiration for Böhme. She soon became his mistress and took up residence with the Ludeman family. Together the healer and his new companion abused Ludeman's wife who eventually ran away in 1721, and five years later their separation was made official. On both occasions (when the mistress moved in and again when Ludeman's wife left) Ludeman's neighbours, angry about his comportment, organized a charivari in front of his house. To defend themselves in the resulting public scandal, Ludeman and Brita wrote a number of pamphlets in which the healer was presented as a *Philosophiae et Medicinae Doctor*. This prompted the *Collegium medicum*, which until then had not taken any notice of his activities, to demand that he presented his university diploma – a qualification which Ludeman, of course, did not have.[13] The healer was then summoned by the *schout* before the court of *schepenen*, the local court of justice,[14] and this seriously threatened his medical practice.

Ludeman then turned to the University of Harderwijk in the province of Gelderland. This institution was widely famed for the ease with which it bestowed the doctorate on its students, especially in those cases where applicants were willing to pay a handsome fee.[15] In March 1728 Ludeman received his doctorate for a dissertation in which he argued that there were seven varieties of dropsy, each of which was governed by one of the seven planets.[16] Eleven days later the new doctor proudly showed his diploma to the *Collegium medicum*.[17]

By then Ludeman's escapades had become the subject of a number of sarcastic libels and even of a farce.[18] The healer was widely exposed as a *mof*,[19] a fraud, quack, money grubber, adulterous hypocrite and wife beater. Nevertheless, patients flocked to Ludeman's door and his business boomed. In 1729 the *Collegium medicum* made one last effort to corner him. When three of his patients lodged a complaint about his huge bills, it decided to examine the case thoroughly. However, the *Collegium* was forced to decide in favour of its unwanted colleague because the patients had agreed to follow the doctor's orders and had accepted the prescribed medicines. They consequently also had to pay their bills.[20] After this incident Ludeman was not further disturbed by his fellow physicians. He became very wealthy. When his possessions were assessed for tax purposes in 1742, he had a yearly income of 8,000 guilders, and compared with the average income of the doctors in Amsterdam at that time – a mere 1,650 guilders per year – his earnings were exceptionally high.[21] On his death in 1757 his possessions were valued at 130,000 guilders.[22]

Ludeman wrote two books in which he described his medical conceptions.[23] Five years before his dissertation, in 1721, he had published his *Key to the Abyss*, in which he explained how every part of the human body had a special relation with one of the planets and that one had to read the Gospel to understand how this affected health.[24] Besides these two books, he must have written thousands of prescriptions. Seventeen of these have been retrieved.[25] They all follow the same pattern. After a few remarks about the conjunctures of the relevant planets, Ludeman gave a brief description of the general character of the patient and then described the nature of the illness and its causes. Eventually he prescribed the medicines that were needed. He was not interested in the names of his patients nor in their social status or family background; indeed the great majority of the people who consulted him must have remained anonymous to him. What mattered to Ludeman was what could be called their 'astrological identity' and his clients seem to have had an infinite trust in his abilities.

A total of only 17 prescriptions is no basis for statistical interpretations, but it is perhaps enough for a sketchy impression. Nine of these prescriptions deal with the problems of male patients and six of them were written for female clients. The sex of one patient is not specified, so although the numerical evidence does not allow any sound conclusion, it does seem that Ludeman found clients among members of both sexes. Most contemporary authors claimed that he was particularly famous among the farmers of North

Holland. Among his clients were Adriaan Vosmaar,[26] a prominent courtier of the *stadhouder* William V, and a Reformed minister.[27]

Through his own efforts Ludeman managed to stake out a place in the medical market of Holland. He did not need any support from his patients to outbalance his disastrous reputation. Although he completely lacked any formal training and despite the fact that the physicians of the *Collegium medicum* strongly disapproved of his therapies, he overcame their opposition by acquiring the impregnable defence that a university degree could offer. Precisely because the physicians had been very effective in securing their privileges by establishing a *Collegium medicum*, they were unable to harm him after his graduation.

## JOHN TAYLOR

John Taylor[28] was born in 1703 in Norwich. After studying surgery in London under the guidance of Cheselden, he began to journey through Britain as an itinerant oculist in 1727. In 1733 he went to the continent for the first time, during which trip he received MDs from several universities. In 1736, back in London, he was appointed royal oculist to George II. Despite this official recognition he kept on travelling for the rest of his life, covering enormous distances and visiting nearly every country in Europe. He died in 1772.

In medical historiography John Taylor is often presented as the quack *par excellence*, a qualification that does not seem to be completely justified. Though his theatrical appearance resembled that of the ordinary mountebank, he did not try to swindle people by selling useless medicines. The majority of his patients suffered from cataracts and he treated them by couching the clouded lens, in his days still the conventional and recognized treatment. It is true that around 1750 the Frenchman Daviel developed a technique to extract the lens, instead of pushing it aside, but one cannot blame Taylor for the fact that he was not yet familiar with this new treatment. Many of his patients contracted severe infections after being operated on by him, because he did not clean his instruments,[29] but then no surgeon at that time made much of an effort to cleanse his instruments.

Taylor visited the Dutch Republic at least three times, in 1734, 1749 and 1758. Virtually nothing is known of his first visit. In 1735 a French as well as a Dutch translation of his *An Account of the*

*Mechanism of the Eye*, originally published in 1727, appeared in Amsterdam.[30] Taylor's claim that he had once assisted the famous Boerhaave seems unfounded.[31] Such a meeting could only have occurred in 1734, when the renowned Dutch physician was still alive. No source besides Taylor's own boasting assertion supports this claim.

On 3 August 1749 it was announced in the *s-Gravenhaegsche Courant*, a newspaper published in Den Haag, that 'Doctor Taylor, oculist to his Great-Britannic Majesty' had

> arrived from London in Den Haag, to make a journey to Italy . . . During the short stay of doctor Taylor in this town, he will, thereby following his ordinary habit in London, help the poor sufferers *gratis*, and the coming week he will continue his journey by way of Leiden, Amsterdam, Paris, Turin etc.

This announcement, presented as if it were a news item, was of course an advertisement paid for by Taylor himself. Shortly afterwards, on 9 August, the same text appeared in the *Amsterdamsche Courant*.

A week after his arrival in Den Haag the *Collegium medicum* discussed the problems caused by the 'English operator named Taylor', who was practising without its permission,[32] though at that stage the *Collegium* refrained from any overt action. According to at least some of its members, Taylor had written a 'treatise about the eyes that has been duly cited and praised by several people'. Furthermore, *stadhouder* William IV of Orange had put Taylor under his protection and the oculist had promised in his advertisements that he would soon leave town.

On 14 August Taylor was received by the wife of the *stadhouder*, Anna of Hannover, a daughter of King George II. The following day the oculist was introduced to the *stadhouder* himself. On that occasion Taylor operated on the eyes of one of the *stadhouder*'s valets and the result impressed the princely couple so much that they conferred on him the title of 'Oculist to their Serene and Royal Highnesses'.[33] This made it very difficult for the *Collegium medicum* to oppose Taylor in public. The third reason for the initial inertia of the *Collegium* was the fact that Taylor repeatedly announced that he would soon leave, though such announcements were always quickly followed by a notice in which Taylor stated that he felt forced to postpone his departure.[34]

These press notices had a dual effect. A potentially powerful enemy was kept at bay and, at the same time, the general public was constantly reminded of Taylor's presence. To get even more publicity Taylor sent some untreated patients ahead to his next stop, which would be Amsterdam. While waiting there, they spread the news of his forthcoming visit to the town. To prepare the public in Amsterdam even further, Taylor put a news item in the *Amsterdamche Courant* of 2 September, in which he claimed that he had treated four or five hundred people in Den Haag. He eventually left Den Haag on 3 September and arrived in Amsterdam two days later.

Three days after his arrival in Amsterdam, the surgeons' guild was convened and discussed the flyers that the oculist had distributed. They decided to summon him before the *schepenen*, but to their dismay the *burgemeesters* would not permit this. The magistrates had heard that Taylor was supported by 'crowned heads' and that 'he was reported to be an able person, perfect for such operations'.[35] Once again the support of the *stadhouder* and his wife helped the oculist to overcome the opposition of his sedentary colleagues.

Taylor stayed in Amsterdam for a period of three weeks. Several times he notified the public that his departure was imminent, contradicting the announcement a few days later because the 'unbelievable . . . huge mass of people' who came to ask his help made it impossible for him to leave.[36] He again claimed that he had helped hundreds of people. In the meantime the *Collegium medicum* of Den Haag had drawn up a list of 29 people who had been treated by Taylor. According to this survey only two of his patients had benefited from his cure. The other 27 had suffered terrible agonies without any result, while the eyesight of some had even deteriorated. This list was published on 26 September and Taylor answered this challenge by publishing a flyer, on which 27 patients figured who had benefited greatly from his treatment.[37]

On 15 October Taylor showed the *Collegium medicum* of Utrecht his diploma from the University of Reims, as well as documents that proved that he had been admitted by the fellow *collegia* of Basel and Cologne. The Utrecht physicians gave him an authenticated note which said that they had indeed received him.[38] Without hesitating, Taylor used this paper as proof that he had been admitted as a full member to the *Collegium medicum* of Utrecht. The *Collegium* quickly put an advertisement in several newspapers in which it announced that it had only examined his diploma.[39] At that moment Taylor had already left Utrecht to go to Leiden and he announced that he would lecture at the University of Leiden on eye diseases. On 19 October he presented himself to the surgeons' guild and to the professors of the faculty of medicine.[40] On their advice the *burgemeesters* prohibited Taylor from practising in their town[41] after which the English oculist then left the Dutch Republic and went to the Austrian Netherlands.

Despite the unfortunate end of this visit, Taylor returned to Holland on one more occasion. In February 1758 he arrived in Amsterdam, but this time the surgeons' guild was ready for him. Before he could put a notice in the newspapers, the guild had requested that the *burgemeesters* prohibit him from practising.[42] A few days later an advertisement was published in which the guild as well as the *schout* cautioned the public against resort to the English oculist. They claimed that in 1734 as well as in 1749 his operations had been detrimental to his patients.[43] At the same time, Taylor and the printer he had hired to print a handbill for him were intimidated by the guild's barrister and a public notary.[44]

Taylor then left for Utrecht, but the Amsterdam surgeons had already notified the physicians in Utrecht about his imminent arrival. When Taylor found out that it was impossible for him to work in Utrecht, he returned to Amsterdam where he requested the *burgemeesters* to allow him to operate. The answer was very short: '*Nihil*'. He was even fined 50 guilders, the usual penalty for illegal medical practice. In a final effort to turn the tide he put a series of advertisements in the *Amsterdamsche Courant* in which four persons declared that Taylor had restored their eyesight.[45] The surgeons retaliated by threatening that they would prosecute anybody who signed such statements.

This was enough to force Taylor to leave Amsterdam. He went to Rotterdam, a town he had never visited before. At first his well-tried tactics had the usual success there. The surgeons seemed to be willing to admit him for, as they wrote to their colleagues in Amsterdam, 'we believe that this man has exceptional capacities to treat those defects [of the eyes] and to do the necessary operations'. Taylor had told them that he was on the best of terms with their colleagues in Amsterdam. However, on 26 April 1758 the Amsterdam surgeons' guild replied furiously that Taylor was nothing more than 'an adventurer who earned his living by wandering about through the country to make money'; not the sort of person with whom the guild wanted to converse.[46] It is not very likely that after receiving this missive the Rotterdam guild allowed Taylor to operate. By then he must have understood that it had become impossible for him to work in the Netherlands and he probably left the country soon after the letter of the Amsterdam guild had arrived in Rotterdam.

It is unusual to find out anything about the patients of a particular healer in this period, but as a result of the sharp conflicts between Taylor and the regular practitioners, a large number of his clients can be identified. Two lists, one drawn up by the *Collegium medicum* of Den Haag, the other by Taylor himself, plus the advertisements that appeared in 1758, together constitute 62 patients. It is of course impossible to establish whether this group is representative of all Taylor's Dutch patients, but it is only through such accidental discoveries that we can find out anything at all about the clients of such healers.

According to this sample Taylor had more male than female patients. Of the 27 persons who figured on the list drawn up by the physicians of Den Haag, 13 were men and 10 women. The sex of 4 persons, all of them children, remained unspecified. Of the 28 patients who supported him in 1749, 18 were male, 9 female and the sex of one person was not given. The four advertisements published in 1758 add to the impression that Taylor found the majority of his patients among men. Three of them were signed by male clients and only one by a woman. This male majority among his patients might be one of the reasons why he managed to hold out so long in his struggle against the organizations of the regular practitioners. Nevertheless, the possibility cannot be ruled out that more men than women were willing to have their name put on such a list.[47]

John Taylor apparently attracted clients from all social strata. Among the people who figure on the Amsterdam list are, for example, three women who were unable to write their own names. In the Dutch Republic, where literacy was very high, this means that they came from the lowest strata of society. But he also treated members of the social elite like Mrs Gerarda Wittert in Den Haag, a lady from a well-to-do Old Catholic family and, in Amsterdam, mister Bosboom, a *schepen* (alderman) of Berg, a town on the Lower Rhine. Taylor also operated upon the servants of high-ranking persons. As already mentioned, he couched the cataract of a valet of the *stadhouder* and in Amsterdam he operated upon the manservant of Baron van Heyden, a prominent member of the Dutch nobility.

The majority of Taylor's patients in 1749 seem to have come from the class of shopkeepers and craftsmen, among whom there were large differences in income and status. The silversmith Frederik Ghijsen, operated upon in Den Haag for an inflammation of the eyelids, was a rich man, whereas the yearly income of the widow Broman, who ran a grocer's shop in Amsterdam, was very modest. Still, it appears that in general the majority of the persons who figured on the lists that were drawn up in 1749 belonged to the middle layer of Dutch society.

When Taylor returned nine years later, he could no longer draw on such an extensive reservoir. In 1758 all his known patients were Sephardic Jews, whereas in 1749 no patient of his was reported to be Jewish. In that year all his patients were Christians, albeit of varied sorts. Apparently Taylor was no longer called upon by Christians in 1758. There is no proof that priests or ministers prohibited members of their flocks from consulting the oculist. It seems therefore that the surgeons' action to isolate him was quite successful. The Jewish community was perhaps less susceptible to this strategy, but this group also backed down when the guild threatened that it would sue anybody who dared to support Taylor.

## JEAN BAPTISTE CHARLIER

In May 1762, at the age of 45, Jean Baptiste Charlier[48] was tried by the *Hof van Holland en Zeeland*, the province's supreme court of law. Born in Poperinge, a small Flemish community not far from Yperen, he had moved to Den Haag around 1743. Since then he had practised there as a healer. Being unable to read or write he had not received any formal medical training but, as he boasted, he had nevertheless treated 22,000 patients, of whom only eight had died. He could cure people because he 'was gifted with the knowledge of the nature of men, as a result of which he was able to detect the basic causes of their illnesses and sicknesses, mostly from the signs that can be seen in the water'.

Charlier had not bothered to ask anybody's consent to practise, but for years nobody had crossed him in any way. Then in 1759, he was summoned by the physicians of the *Collegium medicum* before the *schepenbank* of Den Haag for his illegal medical practice. At first the *burgemeesters* were unwilling to allow this prosecution because they had been petitioned by more than 70 citizens to allow Charlier to continue his good work, but only a little extra pressure from the

*Collegium medicum* was needed to convince the magistrates that the quack healer should be tried and convicted.

Charlier was fined the usual sum of 25 guilders. He refused to pay, however, and he was even stubborn enough to continue his practice. Consequently, he was sentenced a second time and ordered to pay the standard double fine of 50 guilders. Again he refused to pay, which prompted the *schepenen* to imprison him for debt. Charlier finally yielded and paid up, but immediately after his release he started to practise again, despite his solemn promise to leave Den Haag at once. The *burgemeesters* came to the conclusion that he was mad, or as the *Collegium medicum* put it, that 'a screw was loose'. In February 1761 Charlier was put in the municipal madhouse, but as this meant that the town had to pay for his confinement, it was decided to release him on the condition that he would definitely leave town. He moved to Voorburg, a village just outside the jurisdiction of Den Haag and resumed his practice. In 1762 Charlier was again arrested, this time on the orders of the *Hof van Holland en Zeeland*.

The reason for this third arrest was the fact that he had become entangled in a witchcraft scandal. In October 1761 Pieter Hendrik Mesch, an eight-year-old boy, had started to show symptoms of a very strange affliction. At first his parents thought that he was suffering from the aftermath of the measles. His father had consulted an apothecary and a physician, but neither of them could help the boy and father Mesch came to the conclusion that the illness must be of a preternatural nature. Although a devout member of the Dutch Reformed Church, he consulted a Jesuit – Father Bos – who was attached to the household of the Austrian ambassador in Den Haag. The clergyman convinced Mesch that his boy was bewitched, but that he was unable to cure him. Then Pieter's father, who by now was extremely worried, came into contact with Charlier.

On entering the scene, the Flemish healer promised to drive out the evil force that troubled the child. He took the little patient on his lap and hit him very hard on the knees and cheeks. When the child began to scream, Charlier shouted that this was a good sign. 'Go out, you evil one', he yelled and threw large quantities of water in the face of the crying boy. With a loud voice he asked 'the spirit of the Lord to enter into the child and to bless the water, and that he would take away the power of Satan and his following'. He assured Pieter's mother that there was no reason for fear, not even if there were as many devils in the room as there 'flew gnats over the earth'.

By now the case had become a public sensation. This caused the *Hof* to intervene. It came to the conclusion that Charlier was indeed completely mad and put him in an asylum at Delft where, it seems, he spent the rest of his days. The *Hof* also impressed upon Father Bos that he had to refrain from any further magical activities. Pieter Hendrik Mesch recovered completely. He died in 1830 at the age of 76.[49]

In October 1759, when Charlier was trying to ward off the attacks of the *Collegium medicum*, he had several petitions drawn up for the *burgemeesters* of Den Haag in which 77 inhabitants declared that they had benefited greatly from his cures. Each of them gave a brief description of the nature of his or her illness. The illnesses that were mentioned most frequently in these petitions were podagra or gout (nine cases), different sorts of obstruction (five of the uterus, two in the head, two of the blood and one in the entrails), unspecified breast illnesses and problems with the nerves (both seven cases), consumption (six), dropsy (five), fever and headache (both four cases). A score of other problems like 'sharpness through the blood' or discharge were mentioned less frequently.

The majority of Charlier's patients were female: 46 out of 77, 27 were male. The sex of two small children and of two other persons could not be established. In 31 cases it was possible either to find the date of their burial or at least to establish that they were still alive five years after the presentation of the petitions. Only two of Charlier's patients died very soon after the petitions had been drawn up. One of them, a man of 42, died of dropsy at the beginning of December 1758, that is less than two months after he had declared that he was suffering from that illness, but that he was feeling a little better as a result of Charlier's treatment. Another man of 35 died only a few days after the presentation of the petition. He had testified that Charlier had cured him of 'dehydration and dropsy caused by gastric acid'. According to the death certificate he died of consumption. Another two patients died within five years of the 1759 petitions. At least 27 of Charlier's clients were still alive in 1764, so the least one can say about Charlier's therapy is that it was not a mortal danger to his patients.

As to age or religious background, Charlier's patients had little in common. They belonged to at least three generational cohorts. The religion of 36 of his patients could be established: 24 of them were Reformed, 8 Catholic, 2 Lutheran and one was Jewish. It does not seem that Charlier's own religious convictions – he was a Catholic – were of any importance to his clients and in this respect his patients fitted with the religious composition of Den Haag and the rest of Dutch society.

However, the social backgrounds of Charlier's patients differed greatly from the general social structure of Den Haag in that period. An overwhelming majority of them were very poor. Only one of them came from a higher social group: he was a bookseller by profession. About a third of Charlier's clients lived in Scheveningen, the coastal district of Den Haag which was mainly inhabited by poor fishermen, and around a sixth were soldiers or the wives of soldiers who had very low social esteem in the Dutch Republic. The differences in the backgrounds of Charlier's patients and those of Taylor is striking. Where the English oculist found most of his patients among men of comfortable means, the Flemish empiric was mainly consulted by poor fishermen's and soldiers' wives.

## THE IRREGULAR HEALERS COMPARED

There were important differences between the careers of Ludeman, Taylor and Charlier. The astrologist Ludeman was undoubtedly the most successful of the three. Taylor only managed to work in Holland unimpeded for short periods and, while Charlier practised for several decades, his career ended in total failure.

Ludeman gained an unchallenged position by acquiring an MD. Taylor's approach was completely different. His main weapons were his swiftness, his almost limitless impudence, his ability to manipulate the press and above all the support of powerful and influential people. For weeks his opponents were too bewildered to develop an effective counter strategy. As soon as they went into the offensive, he moved out, to another town or, if necessary, to another country. Charlier, by comparison, was unable to counter the attack of the physicians. He could muster the support of more than 70 people, but as almost all of them came from the lowest ranks of society this could only postpone his downfall. Even if his mental powers may not have been as feeble as the physicians claimed they were, the social composition of his defensive forces was simply too weak.

All three of these healers were reproached by regular physicians and surgeons for being a danger to the health of their patients, though it is doubtful whether their results were really that bad.

Ludeman must have treated an enormous number of people, but nowhere do the sources tell us anything about patients who died or suffered severe setbacks as a result of his activities. The strong antipathy of his fellow physicians had probably more to do with the fact that Ludeman was an astrologist.

Until the seventeenth century many physicians and surgeons in Holland had relied on astrology, just as their colleagues elsewhere in Western Europe had done. Still, as early as the 1630s astrology was rapidly losing ground among physicians in the Dutch Republic as an auxiliary science,[50] a development that did not set in until after 1660 in England.[51] It is not, however, very likely that astrology lost its prestige among all Dutchmen at the same pace. In England even Isaac Newton readily acknowledged it as a reliable source of knowledge.[52] During the last decades of the seventeenth century astrology made a comeback in Holland.[53] It might be assumed that many people felt uneasy about the fact that physicians and surgeons refused to continue to use it. Ludeman filled this need. His fellow physicians could call him a witch doctor and a wizard, but this probably only added to his reliability in the eyes of his patients.

Charlier tried to carve out a place for himself in a comparable way. In the eighteenth century, uroscopy had lost much of its former appeal among physicians in Holland yet Charlier still inspected the urine of his patients. On the other hand he also did his best to present himself as an expert in modern methods. Again and again he argued that he knew everything about the laws of nature and in so doing he was probably trying to profit from the enormous prestige that natural science had acquired at that time. It cannot be established whether Charlier's therapy was successful or not, but it seems that it was not dangerous either.

The abilities of the oculist Taylor were debated by the physicians and the surgeons, but the real ground for their enmity does not seem to have been his lack of knowledge and experience. When the *Collegium medicum* of Den Haag tried to find as many examples of his malpractice as it could, it registered no more than 28 cases – 26 of which were presented as failures. At first sight this seems to be a considerable proportion, but is it really such a disastrous result? After all, Taylor had worked a whole month in Den Haag. If this list indeed contained all the names of the patients he treated there, he would have performed on average only one operation a day. This is not very plausible. It is possible that Taylor's own figures – he claimed that he had cured three or four hundred people in Den

Haag – were exaggerated, but he may well have treated about ten clients a day. In that case a total of 26 failures is not really such a bad result.

On other occasions Taylor's qualities were not contested at all. Petrus Camper, for instance, who worked as a professor of anatomy and surgery at several Dutch universities,[54] repeatedly commended the Englishman as an able oculist. In 1746 he wrote in his *Dissertatio optica de visu* that Taylor had shown one of Isaac Newton's theses on optics to be true.[55] In Camper's eyes Taylor was an authority of the same standing as De la Hire, Porterfield and Pemberton – physicians whom he considerably admired.[56] About 20 years later Camper referred to Taylor as an expert in the couching of cataracts.[57] Between 1757 and 1761, when Camper lectured in Amsterdam, he was often asked by the surgeons to conduct dissections on corpses. They undoubtedly held him in high esteem, but in 1758, when Taylor visited Amsterdam, the surgeons did not ask Camper for advice. If the expertise of Taylor had been the real issue, Camper's sympathetic opinions about this oculist would certainly have mattered a great deal. So the animosity of the Amsterdam surgeons was not caused by Taylor's lack of skills, but by his refusal to adjust himself to their whims. It was his insolence that prompted the regulars to drive him off the market, not his alleged clumsiness.

The organizations of physicians or surgeons probably did not object much to an irregular healer who practised in their jurisdiction without their approval, so long as he showed enough signs of submission, did not blunder too much and was no serious competitor. Some irregulars managed from time to time to be accepted by the *Collegia medica* or the surgeons' guilds, provided they were willing to suffer their arbitrariness. The oculist Daniel Schouwerman, for example, was admitted in 1724 by the *Collegium medicum* of Amsterdam, though in 1734 the Amsterdam surgeons' guild advised the *burgemeesters* to refuse him admittance on the ground that he was 'a cheat . . . and only fit to . . . act as principal of the quacks'.[58] In January 1735 the surgeons again advised turning him away, but only four months later he was admitted on the recommendation of the *Collegium medicum*.[59] Schouwerman remained polite and eventually this attitude brought his family the desired result. Although in 1769 his daughter Izabella was refused admittance to practise in Groningen,[60] another daughter, Catharina, was appointed municipal oculist of Dordrecht, Haarlem and

Rotterdam.[61] In 1756 she was also allowed to work in Amsterdam[62] and she even became a model for other healers. In 1755 the surgeon Arnoldus Mensinck requested to be appointed municipal oculist of Den Haag like 'the daughter of the former quack Schouwerman' in the three said towns.[63]

For an itinerant healer like Taylor, explicit support from his patients was indispensable. By producing a stream of testimonies from satisfied patients he managed at least for a while to keep the regular physicians and surgeons at bay. The communication with his patients therefore had a reciprocal character. When the *burgemeesters* had to decide whether they would allow a particular irregular healer to practise in their jurisdiction, they were clearly susceptible to pressure from their citizens, so irregular healers were ready to stir up such support when necessary. As a result great numbers of such lists drawn up to sanction particular healers are preserved in the archives of the *Collegia medica* and the surgeons' guilds.[64] Taylor was clearly well aware of the importance of such help and, by winning the express sympathy of prominent people, he managed to ward off the *Collegia medica* and the guilds for several weeks.

Charlier tried to secure his practice in the same way. He enlisted the support of even more people, but as none of them was very rich or powerful, this manoeuvre only delayed his trial for a few days. However, it is doubtful whether he would have saved his position even if he had also won the sympathy of influential people because Charlier was, unlike Taylor, not an itinerant. The *Collegium medicum* would perhaps have been obliged to use more energy and patience, but eventually it would have overcome Charlier's resistance.

A sedentary irregular healer could only hope to keep a hostile *Collegium medicum* or surgeons' guild at bay for a while by stirring up the support of patients, but a short span of time was all that an itinerant irregular needed. He could assume that he would be gone before the regulars could undo the effects of his publicity campaign. Paradoxical as it may seem, it is evident that the shorter a healer stayed in a particular town, the more he needed the express sympathy of his patients. Their support in this socio–cultural encounter could be of vital importance, as it was often the only way for an itinerant healer to overcome the barriers thrown up by the town magistrates to protect the position of the sedentary regular healers on the local medical market. The irregulars had to use the sympathy and influence of their patients if they wanted to break these boundaries.

## ABBREVIATIONS

| | |
|---|---|
| ACM | Archief van het Collegium medicum |
| AG | Archieven van de Gilden |
| AHvH | Archief van het Hof van Holland en Zeeland |
| GAA | Gemeente Archief van Amsterdam |
| GADH | Gemeente Archief van Den Haag |
| GAL | Gemeente Archief van Leiden |
| GAR | Gemeente Archief van Rotterdam |
| GAU | Gemeente Archief van Utrecht |
| UBA | Universiteits Bibliotheek Amsterdam |

## NOTES

1 Matthew Ramsey, *Professional and Popular Medicine in France, 1770–1830: The Social World of Medical Practice* (Cambridge, 1988), pp. 129–264; Roy Porter, *Health for Sale: Quackery in England 1660–1850* (Manchester, 1989). A great number of examples of the attitudes of irregular healers are to be found in W.F. Bynum and Roy Porter (eds), *Medical Fringe and Medical Orthodoxy 1750–1850* (London, 1987).

2 Hans de Waardt, *Toverij en samenleving. Holland 1500–1800* (Den Haag, 1991), pp. 245–76.

3 Frank Huisman, 'Itinerant medical practitioners in the Dutch Republic: the case of Groningen', *Tractrix: Yearbook for the History of Science, Medicine, Technology and Mathematics*, 1 (1989): 63–83; *idem*, 'Gevestigden en buitenstaanders op de medische markt. De marginalisering van reizende meesters in achttiende-eeuws Groningen', in W. de Blécourt, W. Frijhoff and M. Gijswijt-Hofstra (eds), *Grenzen van genezing: Gezondheid, ziekte en genezen in Nederland, zestiende tot begin twintigste eeuw* (Hilversum, 1993), pp. 115–54.

4 Roy Porter, 'The patient's view: doing medical history from below', *Theory and Society*, 14 (1983): 175–98.

5 Lucinda M. Beier, *Sufferers and Healers: The Experience of Illness in Seventeenth-Century England* (London and New York, 1987), pp. 51–96.

6 Roy Porter, 'The language of quackery in England, 1660–1800', in P. Burke and R. Porter (eds), *The Social History of Language* (Cambridge, 1987), pp. 73–103, esp. pp. 79–80.

7 Johan Christoph Ludeman, *Pedum pastorale, contra magistratum Harburgensem erectum* (Amsterdam, 1727); *idem*, *De herder-staf, gebruikt tegen de magistraat der Stad Harburg* ([Amsterdam], 1727).

8 Brita Beyer, *De middernachtskroon: Door de weedergeboorte erkampt en beschreven* ([Amsterdam], 1723); *idem*, *De gekroonde morgenstond, na een veertienjaarige verdrukkinge verscheenen en beschreeven* ([Amsterdam], 1727).

9 Willem van Swaanenburg, *De vervrolykende Momus, of koddige berisper, opgedragen aan Hans Christoffel Ludeman, doctor, zonder promotie*

(Amsterdam, 1726); *idem*, *Hans Christoffel Ludeman, afgerost door zyn eigen harderstaf, die hy gebruikt heeft, tegens de magistraat der stad Haarburg* (Amsterdam, 1727); [J.W. Claus van Laar], *Zeldzaame Levens-gevallen van de alom beruchten J.C. Ludeman, vermaard philosooph en medicine doctor* ([Amsterdam], 1757).

10 Arno van der Plank (ed.), *Nieuws tyding uit de andere waereld of samenspraak tusschen den beroemden schilder en schryver Jacob Campo Weyerman en den beruchten doctor en astrologist Ludeman* (Deventer, 1986), pp. i–viii.

11 On the similarities between the ideas of Paracelsus and those of Böhme, see Arlene Miller-Guinsburg, 'Von Paracelsus zu Böhme. Auf dem Wege zu neuen Bestandtsaufnahmen in der Beeinflussung Böhmes durch Paracelsus', in Sepp Domandl (ed.), *Paracelsus in der Tradition. Vorträge Paracelsustag 1978* (Vienna, 1980), pp. 96–118.

12 On the influence of Paracelsus's ideas in Germany in this period, see Siegfried Wollgast, 'Zur Wirkungsgeschichte des Paracelsus im 16. und 17. Jahrhundert', in Peter Dilg and Hartmut Rudolph (eds), *Resultate und Desiderate der Paracelsus-Forschung* (Stuttgart, 1993), pp. 113–44; Rudolf Schlögle, 'Ansätze zu einer Sozialgeschichte des Paracelsismus im 17. und 18. Jahrhundert', in *ibid.*, pp. 145–62.

13 GAA ACM inv. nr. 3, fos. 137, 138.

14 GAA ACM inv. nr. 47.

15 Willem Frijhoff, *La Société Néerlandaise et ses gradués, 1575–1814. Une recherche sérielle sur le statut des intellectuels à partir des registres universitaires* (Amsterdam and Maarssen, 1981), p. 34.

16 Johan Christoph Ludeman, *Disputatio medica philosophica inauguralis de septem morborum hydropicorum generibus* (Harderwijk, 1728); *idem*, *Genees en wysgerige inwydings twist-reden over zevenderley zoorten van waterzuchtige ziektens* (Amsterdam, 1728).

17 GAA ACM inv. nr. 3, fo. 157.

18 *De doctor, zonder promotie, of de geanotomiseerde courant* (Amsterdam, 1726); Van Swaanenburg, *Hans Christoffel Ludeman*; [G. Tysens], *Doctor Hans gepromoveert tot de narrekap van Esculapius op het uilebord van Mercurius* ([Amsterdam, 1727]).

19 Dutch invective for Germans.

20 GAA ACM inv. nr. 33, fo. 139$^{v}$; inv. nr. 35.

21 W.F.H. Oldewelt, *Kohier van de personeele quotisatie te Amsterdam over het jaar 1742* (Amsterdam, 1945), vol. 2 , p. 140. Regarding annual earnings for doctors, see Willem Frijhoff, 'Non satis dignitatis . . . Over de maatschappelijke status van geneeskundigen tijdens de Republiek', *Tijdschrift voor Geschiedenis*, 96 (1983): 379–406, on p. 402.

22 GAA Archief Collaterale Successie inv. nr. 34, fos. 166–7.

23 Before 1713, in Germany, he had already published several pamphlets, though they were not devoted to medicine.

24 Johan Christoph Ludeman, *De sleutel des afgronds: Apocalypsis XX.1* ([Amsterdam], 1721).

25 A small number of his prescriptions has been saved: see UBA MS KNMG Aq 3, Ec 70, IJ 81 a, b, c, d, e; GAA Hs. F/Ludeman; *ibid.*, a prescription put in a copy of Franciscus Lievens Kersteman,

*Gedenkwaardige Levens-Beschryving van den Wereldberoemden Johan Christophorus Ludeman* (n.p., 1785). See also A.D. Schinkel, *Geschied- en Letterkundige Bijdragen* ('s-Gravenhage, 1850), pp. 113–16; A.J. Servaas van Rooijen, 'Dr. Johan Christophorus Ludeman', *De Navorscher*, 33 (1883): 145, 192; *idem*, 'Dr. J.C. Ludeman', *De Navorscher*, 35 (1885): appendix N; G.D.J. Schotel, *Vaderlandse volksboeken en volkssprookjes van de vroegste tijden tot het einde der 18e eeuw* (Haarlem 1874), vol. 1, p. 136.

26 Schotel, *Vaderlandse volksboeken*, p. 136.

27 S. Cuperus, *Kerkelijk leven der hervormden in Friesland tijdens de Republiek* (Leeuwarden, 1916), vol. 1, p. 199.

28 This section deals almost exclusively with Taylor's itinerarium and exploits in the Dutch Republic. I have not been able to consult his autobiography, which was published in 1761, or the short biography by Coats, which appeared for the first time in 1917. For details about his life in general I rely on the sections about him, his son and his grandson in Sidney Lee (ed.), *Dictionary of National Biography*, (London, 1898), vol. 55, pp. 441–2, 445–6; and in Porter, *Health for Sale*, pp. 66–80. I would like to thank Peter Paul Chaudron, Menno Heetveld, Cécile Mekes, Theo van Noord, Anje Romein, Hiska Wiersma and Bart Wijmans, students who participated during the winter term of 1992–93 in a seminar on the history of quackery. This section is partially based on their research.

29 A well-known example of this is the case of Johann Sebastian Bach who, after having been operated on by Taylor, contracted a very severe infection that spread to his brain. After a few weeks the composer died, by then stone blind: see David M. Jackson, 'Bach, Handel and the Chevalier Taylor', *Medical History*, 12 (1968): 385–93; William B. Ober, 'Bach, Handel and "Chevalier" John Taylor, M.D. ophthalmiater', *New York State Journal of Medicine*, 69 (1969): 1797–1806.

30 John Taylor, *Traité sur les maladies de l'organe immediat de la vue* (Amsterdam, 1735); *idem*, *Vertoog over de ziektens van het onmiddelyk werktuig des gezichts* (Amsterdam, 1735).

31 See Porter, *Health for Sale*, pp. 69–70.

32 GADH ACM inv. nr. 2, fos. 59–60.

33 *'s-Gravenhaegsche Courant*, 18 and 25 Aug. 1749.

34 *'s-Gravenhaegsche Courant*, 11, 13 and 25 Aug. 1749.

35 GAA AG inv. nr. 218, fos. 239–41.

36 *Amsterdamsche Courant*, 9, 11, 13, 18, 20 and 23 Sept. 1749.

37 For a copy of this flyer together with many other data about Taylor: GADH ACM inv. nr. 6: nrs. 9–18, 45–8.

38 GAU Archief nr. 3.A.1, *Supplement Stads-archief* inv. nr. 144 vol. 1, fos. 119–120$^v$, 121.

39 *'s-Gravenhaegsche Courant*, 25 Oct. 1749.

40 GAL AG inv. nr. 316, fo. 159; P.C. Molhuijsen (ed.), *Bronnen tot de geschiedenis der Leidsche universiteit* (Den Haag, 1921), vol. 5, pp. 305–07.

41 *Ibid.*, pp. 311–12.

42 GAA AG inv. nr. 218, fos. 588–604.

43 *Amsterdamsche Courant*, 2 March 1758.
44 GAA notarial archive inv. nr. 10283: nrs. 147, 173.
45 *Amsterdamsche Courant*, 13, 15, 18 and 20 March 1758.
46 GAR AG inv. nr. 24, 26 April 1758.
47 A detailed analysis of the many lists of patients that were drawn up by irregular healers in similar situations is needed to solve problems such as this one.
48 On this case, see GADH ACM inv. nr. 2, fos. 93–8, 102, 103; *ibid.* inv. nr. 6: nrs. 51, 53–4, 57; AHvH inv. nr. 5479: nr. 7; *ibid.* inv. nr. 316, 1762, 12 and 13 March, 30 June, 26 July.
49 C. Postma, 'Een geval van St. Vitusdans in 1761 te Voorburg, geconstateerd door een Delftse medicus, en wat de kwakzalvers er van maakten: bijdrage tot de geschiedenis der geneeskunde in de achttiende eeuw', *Nederlands Tijdschrift voor Geneeskunde*, 96 (1952): 3205–9, esp. p. 3208.
50 This information was supplied by Jeroen Salman, who includes views on astrology in his research on seventeenth-century Dutch almanacs.
51 Patrick Curry, *Prophecy and Power: Astrology in Early Modern England* (Cambridge, 1989), pp. 55–6, 99–100.
52 Charles Webster, *From Paracelsus to Newton: Magic and the Making of Modern Science* (Cambridge, 1982), pp. 10–11.
53 Towards the end of the seventeenth century writers of Dutch almanacs again inserted stories in which astrology featured as an important source of knowledge. However, they no longer published long lists of dates and astrological conjunctions for physicians and surgeons as they had done about half a century earlier. Once again I thank Jeroen Salman for this information.
54 From 1749 to 1757 at the University of Franeker, from 1757 to 1761 at the *Athenaeum Illustre* in Amsterdam and from 1763 to 1773 at the University of Groningen.
55 G. ten Doesschate (ed.), *Petrus Camper's Optical Dissertation on Vision 1746* (Nieuwkoop, 1962), pp. 12–13.
56 *Ibid.*, p. 11.
57 Petrus Camper, *De oculorum fabrica et morbis*; [W.P.C Zeeman (ed.)], *Opuscula selecta Neerlandicorum de arte medica* (Amsterdam, 1913), vol. 2, p. 271.
58 GAA AG inv. nr. 216, fo. 13.
59 *Ibid.*, fo. 17; ACM inv. nr. 3, fo. 293; J.J. Haver Droeze, *Het collegium medicum Amstelaedamense, 1637–1789* (Haarlem, 1921), pp. 120–3.
60 Huisman, 'Gevestigden en buitenstaanders', p. 144n.
61 GAR GAA inv. nr. 24.
62 Haver Droeze, *Het collegium medicum Amstelaedamense*, p. 130.
63 GADH ACM inv. nr. 6: nrs. 33, 34, 35.
64 In particular the archives of Den Haag and Amsterdam have much to offer in this respect. These documents are a rich basis for systematic research on the relations between patients and irregular healers in eighteenth-century Holland.

Chapter 8

# Conversions to homoeopathy in the nineteenth century

## The rationality of medical deviance

*Marijke Gijswijt-Hofstra*

The history of homoeopathy is partly a history of conversions. This is especially true of homoeopathy's early stages, from the 1820s until the end of the nineteenth century, although examples of conversions are by no means absent in the twentieth century. Conversion narratives form part and parcel of nineteenth-century homoeopathic writings and accounts reflecting back on that period, as they do in the history of sainthood or religious sects.[1] Indeed, conversion has so far been mostly associated with religion, but religion has no monopoly of conversions; medicine and science have had their conversions as well.

In fact, any profound change of conviction or way of life may be called a 'conversion', all the more so if it was named and propagated as such by the people involved. That is exactly what homoeopaths were doing when they described their transition from orthodox medicine to homoeopathy in terms of a conversion. This did not stay unobserved by their medical adversaries, who in their turn accused homoeopaths of sectarianism and of blindly following their (false) prophet Hahnemann. Obviously, religious metaphors were popular at that time, though they were used with different connotations and for different purposes.

My discussion of conversions to homoeopathy is intended to be a contribution to the analysis of the complex relations between healing and 'belief', interpreted as the trust doctors or patients have in someone or something: in this case trust in the healing powers of Hahnemann, his disciples and homoeopathic therapy. I intend to concentrate on the rationality of conversions, the propagandistic and, in the case of doctors, apologetic use of conversion narratives, and the reactions they provoked. Whether or not a particular transition from orthodox medicine to homoeopathy was called a conversion, it is clear that medical deviance was involved and, for that reason, tolerance or intolerance on the part of orthodox medicine (and vice versa). While conversions to homoeopathy are to be considered as medical deviance – at least if doctors are involved – there is another type of deviance which requires attention, namely the relative lack of homoeopathic conversions and conversion narratives in the Netherlands.

## HAHNEMANN AND HIS DISCIPLES

Samuel Hahnemann (1755–1843) of Saxony was the founder of homoeopathy. In his *Organon*, first published in 1810, he qualified his new therapeutic system as gentle, prompt, certain and lasting.[2] This was to become homoeopathy's slogan, reiterated time and again. Likewise, Hahnemann's appeal to imitate his therapy, stressing the need to do so accurately, was eagerly adopted by his followers – at least by the most faithful among them.[3]

What was special about Hahnemann's therapy? The basic principle was and is the so-called *similia similibus curentur*, meaning: like can be cured by like, or, in other words, patients can be cured by drugs that would produce the symptoms of the disease in a healthy person. In contrast, allopathy, as Hahnemann labelled orthodox medicine, generally prescribed treatment based on principles other than symptom similarity. Additionally, Hahnemann and his followers prescribed highly diluted medicines and special diets. Compared with orthodox medicine's 'heroic therapy' at that time – bloodletting, purging and strong doses of medicine – homoeopathy was rightly propagated as a gentle therapy.

In the 1820s and 1830s many European countries and the United States had their first experience of homoeopathy. The way in which this therapeutic system was introduced varied and its subsequent popularity differed even more. Homoeopathy attracted most converts in the United States, but other countries including England, France, Belgium and Italy did not lag very far behind. The Netherlands proved to be much less receptive. Hahnemann's *Organon* was translated into Dutch as early as 1827 and several Dutch physicians took the trouble of publishing on the pros and cons of homoeopathy – though more often on the cons. Still, it was not until 1886 that Dutch homoeopaths organized themselves nationally, much later than elsewhere. Even then, homoeopathy's share of the Dutch 'medical market' remained modest.

Although research on the introduction and reception of homoeopathy in various countries still has a long way to go and conversions to homoeopathy have so far received no special attention, the existing literature seldom fails to provide us with one or more conversion narratives, however poorly worked out and documented they usually prove to be.[4] By no means claiming to be exhaustive, I will first present five conversion accounts from the 1820s. Except for one, these early accounts are 'second hand' and they all relate to Hahnemann's best-known disciples. Most of these accounts follow what may be called the dramatic line: the hero's wife or perhaps his patient is critically ill and orthodox medicine is unable to bring relief. The hero happens to come across homoeopathy, generally in the form of a homoeopathic practitioner who miraculously (as it were) effects a cure. The unexpected cure makes a deep impression on our hero. He decides to find out what homoeopathy is about, starts reading Hahnemann's works, corresponds with the master and usually visits him as well. At that stage, one might say, the process of conversion is completed. What then follows is the convert's long and successful career as a homoeopathic practitioner.

The earliest conversion story I have found relates to Constantin(e) Hering (1800–80), who became America's most influential proponent of homoeopathy from the mid 1830s.[5] Like Hahnemann, Hering was born in Saxony. After attending the Surgical Academy at Dresden and privately studying mathematics and Greek, Hering began his medical studies at the University of Leipzig in 1820. There he became a pupil and assistant of the surgeon Jakob Robbi. At that time Hahnemann was lecturing at Leipzig, but his ideas had already become highly controversial, which is not surprising since he seized every opportunity to express an extremely unfavourable opinion on 'allopathy'. Robbi was asked to write a book criticizing homoeopathy, but as he was short of time he gave the job to Hering. While doing research for the book, Hering started to experiment with homoeopathy himself, then he injured one of his hands which became infected. When orthodox medicine failed to cure him and an amputation seemed to be the only alternative, Hering decided to use homoeopathic remedies. This saved his hand, but not the book, which remained unfinished as Hering from then on became an adherent of homoeopathy. Hering's conversion is somewhat atypical; instead of beginning to read about homoeopathy after the crisis and the successful homoeopathic cure, Hering did so in advance, as an antagonist. His own reading and experiments, and finally the cure, turned him from a sceptic into a believer.

While Hering was still a student at the time of his conversion, circumstances were different for his British peer, Frederick Foster Hervey Quin (1799–1879) who, in 1832, became the first established homoeopathic practitioner – and a prominent one as well – in Britain. Quin's conversion took place about five years after his graduation from the University of Edinburgh in 1820.[6] As personal physician to the Duchess of Devonshire he had accompanied her on her travels through Italy, and in 1824 he was appointed physician to Prince Leopold, the future King of the Belgians. According to Nicholls's version, it was during this period that Quin came into contact with homoeopathy. A member of the prince's household had fallen sick and after Quin had given up the patient, a homoeopath effected a cure. This made a deep impression on Quin, and from then on he started to study and practise homoeopathy himself. He also studied for nearly two years with Hahnemann. According to Goetze's version, however, Quin first learned about homoeopathy in Italy from the personal physician of an Austrian general. He then – in 1826 – went to Leipzig to study homoeopathy, but the professors whom he questioned about it put him off and ridiculed him. Soon after this, Quin developed severe pneumonia for which he received homoeopathic treatment. Again the results were excellent and Quin was all the more convinced of homoeopathy's promise. He then visited Dr J.E. Stapf (1788–1860), Hahnemann's most loyal friend, and Hahnemann himself, and made an intensive study of homoeopathic literature before establishing himself in London in 1832. Quin's conversion to homoeopathy certainly did not effect his career adversely for his services proved to be extremely popular among royalty and high society in general.

The conversion of Baron Clemens Maria Franz von Bönninghausen (1785–1864) came at a much later stage of his life, in 1827 when he was 42 years old.[7] He was not even a doctor at that time, but only became one as a consequence of his conversion to homoeopathy. Bönninghausen had been raised at his father's country estate, Herinkhave, in the Dutch province of Overijssel, and studied law at Groningen. After a brief career as a lawyer, and having filled various functions at the court of King Louis Napoleon until the end of his reign in the Netherlands in 1810, Bönninghausen retired to Herinkhave. Then in 1814 he moved to his own country estate Darup near Münster where he first became commissioner for land tax reform and in 1822 was appointed general commissioner of the land register. He was also an enthusiastic botanist.

In 1827 Bönninghausen developed severe consumption. When he had given up all hope of recovery, he wrote a farewell letter to his botanical friend, the physician Dr A. Weihe, who had taken up homoeopathy without Bönninghausen being aware of it. On Weihe's advice Bönninghausen took homoeopathic medicines and he quickly recovered. This led him to study Hahnemann's books and he soon began to practise homoeopathic medicine himself. Thereafter, Bönninghausen became Hahnemann's favourite disciple. In 1843 the Prussian King Wilhelm Friedrich IV gave him permission to practise and the Münster doctor went on to acquire a large and international clientele, including the French Empress Eugénie and many Dutch patients.[8] He also wrote a number of books on homoeopathy and furthered the homoeopathic cause in various other ways.

About a year after Bönninghausen's conversion it was the turn of the then nearly 60-year-old physician Count Sébastien des Guidi (1769–1863).[9] Des Guidi's first introduction to homoeopathy took place in Italy. Des Guidi had been born in Naples. Because of his revolutionary activities he had been banished from Naples in 1799 after which he took refuge in France. There he became first a physics teacher and later a school inspector. In 1820, at the age of 51, he acquired a doctorate in medicine after having gained one in science the year before. According to Des Guidi himself – the other conversion stories so far presented have been 'second hand' – his wife had been ill for years and every possible treatment had been tried, but none had effected a recovery. As a last resort Des Guidi had taken his wife to the baths at 'Pouzzoles', near Naples. There she developed a cerebral fever which endangered her life. Des Guidi immediately sent for the hospital doctor and had him join the doctor of the baths, for he wanted to hear the advice of them both. The hospital doctor proved to be an old friend of his, a doctor Cimone, who had recently discovered homoeopathy. He told Des Guidi that homoeopathy had been introduced to Naples by a physician from the occupying army, a doctor Necker. Cimone urgently advised Des Guidi to consult Francesco Romani, a doctor of great renown as well as being a man of literature and a philosopher (Romani had translated several of Hahnemann's books). Cimone also informed Des Guidi that the court physician, Cosmo Maria de Horatiis, had become a further adherent of homoeopathy.

Des Guidi followed his friend's advice – he had little choice anyway – and sent for Romani, who effected Madame des Guidi's recovery. Like her husband she would live to a great age. Of course, Des Guidi then wanted to study homoeopathy himself. He stayed on for two years while being initiated into this therapy by Romani and De Horatiis. In 1830 he completed his studies after having spent some time at Köthen with Hahnemann himself. In that same year he established himself in Lyon and from then on Des Guidi not only had a successful practice, but he effectively propagated homoeopathy in France, converting in turn many French physicians.

The last of these early converts I want to introduce is Georg Heinrich Gottlieb Jahr (1800–75).[10] Being much younger than Des Guidi, this German physician would also greatly further the homoeopathic cause in France, as well as in Belgium. Gottlieb Jahr must have been a young man when he was converted to homoeopathy, maybe even younger than Hering was at the time of his conversion. The story tells us that Jahr's conversion was the result of a miraculous recovery. The physician who had effected this recovery was Dr Aegidi, one of Hahnemann's disciples at Düsseldorf. Jahr then studied medicine and, supposedly, homoeopathic medicine in particular. After his studies he became a personal physician to aristocratic families whom he accompanied to French thermal resorts. When Hahnemann established himself in Paris in 1835, Jahr also moved there to become his collaborator, after having spent a year in Liège. Jahr would stay in Paris until 1870, when he had to leave because of the Franco–German War. He then returned to Belgium and set up in practice in Brussels. Like Bönninghausen and Hering, Jahr wrote many books on homoeopathy. Moreover, all the aforementioned converts did much to get homoeopathy organized and accepted. Apart for Hering, who went to the United States, all of them moved in the highest circles – the two eldest of them being a count and a baron – which certainly helped homoeopathy become fashionable.

## MODES OF CONVERSION

The conversion accounts of these early disciples of Hahnemann all follow the same form and take a dramatic line. At the time of their conversion these individuals were already medical practitioners

(Quin, Des Guidi), or a medical student (Hering), or they would later become doctors (Bönninghausen, Jahr). However this was not the only path to homoeopathy for (future) doctors. The other one was, as I will demonstrate, the route of experiment. This was brought about not by a dramatic turning point resulting from sudden crisis, but by dissatisfaction with orthodox medicine in general, or an open, eclectic attitude – sometimes combined with the advice of a relative or friend – or maybe even an express distrust towards homoeopathy. This less spectacular route of the experiment is likely to have been, and certainly was to become, the common one which led doctors to study and eventually adhere to homoeopathy.

Of course, not only (future) doctors were converted to homoeopathy.[11] There were also lay persons, not to be confused with lay healers. Apart from the dramatic line, their conversion could follow a (partially) different route, which may be called the 'happy ending' variant. Following this formula, the patient had a serious, but not necessarily acute disease. The failure of orthodox medicine to cure the patient was followed by an impressive, though not always quick recovery thanks to homoeopathic therapy. From then on the patient would remain loyal to homoeopathy. Lay persons could also turn to homoeopathy for pragmatic reasons, such as the absence of nearby orthodox medical practitioners, the cheapness of homoeopathic medicines or free homoeopathic treatment, and in due time become 'converts'. Convenience thus paved the way for conversion (or not, for lay persons could and often did shop around on the medical market without converting to homoeopathy or any other therapy).

It should be noted that the conversion of lay persons is of a different order than the conversion of doctors, even though the paths to conversion could be the same. Lay persons did not risk any form of social exclusion by converting to homoeopathy, whereas doctors often had, and still have, to pay for their 'apostasy' with professional isolation from their orthodox colleagues.

This being said, one might well ask to what extent religious and medical conversions are similar to each other, and which theoretical insights concerning religious conversions might contribute to our understanding of medical conversions. Literature on religious conversions distinguishes between various types of conversion.[12] Internal conversions, that is conversions within one and the same belief system are, for example, contrasted with external conversions, involving a transition to a different belief system. Conversion of medical practitioners to homoeopathy can be classified under this second category, though it should be noted that homoeopaths never distanced themselves from orthodox medicine in every respect or to the same degree. Likewise, for lay persons a conversion to homoeopathy could mean that they would from then on only consult homoeopathic doctors and use homoeopathic medicines, or they might opt for a more eclectic strategy.

Just as conversions to homoeopathy follow different routes and have different consequences, similar patterns can be found for religious conversions. Religious conversions can also come about suddenly and dramatically, or gradually. They can be preceded by a crisis, which may even take the form of a fatal illness. The crisis results in insight into the truth and thus the conversion comes about, and as a rule the convert joins a church or sect. In fact doctors too may join a sect, providing sect formation has already taken place. Within homoeopathy this was sometimes the case.

This brings me to the consequences, especially those connected with the scope and intensity of the conversion. In principle medical conversions only bear upon the domains of profession and science in the case of doctors and on the field of medical consumption where patients are involved. Religious conversions, on the other hand, can also affect one's life more completely, for example if one enters a convent or becomes a member of a demanding sect. The heuristic value of religious conversion models for medical conversions therefore tends to remain limited to conversion routes, or part of them, and even then one has to be careful not to abstract from the scope and intensity of the conversion.

Rambo, for example, has presented a stage model of religious conversions, consisting of macro- and microcontext, crisis, quest, the encounter between advocates and potential converts, interaction, commitment and consequences. If this stage model is applied to conversions to homoeopathy, it is striking that doctors who experience a dramatic conversion pass over the quest after the crisis, for they already know where to look for the truth. Also, the reading of homoeopathic literature could be at least as important to them as meeting advocates of homoeopathy, certainly if the route of experiment was followed. In fact, quest and encounter could very well coincide. On the other hand, for patients following the happy ending variant, Rambo's scheme is quite adequate, at least until the stage of interaction. Comparisons become problematic when we arrive at interaction and commitment, certainly when it concerns the early period of homoeopathy, or when patients are involved. For Hahnemann's early disciples there simply was no group of homoeopaths who could receive them into their midst. Nor would homoeopathic group formation and institutionalization in the period thereafter take place with equal momentum in different countries or regions.

## THE CONVERSION NARRATIVES OF DOCTORS AND LAY PEOPLE

Most conversion stories, whether of doctors or lay people (especially lay women) will remain hidden to posterity. Few have been published, and while some more can be uncovered from diaries and letters, the majority of the converted have left no traces. Most published conversion accounts are 'second hand' and they were quite frequently published for propaganda purposes. 'First hand' conversion accounts could be published for the same purpose and might also, or even primarily, be intended as an apologetic gesture towards the author's orthodox colleagues. Although dating from a much later period, it is interesting to mention the conversion stories of the *Groupement Hahnemannien de Lyon*, published in the 1960s and 1970s. The Genevan organizer of this group of professedly Kentian homoeopathic practitioners, Pierre Schmidt, urged the members to public confessions (as a reluctant member called them).[13] In fact, these public testimonies and the ensuing comments by the master had a dual function. It helped new group members strengthen their commitment and it also confirmed and reminded this sect-like group of the validity of their interpretation of homoeopathy. Most of the related conversions were of the experimental type. Conversions of the dramatic genre, including the only conversion story by a female physician which I have come across, were exceptional.

Conversion narratives of the dramatic type are mainly connected with the early stages of homoeopathy. A few more examples can be added to those outlined above, dating from the 1820s and 1830s, such as the conversions of the Germans Karl Gottlob Franz (1795–1835) and Karl Julius Aegidi (1795–1874), who were both 'saved' by Hahnemann himself, the Belgian Louis Joseph Varlez (1792–1874), who would become personal physician to the Dutch King Willem I, and the Frenchman Benoît-Jules Mure (1809–?), whose cure was effected by Sébastien des Guidi and who would introduce homoeopathy to Brazil.[14] Thereafter dramatic conversion accounts became much scarcer. Examples are the autobiographical account of the Dutch homoeopathic physician Stephanus Jacobus van Roijen (1828–1909), published in 1859, and the conversion story of the American physician James Tylor Kent (1849–1916), probably dating from the 1890s.[15]

The great majority of conversions by doctors, even in the 1820s and 1830s, seem to have been of the experimental type. An interesting, but rather unusual story, is that of Fewster Robert Horner, former president and later vice-president of the British Medical and Surgical Association, and the former senior physician to the Hull General Infirmary.[16] After his conversion to homoeopathy in 1857 he published a letter to the governors of the infirmary.[17] To summarize the story, Horner had been an opponent of homoeopathy and under his presidency an amendment had been passed stating that homoeopaths would not be accepted as members of the British Medical and Surgical Association. Thereafter Horner began to study – at first in order to expose homoeopathy as an error – and then (privately) to practise it himself. Having become convinced of homoeopathy's excellence, he wanted to treat his hospital patients using homoeopathic methods. His request to the president of the hospital for the means to do so – two nursing assistants and homoeopathic medicines – was not granted. Horner's colleagues were horrified at his desertion to homoeopathy and he was compelled to resign. His open letter is a passionate testimony of his conversion: he had gained sight after having been blind and he had become convinced of homoeopathy's great and mighty truth, which from a scientific point of view should be considered as the greatest discovery of the (nineteenth) century. Interestingly, the author did not condemn the traditional therapies completely, but he did complain about the extreme intolerance of his former colleagues.

Similar complaints were uttered by others, for example by the Dutch homoeopathic physician Johann Frederik Petrus Schönfeld (1792–1861) in the early 1830s (his story will be presented later) and by the American homoeopath and defender of slavery, William Henry Holcombe (1825–93). Being the son of an orthodox physician, Holcombe converted to what he used to regard as 'the most gigantic humbug of the day – Homoeopathy', after having successfully experimented with homoeopathic treatment during the cholera outbreak of 1849.[18] Autobiographical publications such as these are fairly scarce. 'Second hand' conversion accounts of the experimental type are much more numerous.[19]

Lay persons also had their conversion stories published occasionally, whether written by themselves or by someone else. Homoeopathic journals, especially those with a strong lay influence, contain accounts of dramatic conversions and conversions of the happy-ending variant – of which a Dutch example will be presented in the next section – as well as conversions of a more pragmatic type. An example of the latter is the story told by the widow of a Württemberg parson. She and her husband had already heard about homoeopathy when they moved to a new parsonage in 1864. Feeling anxious about having to cope without the advice of their allopathic doctor, whom they had frequently consulted both for themselves and their children, they made enquiries about homoeopathy. The parson quickly became enthusiastic and purchased his own homoeopathic medical kit and two homoeopathic domestic guides. They had both studied the books conscientiously and they were delighted that they achieved good results in their own family and also in the parish, especially among children.[20]

Another German story, which took place a few decades later, combines elements of the happy-ending variant with pragmatic considerations. A village mayor reported on his own illness and the fact his late wife had given birth to five children. Every year he had needed about 100 guilders for the doctor and for medicines, and every year he had had a dead body in his house. In the end he was without a wife or children. He had also suffered great losses in his stable, despite paying high bills for the vet and medicines. Being desperate, he had bought a homoeopathic medical kit and a book. He had remarried, and again had a wife and five children. There had been no more expenses for a doctor or medicine, no more 'dead bodies' in the house, no more losses in the stable and he had become healthier as well.[21]

Clearly, the publishers of these stories were convinced of their propagandistic value. It would be interesting to examine more systematically the use that has been made of the various types of conversion stories over the course of time and in different countries, and the effects these testimonies had.

## DUTCH CONVERSIONS TO HOMOEOPATHY

Homoeopathy's lagging popularity in the Netherlands is reflected in the scarcity of Dutch conversion accounts. Only three of these have been found.[22] The first Dutch homoeopathic practitioner who published on homoeopathy, J.F.P. Schönfeld of Winschoten in the north-eastern province of Groningen, did not develop into a leading homoeopathic figure. If this had been otherwise, and Schönfeld had been able to convert colleagues and to recruit a high-class clientele, then homoeopathy may well have become more popular in the Netherlands.[23]

Schönfeld's conversion was of the experimental type. I have come across two sources which reveal part of the story: a letter from Schönfeld to Hahnemann, dated 27 September 1832, and an introduction by Schönfeld to his translation of Hahnemann's *Geist der Homöopathischen Heil-Lehre* which was published in 1834.[24] In his letter Schönfeld explained that he had bought and read Hahnemann's books and studied them thoroughly, as far as his work allowed him. He had become convinced that Hahnemann's theory contained medicine's only true method. While reading Hahnemann's books he had pondered about how the truth could have remained hidden for such a long time and, now it had been revealed, how it could still be denied – for this was the case in Schönfeld's own country. None of his Dutch colleagues shared his conviction and he could therefore not turn to them for advice, which was the reason why he called on Hahnemann for help.

In May 1834 Schönfeld wrote in his introduction to Hahnemann's translation that he had continuously been doing research on homoeopathy for nearly two years, as well as practising homoeopathic therapy. He had become convinced of its great merits for both acute and chronic diseases. With this translation he hoped to draw his colleagues' attention to this 'wholesome and wellnigh miraculous therapy' and to exhort them to examine it themselves. These sources do not clarify why Schönfeld wanted to read Hahnemann's books in the first place, though it is unlikely that Schönfeld's conversion – he does not use the term himself – was triggered off by a critical illness and unexpected recovery thanks to homoeopathic treatment. If his conversion had followed the dramatic line, he would certainly have mentioned it.

The other two Dutch conversion accounts were published in Rotterdam in the late 1850s. They concern a doctor and a lay person. In 1857 a Society of Champions of Homoeopathy (*Vereeniging van Voorstanders der Homoeopathie*) was founded in this industrial harbour town by patients of the Münster homoeopath Clemens von Bönninghausen.[25] The society exerted itself for the homoeopathic cause by attracting three homoeopathic practitioners to Rotterdam – two Germans and the already mentioned Dutch homoeopath and doctor of medicine, S.J. van Roijen – and by establishing dispensaries where the poor could receive free homoeopathic treatment.

When Van Roijen set up in practice in Rotterdam in 1859 he deemed it wise to give a full explanation of his conversion to homoeopathy to his allopathic colleagues. This he did in a brochure entitled: 'Why I have become a homoeopath'.[26] Van Roijen's account is the one Dutch example of a doctor following the dramatic conversion line. Unlike Schönfeld, Van Roijen described his transition to homoeopathy in terms of a conversion. The story goes as follows. In October 1855 Van Roijen received a letter from a Dr Windemuth at Cassel who informed him that his brother, while stopping off there, had fallen seriously ill. Dr Windemuth deemed it necessary that a member of the family should come immediately. Van Roijen started on his journey at once and found his brother, according to the doctor's diagnosis, suffering from *phlebitis venae saphenae*. Although he had not yet studied medicine, Van Roijen was familiar with the subject because he had studied physics and had also heard much about medicine from his friends, most of whom were physicians. Moreover, he was acquainted with this particular disease, since another of his brothers had died of phlebitis some years earlier.

Dr Windemuth told Van Roijen that the danger was over, thanks to the administration of large and repeated doses of calomel and jalap (a purgative). Even so, while the phlebitis was cured the patient was not at all well. He developed a severe *neuralgia ischiadica* which forced him to keep his leg still. Van Roijen had to return home to look after his affairs and another brother came to stay with the patient. When things got worse and the patient developed a gangrenous spot, Dr Windemuth decided to have him moved to the hospital of Dr Bonhoff at Münden, situated on a mountain. Very soon Dr Bonhoff was able to effect a cure by treating the patient homoeopathically and when Van Roijen returned a few days later, Dr Bonhoff explained homoeopathy to him. Until then, Van Roijen confessed, he had only heard of homoeopathy being ridiculed and he had shared in this negative assessment. However, after his brother's recovery, his own medical degree at Leiden and studies of homoeopathy at Leipzig, Van Roijen had become quite convinced that 'homoeopathy is truth'.

Van Roijen would contribute much to the homoeopathic cause. He not only published on homoeopathy, but in 1898 he also took the initiative of founding the Society of Homoeopathic Physicians in the Netherlands (*Vereeniging van Homoeopathische Geneesheeren in Nederland*).

The third Dutch conversion account is by the Rotterdam baker Samuel Willem van der Velde (1816–80). It is the earliest – and the only Dutch – conversion story by a lay person that I have come across, and an example of the happy-ending variant. The account has been included in a Rotterdam series of contributions on homoeopathy, which were edited by the three Rotterdam homoeopathic practitioners and published between 1859 and 1861.[27] An interesting detail is that the editorial introduction to this series ends with a call to all adherents to homoeopathy to make the history of their conversion known. Such communications frequently have the greatest impact, said the editors, and everyone who is acquainted with homoeopathy from experience knows how to value homoeopathy as one of the greatest blessings of humankind.

Samuel van der Velde had his conversion story – again he did not use this term himself – published anonymously, though he told the reader that he was prepared to disclose his identity to anyone who had an interest in the matter, and to give them further information if requested. Elsewhere I have explained how I identified the anonymous author as Van der Velde, a fairly well-to-do baker who, in 1843, became Bönninghausen's first Rotterdam patient and who, in 1857, became secretary of the committee of the newly founded Rotterdam Society of Champions of Homoeopathy.[28]

Since the spring of 1840 Van der Velde had been suffering from a bad cough and had also started coughing up blood. Bloodletting, footbathing, internal medicines and complete rest had been recommended, and he had followed all this advice. There had been a temporary improvement, but by spring 1841 his condition had deteriorated. In the summer of 1842 and thereafter, Van de Velde suffered from shortness of breath and palpitations, and none of the prescribed medicines had helped. While in this deplorable condition he had, in January 1843, become related via the marriage of a family member, to J.G. Lee, a country doctor at Overschie near

Rotterdam. When Lee heard about the author's disease, he advised him to consult Bönninghausen at Münster. Lee told Van der Velde that he had been practising homoeopathy himself for some time, and that he had witnessed 'miraculous' healing in other countries, especially in Germany – even of consumptive patients. Van der Velde then consulted his own doctor, but this doctor had ridiculed the small doses prescribed by homoeopaths. Lee advised Van der Velde to read a few of Hahnemann's books and judge for himself, and this resulted in Van der Velde's decision to consult Bönninghausen. Before travelling to Münster he corresponded with Bönninghausen. The consultation and the advice to try a certain medicine had inspired confidence. He went on consulting Bönninghausen by letter and slowly but surely the cure made progress, until after four years his recovery was complete. Needless to say our baker's conversion was complete as well, and he was immensely thankful for having become acquainted with homoeopathy and having been treated by Bönninghausen.

Van der Velde also gave the reason why he published his story. This was partly because he felt obliged to homoeopathy and its practitioners, but mostly to highlight the benefits of the therapy to his fellow Dutch sufferers for whom homoeopathy had, until recently, only been known by name, though it had been successfully practised in other countries for many years. Van der Velde pointed out that since many sick people who had been given up by ordinary Dutch physicians had been completely cured by homoeopathic treatment, it was important that anyone who had been cured in this way should give a truthful account of his experience to his fellow countrymen.

In the meantime the popularity of homoeopathic treatment had been increasing in the Netherlands, albeit on a modest scale. Although the demand for homoeopathy had increased further in the 1880s and 1890s, relatively few practitioners had converted to it. The modest increase in the number of homoeopathic practitioners – from four in 1887 (one year after the founding of the Society for the Advancement of Homoeopathy in the Netherlands) to 14 in 1900 – was partly self generated (the son following in his father's footsteps) and financially supported by the society. Like S.J. van Roijen, these homoeopaths had taken a medical degree at a Dutch university, thereafter studying homoeopathy abroad in Leipzig, Prague or, from the 1870s onwards, Budapest. There was no chair of homoeopathy at a Dutch university – nor would there be one until the early

1960s – and the first Dutch homoeopathic hospital was opened only in 1914. The absence of homoeopathic training in the Netherlands and the predominantly scientific orientation of the Dutch medical faculties hardly formed a stimulating climate for medical students to opt for homoeopathy as it would force them to become medical outsiders. Although the Medical Act of 1865 raised no barrier to homoeopathy, it did make homoeopathic practice more difficult because medicines could no longer be freely distributed. A way out of this problem was to persuade pharmacists to sell homoeopathic medicines prepared by the Leipzig pharmacist Wilmar Schwabe.

This was the situation towards the end of the nineteenth century. One of the means to promote homoeopathy was of course through propaganda. The Rotterdam Society of Champions of Homoeopathy had set an example, but there was no sequel to the Rotterdam series of contributions on homoeopathy which had stimulated readers to present their conversion stories. The publication of Dutch or foreign conversion accounts, whether by doctors or laymen – women never featured as the converted star during this period – never contributed significantly to the propaganda of the Dutch Society for the Advancement of Homoeopathy. Its policy was rather to inform the public – primarily their members, but presumably also a wider lay and professional public – in a more general, less personal way about homoeopathy; to present statistics on the superior results of homoeopathy and to counter unjustified attacks by 'allopaths'. Great pains were taken to point out the 'scientific' status of homoeopathy, as 'scientific' was the magic word for allopaths and homoeopaths alike.

Some attempts at conciliation were in fact made. One homoeopathic practitioner went so far as to claim that homoeopathy was part of general medicine and he even admitted that scientific proof of the truth of the *similia* principle was still lacking.[29] Compromise, not conflict, was what most Dutch homoeopaths were after and it is thus hardly surprising that conversion accounts did not figure prominently in the *Homoeopathisch maandblad*. It is also likely that the intolerance of orthodox practitioners contributed to homoeopathic reticence.

## MEDICAL DEVIANCE AND INTOLERANCE: 'ALLOPATHIC' REACTIONS TO HOMOEOPATHIC CONVERSIONS

Conversions to homoeopathy did not go unnoticed, especially if they concerned colleague physicians. Both early and later conversions to Hahnemann's truth provoked negative reactions from orthodox practitioners. Everywhere converts to homoeopathy met with incomprehension, scorn, ridicule or even ostracism. Hering and Quin were ridiculed by the Leipzig professors of medicine and Horner was even compelled to resign.

The Dutch converts were hardly better off.[30] Hahnemann's early Dutch disciple, J.F.P. Schönfeld, had to endure heavy criticism that was published by three of his Groningen colleagues. One of them, B. Eekma, even tried to persuade his friend Schönfeld to give up homoeopathy and come back to the 'old school', for, as he wrote: 'Today you are still being worshipped because of some so-called miracle cures, but tomorrow you may well be misunderstood, cursed and placed on the same level as the quacks of former and later times.'[31]

Less personal attacks were also launched at that time in the Netherlands. Homoeopathy's fiercest opponents scornfully called Hahnemann 'the prophet', and designated his followers a sect of credulous people who much too easily believed in the miraculous. Some denounced them as quacks. However, there were also moderate critics who offered a less biased opinion. Although they remained true to orthodox medicine, they were inclined to pass a favourable judgment on the less essential aspects of homoeopathy, like the homoeopathic diet and the highly diluted medicines, which they considered to be less harmful than some of orthodox medicine's prescriptions. They argued that, in this way, the healing power of nature could do its work.

Both fierce and moderate arguments were taken up again, especially in the 1880s and 1890s. Whereas in the 1850s S.J. van Roijen had apparently endured few severe attacks from his colleagues for having converted to homoeopathy, his son J.I.A.B. van Roijen was treated most unpleasantly in 1896 by his orthodox Rotterdam colleagues, though this seems to have been the only serious personal attack in those years. Most criticism was directed at homoeopathy as such, and at homoeopaths for claiming a monopoly of the truth. This caused irritation, for the critics were often no less convinced of their own rightness, supported by scientific truth. They considered homoeopathy to be a scientific error.

Of course, this did not make it easy for medical students or practitioners to choose homoeopathy. They risked criticism and marginalization. In a small country like the Netherlands, with only a few homoeopathic practitioners to give moral and practical support, conversion to homoeopathy was indeed a serious matter. Those converted to homoeopathy pursued two seemingly incompatible aims: propagating homoeopathy as such and, at the same time, conciliating 'allopathy' by keeping a relatively low profile. The publication of conversion accounts hardly contributed to the second aim but, if published, the 'ordinary' type of conversion with its scientific pretensions was clearly considered to be more suitable than the dramatic type. Nor were patients' conversion accounts of the happy-ending type extensively published.

## HEALING, 'BELIEF' AND THE RATIONALITY OF CONVERSIONS TO HOMOEOPATHY

Doctors and patients alike expressed their belief in homoeopathy. Hahnemann himself had set the tone, for he called all allopaths unbelievers.[32] Hahnemann's disciples imitated his choice of words. In his introduction to the Dutch translation of Hahnemann's *Organon*, the anonymous translator even compared the master's doctrine with the only true religion, for both had spread more and more, notwithstanding the most terrible persecutions. Hahnemann and his disciples all 'believed' in homoeopathy's truth and miraculous effects, though dissension would soon arise among them about what exactly this truth consisted of. Some of them remained truly faithful to Hahnemann, others more or less went their own way. However, none of them questioned the *similia* principle. One had to believe in this basic principle, or one could no longer belong to homoeopathy's following. Indeed, as Kallenbach admitted in 1888, one *could only* believe for, as already mentioned, he stated that the scientific proof of this principle was still lacking.

Orthodox physicians – the unbelievers according to Hahnemann and his disciples – in their turn expressed their scepticism and in doing this they used comparable metaphors, though with different connotations. Homoeopathy's so-called miraculous effects were ridiculed by them and ascribed to the credulity of its believers. Hahnemann was labelled a false prophet, while his followers were called a sect. Interestingly, from the 1850s onwards both sides in the Netherlands became increasingly fascinated by what they called science and scientific. It could be said that they believed in science and worshipped the scientific. Whatever they meant by scientific, it may be concluded from the Dutch debate on homoeopathy during the 1880s and 1890s that the god of science revealed different truths to allopathic and homoeopathic believers.

It is within this verbal and mental context that conversions to homoeopathy should be understood, but there was more to it. Because of orthodox medicine's shortcomings both physicians and patients could be driven to try a different type of therapy. This could lead to their conversion, no matter which route was followed. The dramatic line figures prominently in the conversion accounts of Hahnemann's early disciples, while some of them were seriously ill themselves at the critical moment. Of course, the dramatic route could also be followed by lay persons, but their conversion accounts had much less chance of being published. This appears anyhow to have been the case from the middle of the nineteenth century onwards; dramatic conversion accounts might well have become less effective at a time when the miraculous had to give way to the scientific. The path of the experiment was followed by doctors. This route became the dominant one in the later conversion accounts and many fewer accounts seem to have been published of happy-ending conversions, perhaps because these were primarily experienced by patients.

Whether conversion accounts were published or not, all conversions to homoeopathy marked the line between life and death or, less dramatically, between health and illness – for homoeopathy had succeeded where allopathy had failed. From this point of view conversion to homoeopathy was a rational move, for doctors and patients alike; people had become convinced that Hahnemann's therapy was the only reliable way to salvation. For doctors, however, there was the other side of the coin – their marginalization in the medical world. With regard to their medical career and prestige a conversion to homoeopathy could hardly be called a rational step. This was the dilemma doctors and medical students were confronted with. Medical deviance had its price and only a few Dutch doctors were prepared to pay it.

## ACKNOWLEDGEMENT

With thanks to Eberhard Wolff for his assistance.

## NOTES

1 See on saints Donald Weinstein and Rudolph Bell, *Saints and Society. The Two Worlds of Western Christendom, 1000–1700* (Chicago, IL, and London, 1982). See on conversion in general Lewis R. Rambo, 'Conversion', in Mircea Eliade (ed.), *The Encyclopedia of Religion* (New York and London, 1987), vol. IV, pp. 73–9 and the literature there mentioned.

2 In German *sanft, schnell, gewiss und dauerhaft*. Samuel Hahnemann, *Organon der rationellen Heilkunde nach homöopathischen Gesetzen* (Dresden, 1810). The later editions, published after 1819, were called *Organon der Heilkunst*.

3 In German *Macht's nach, aber macht's genau nach*.

4 Compilations of biographical data of homoeopaths can be found in Thomas Lindsey Bradford, *The Pioneers of Homoeopathy* (Philadelphia, 1897); Rudolf Tischner, *Geschichte der Homöopathie*, vol. III, *Ausbreitung der Homöopathie (bis 1850)* (Leipzig, 1937) and vol. IV, *Die Homöopathie seit 1850* (Leipzig, 1939); William Harvey King, *History of Homoeopathy and its Institutions in America* (New York and Chicago, IL, 1905).

5 See Bradford, *The Pioneers of Homoeopathy*, pp. 344–9; Tischner, *Geschichte der Homöopathie*, vol. IV, p. 783; Anthony Campbell, *The Two Faces of Homoeopathy* (London, 1984), p. 84; and esp. Reinhart Schnüppel, 'Constantin(e) Hering's influence on (American) homoeopathy and medical education', unpub. paper, conference *Culture, Knowledge and Healing: Historical Perspectives of Homeopathic Medicine in Europe and North America*, 5–7 April 1994 at the University of California, San Francisco.

6 See Bradford, *The Pioneers of Homoeopathy*, pp. 532–48; Phillip A. Nicholls, *Homoeopathy and the Medical Profession* (London, 1988), p. 108; O.E.A. Goetze, 'Geschiedenis van de homeopathie', in H.G. Bodde, O.E.A. Goetze and E.S.M. de Lange-de Klerk (eds), *Leerboek homeopathie* (Utrecht, 1988), pp. 3–28, esp. pp. 19–20.

7 See Bradford, *The Pioneers of Homoeopathy*, pp. 167–91; Tischner, *Geschichte der Homöopathie*, vol. IV, p. 499; *ibid.*, vol. III, p. 499; Friedrich Kottwitz, *Bönninghausens Leben. Hahnemanns Lieblingsschüler* (Berg am Starnberger See, 1985).

8 See Marijke Gijswijt-Hofstra, 'Homeopathy's early Dutch conquests: the Rotterdam clientele of Clemens von Bönninghausen in the 1840s and 1850s', *Journal of the History of Medicine and Allied Sciences*, 51: 2 (1996): 155–83.

9 See Sébastien des Guidi, *Lettre aux médecins français sur l'homéopathie* (Lyon, 1988), pp. 22–4; Bradford, *The Pioneers of Homoeopathy*, pp. 331–5; Marc Haffen, *Structures de l'homéopathie en France*

*(1919–1982)* (Paris, 1982), p. 21; Maurice Garden, 'L'Histoire de l'homéopathie en France, 1830–1940', in Olivier Faure (ed.), *Praticiens, patients et militants de l'homéopathie aux XIXe et XXe siècles (1800–1940)* (Lyon, 1992), pp. 59–82, esp. pp. 63–5; Olivier Faure, 'The introduction of homeopathy into France in the nineteenth century (1830–1870)', unpub. paper, conference *Culture, Knowledge and Healing*.

10 See Bradford, *The Pioneers of Homoeopathy*, pp. 366–86; Tischner, *Geschichte der Homöopathie*, vol. III, pp. 499–500; Garden, 'L'Histoire de l'homéopathie en France', pp. 65–6; Faure, 'The introduction of homeopathy into France'.

11 Because it is difficult to come by conversion accounts of other types of homoeopathic healers (those without a university degree), I have decided not to discuss them here.

12 Rambo, 'Conversion'.

13 *Cahiers Groupement Hahnemannien de Lyon: Compte rendue des reunions animées par le docteur Pierre Schmidt de Genève*. Over 20 conversion accounts have been included in the undated series 2, 3, 6, 8 and 9, and in the series 10 to 12 (1973–5), and 15 to 17 (1978–80). Like the American homoeopathic physician and Swedenborgian James Tylor Kent (1849–1916) the *Groupement Hahnemannien* were inclined towards the occult. Schmidt, for example, made much of astrology.

14 See Tischner, *Geschichte der Homöopathie*, vol. IV, pp. 769–70 (Aegidi); Bradford, *The Pioneers of Homoeopathy*, pp. 14–20 (Franz), 638–9 (Varlez), 493–501 (Mure).

15 S.J. van Roijen's conversion will be discussed in the next section of this chapter. On Kent, see Anthony Campbell, *The Two Faces of Homoeopathy* (London, 1984), p. 96.

16 Horner's dates of birth and death are unknown to me.

17 Fewster Robert Horner, *Homoeopathy: Reasons for Adopting the Rational System of Medicine* (London, 1857).

18 William H. Holcombe, *How I Became a Homoeopath* (Philadelphia, PA, 1866), pp. 7, 12.

19 Homoeopathic journals and biographical compilations (see n. 4) contain many of these stories.

20 See Eberhard Wolff, ' "Eine gesunde Concurrenz sei für das Publicum stets von Vortheil": Der homöopathische Arzneimittelmarkt als Kräftemessen zwischen Apotheken und Laienvereinen', unpub. paper, conference *"Bilanz der Forschung": Homöopathiegeschichte 200 Jahre nach Entdeckung des Simileprinzips*, 3–4 April 1995, Institut für Geschichte der Medizin der Robert Bosch Stiftung, Stuttgart.

21 Eberhard Wolff, ' " . . . nichts weiter als eben einen unmittelbaren persönlichen Nutzen . . . " – Zur Entstehung und Ausbreitung der homöopathischen Laienbewegung', *Jahrbuch des Instituts für Geschichte der Medizin*, 1 (1987): pp. 61–97, esp. p. 72.

22 My material consists of Dutch books and brochures on homoeopathy – both from adherents and adversaries – and the *Homoeopathisch maandblad*, the monthly journal of the Society for the Advancement of Homoeopathy in the Netherlands (*Vereeniging tot Bevordering van*

*de Homoeopathie in Nederland*), which was published from 1890 onwards.

23 See on this topic Marijke Gijswijt-Hofstra, 'Compromise, not conflict. The introduction of homoeopathy into the Netherlands in the nineteenth century', *Tractrix*, 5 (1993): 121–38.

24 The letter is kept in the Homöopathie-Archiv, A 367, Institut für Geschichte der Medizin der Robert Bosch Stiftung, Stuttgart. The translated book is: Samuel Hahnemann, *Geest der homöopathische geneesleer* (Winschoten, 1834).

25 See Gijswijt-Hofstra, 'Compromise, not conflict', and *idem*, 'Homeopathy's early Dutch conquests'.

26 S.J. van Roijen, *Waarom ben ik homoiopaath geworden* (Rotterdam, 1859).

27 'Mededeeling van een niet-geneeskundige', in A.J. Gruber, F.W.O. Kallenbach and S.J. van Roijen (eds), *De homoiopathische geneeswijze* (Rotterdam, 1859–61), pp. 7–8.

28 See Gijswijt-Hofstra, 'Homeopathy's early Dutch conquests'.

29 F.W.O. Kallenbach, *De aanval afgeslagen: Antwoord op de door H.H. Prins Wielandt en Dr. B.J. Stokvis tegen de homoeopathie gerichte brochures* ('s-Gravenhage, 1888).

30 See Gijswijt-Hofstra, 'Compromise, not conflict'.

31 B. Eekma, *De rationeel-empirische geneeswijze in de geneeskunst verdedigd tegen Dr. J.F.P. Schönfeld en De geest der homöopathische geneesleer van Dr. S. Hahnemann, getoetst naar rede en ervaring* (Groningen, 1836), p. 14.

32 See a letter from Hahnemann to Clemens von Bönninghausen (c.1840), quoted in Kottwitz, *Bönninghausens Leben*, pp. 99–100.

Chapter 9

# Abortion for sale!

## The competition between quacks and doctors in Weimar Germany

*Cornelie Usborne*

> Don't be stupid, woman! Don't go, woman, where you will be given potassium cyanide or syringed with carbolic soap or infected by dirty instruments and you will be sure to die in the convulsions of puerperal fever, don't go there, I warn you!

With these words a doctor pleads with a young woman not to seek a back-street abortion when he cannot help her. The scene is taken from Friedrich Wolf's play *Cyankali* (*Potassium Cyanide*) which caused a sensation when it was premiered in 1929 in Berlin and on its subsequent tour through Germany.[1] The central character is the working-class Hete. Finding herself pregnant by her boyfriend who has just lost his job during the Depression, she seeks an abortion. Although her boyfriend agrees, she does so alone. Hete's journey of pain and humiliation takes her from the cynical doctor and a pathetic attempt at self-help into the clutches of Madame Heye, a so-called wise woman (*weise Frau*). Just as the doctor had predicted, Madame Heye poisons Hete with potassium cyanide and she dies in agony in her mother's arms.

Wolf, a member of the German Communist Party, gave his play a clear political message: because the abortion law discriminated against the lower classes it should be abolished, or at least radically changed. Women should have the right (on any grounds) to an 'expert' termination of their pregnancy by a qualified doctor. Like many on the Left he argued that, after 1927, when doctors were permitted to terminate pregnancies but only on narrowly defined grounds that were often difficult to justify after the event, they normally assisted only the rich who made the risk worthwhile. The poor, it was said, were driven to approach unskilled operators, with terrible consequences. The play's impact was heightened by Wolf's own passionate involvement. As a socialist he had actively campaigned for abortion law reform, and he was also a doctor who regularly referred women for termination of pregnancy to a female colleague who shared his pro-abortion stance. In hindsight the play is particularly poignant since, in 1931, Wolf himself became a victim of the law. He was arrested (though later released) on suspicion of abetting abortions on social grounds, an offence carrying a maximum penalty of five years imprisonment.[2]

## 'QUACK ABORTIONISTS' IN THE MEDICAL DISCOURSE

*Cyankali* was a literary attack on the abortion clause, paragraph 218 of the penal code, though because she exploits the unjust law, Wolf made Madame Heye the real villain. She was one of those back-street practitioners who were accused at the time of having driven every year 'hundreds of thousands of poor women into their dirty dives'.[3] Wolf portrayed her as greedy, dirty, ignorant and dangerous. He leant heavily on the stereotypical image created in newspapers, medical journals, legal tracts and other agit-prop plays and fiction.[4] Whether male (more rarely) or female, this was always negative. A back-street abortionist was seen as posing a double threat to society, first by exploiting the least privileged and even inciting them to abortion, and second by endangering women's lives and health. Such abortionists were accused of taking from a poor woman her foetus, her money and often her life.

This public notion of the dangerous and greedy amateur was vitally influenced by the medical discourse. Although the profession was notoriously divided on the subject of abortion reform,[5] it was united in its strong disapproval of 'quack abortions' (*Pfuscherabtreibungen*). It is true that doctors did denounce colleagues who brought the profession into disrepute by 'abortion-mongering', but it was really the 'unskilled operators' they wanted to eradicate. They alleged that 'quacks' (*Kurpfuscher*) had little, if any, knowledge of gynaecology or hygiene and were only interested in profit. Conservative doctors warned that all abortions were potentially life threatening, but none more so than those performed by unqualified practitioners. Left-leaning doctors generally believed that abortion in the hands of an experienced doctor was not risky and they campaigned for the legalization of abortion by registered doctors, ostensibly in order to save the lives of 'thousands of young persons especially proletarian women' since 'only quacks will destroy foetal life and that of mothers, too!'[6] Socialist doctors usually underplayed the risk of a medical termination and exaggerated that of 'quack abortions'.[7] For example, a well-known communist physician cited '20,000 deaths in Germany annually as a result of self-help abortions and quack interventions and a further 100,000 cases of morbidity'.[8] 'Quack abortions' were also held responsible for the embarrassingly high level of maternal mortality. This served to obscure the uncomfortable fact that obstetrics itself was in urgent need of improvement and before the advent of sulphonamides in the mid-1930s, childbirth – especially when medical intervention took place – was never risk free.[9]

Socialist abortion law reformers were also strongly influenced by Soviet laws which permitted abortion so long as it was performed by qualified and experienced doctors. Although the early petitions to decriminalize abortion tabled by members of the German Communist Party (KPD) and Social Democratic Party (SPD) did not seek to restrict the right to perform the operation to registered doctors, this proviso was introduced in all parliamentary motions after 1925, almost certainly because of pressure from socialist physicians, some of whom had become members of parliament.[10]

## THE ODIUM OF COMMERCIAL ABORTIONS

The widespread public concern about 'back-street abortionists', felt right across the political spectrum from the moral Right to the reforming groups on the Left, has to be seen in the context of the general preoccupation with the rapidly declining birthrate and its effect on national reconstruction after the heavy losses of life in the First World War. Anxieties were fuelled by the scale of the estimated annual abortion figures, which ranged from 250,000 in the early 1920s to one million in the last years of the Weimar Republic, when they exceeded the birthrate. Abortion estimates were notoriously unreliable and differed widely but to contemporaries they conveyed a powerful message, that Germany was swept by a veritable abortion epidemic and that this was worse than elsewhere.[11]

In the early 1920s there was an important shift in the moral perception of abortion. While in Imperial Germany the alleged demographic crisis was blamed on the aborting woman, in the new Republic the blame shifted to the abortionist. In the Wilhelmine authoritarian climate women who had rid themselves of unwanted pregnancies had been accused of immorality, selfishness and neglecting their primary duty as mothers. But the political dislocation and economic hardship after the First World War meant that abortion on socio–economic grounds was condoned by more and more people as a necessary, if desperate, measure. This shift in moral judgement coincided or was possibly reinforced by a perceived trend away from self-help to abortions procured by a third party, a friend, a neighbour, a wise woman, midwife, quack (*Kurpfuscher*) or doctor.[12] These accomplices became the new target for public condemnation as they seemed to be on the increase and exploiting women's predicament in a ready market.

The financial aspect of abortion was of great importance since the German abortion clause had identified those who performed the operation for 'financial gain', that is the commercial abortionists (*Lohnabtreiber*), as a separate category. The penal code of 1871 distinguished between a 'simple abortion' performed by the pregnant woman herself (with or without the aid of an accomplice) and a 'commercial abortion' (*gewerbsmäßige Abtreibung*) performed by an accomplice for money – a distinction unknown in most other European countries.[13] Simple abortion carried a maximum penalty of five years, commercial abortion up to ten years penal servitude. In 1926 the gap widened. Penal servitude was now abolished for the aborting woman and her accomplice. Although the aborting woman continued to face trial – which was unusual in most other European countries[14] – in extenuating circumstances the penalty for the woman and her accomplice who helped without payment could be commuted to a small fine, which was often suspended. This made it the most lenient law in Western Europe. In contrast, the maximum penalty for the commercial abortionist was substantially increased to 15 years penal servitude and came to be on a par with that for the abortionist who had caused death.

This meant that the commercial operator had replaced the aborting woman as scapegoat for what was widely referred to as Germany's 'abortion scourge'. Although theoretically this category included doctors who induced miscarriages for ready money (and there were many of these), medical and public disapproval was directed against wise women and the male quack. Medical circles regularly published damning evidence of their activities and sensational trials were widely reported, revealing the extent of back-street practices and their apparently damaging effect on young women's lives.

Sentencing practice reinforced the tendency to demonize

amateurs and condone renegade doctors who had performed abortions as a trade. Penal servitude was usually reserved for non-doctors. Doctors were generally spared this degrading sentence (which stripped the convict of all civic rights and prevented them practising as healers), even in cases where they had caused the death of their patient. It demonstrated that the definition of 'commercial abortion' was generally reserved for laymen and women.

There were many other reasons why doctors fared better in trials than their lay counterparts. For example, they benefited from the use of medical experts in court, who did not find it easy to expose a colleague in the dock.[15] Doctors also seemed able to impress the jury and judge with their scientific and professional standing, which blinded the courts to some doctors' unprofessional and unskilled behaviour on a number of occasions. The principle of professional ethos, the belief that those who practised medicine as state-registered physicians were guided by humanitarian and not commercial principles, gave doctors an immeasurable advantage over non-doctors who were, after all, in the business to earn their living openly by their healing trade. Thus doctors never tired of stressing the crucial distinction between their 'professional' conduct of 'saving and prolonging life' according to the Hippocratic oath and that of the 'commercialism' of back-street operators, whom they accused of touting for criminal business and charging poor women over the odds for bungled operations. Doctors were able to obscure the fact that they did charge for terminations either directly from their patients or indirectly when they claimed the costs from health insurance funds for fictitious treatments, since these funds only paid for terminations on narrowly defined medical grounds, and only if a second doctor had endorsed the decision. Finally, doctors' misdemeanours were less open to public scrutiny since they were often tried before a medical tribunal quite independently of the state judicial system – a crucial privilege attached to doctors' professional status[16] – and the abortions of their patients, usually of a relatively high social status, were less detectable than those of poorer sections of the community.

Given all these factors, it is not surprising that contemporary social commentators tended to regard doctors' abortion practice leniently, but looked upon that of non-doctors with at best suspicion, and at worst detestation. It is, however, more surprising that historians should share this attitude either explicitly or implicitly.[17] There is abundant evidence that the picture was less clear cut.

Judicial sources suggest that it is quite wrong to draw the dividing line between qualified doctors and unqualified practitioners when distinguishing the skilled from the incompetent, the professional from the unprofessional and the humanitarian from the commercially motivated.[18] Abortion practice attracted a vast array of lay operators – from the experienced nature therapist to the unscrupulous adventurer, out to make money by any means available – yet the group of doctors involved in terminating unwanted pregnancies was just as heterogeneous as far as skill, professional, ideological and commercial attitudes were concerned.

## THE ADVANTAGES OF 'QUACK ABORTIONISTS'

It is clear that the stereotypical negative picture of the back-street abortionist needs revising. Contrary to the official image, court files show that a large proportion of lay abortionists were genuinely concerned to help and were perceived as being helpful by their patients. A sizeable proportion were skilled and interested in healing. Since they included many midwives or former midwives, they could have a strong interest in women's reproductive health. Abortions by midwives were commonly referred to as quack abortions, despite the fact that midwives were both qualified and registered. This was because midwives were barred from inducing artificial miscarriages, even from examining pregnant women internally: if they performed an abortion, they were therefore accused of 'quackery', defined in this case as illegitimate medical practice. Midwives struck off the register following a conviction for criminal abortion who continued to deliver children were also considered quacks, whether they performed abortions or not. But since disgraced midwives were deprived of their livelihood, they often had no other option than to become abortionists in order to survive.[19] In reality they might have played an even larger role since it is not always clear whether a defendant who proved to be surprisingly knowledgeable in gynaecology was, in fact, a trained but deregistered midwife.[20]

Even among genuine lay practitioners a surprising number were found to have been involved in other forms of healing, be it as nature therapists, fortune tellers or simply pharmaceutical salesmen.[21] Although there is no specific reference to this in legal files, it is quite possible that women consulted some of them not just for fertility control, but also for problems of infertility.

Certainly fortune tellers who were also active as abortionists often started their consultations by telling their clients that they were pregnant.[22]

According to criminal files and experienced doctors' opinion, lay abortionists were popular with women and more popular than doctors. For example, in the cases tried by the *Landgericht* Mönchen-Gladbach as many as 80 per cent of all illegal abortions which came to trial had been procured by 'commercial abortionists', the great majority by non-doctors. Levy-Lenz who ran the sex and birth control clinic of Magnus Hirschfeld's Institute of Sexual Science (*Institut für Sexualwissenschaften*) claimed that in Berlin in 1928 at least half of all abortions were procured by lay practitioners, 30 per cent by women themselves and only about 20 per cent by doctors.[23] Gender was an obvious reason for the popularity of lay abortionists: many of them were female whereas there seem to have been very few women doctors prepared to risk their reputation by performing illegal operations. Moreover, many female abortionists were married and had children which might well have instilled trust in their patients.[24]

The popularity of lay men and women abortionists also suggests that they had a good safety record. Max Hirsch, a Berlin gynaecologist and a government adviser, asserted to the Prussian Medical Council that the majority of lay abortionists acted safely. He believed the majority of cases never came to light precisely because nothing went wrong.[25] Indeed, cases which were detected because of a death or serious injury then revealed a large number of unproblematic abortions.[26] Hirsch's opinion is validated by the legal records, as we will see below. Not only midwives, but also many wise women and quacks, had a good 'safety' record. A surprising number of non-doctors carried out their abortion practice systematically and responsibly in a way which was usually only associated with doctors: they kept records, proceeded methodically, used antisepsis and asepsis (by sterilizing their hands or their instruments and applying antiseptic creams or liquids) and displayed considerable gynaecological skill.

One of the most famous abortion trials during the Weimar Republic concerned the Berlin pharmacist Heiser in 1924. It revealed not only an abortion practice far larger than previously thought possible, but also surgical standards which put many a clinician to shame. Although he was convicted for having performed three hundred abortions, Heiser had confessed to 11,000 and these had been 100 per cent successful, leading to terminations of pregnancy with not a single case of injury or death. Like a conscientious physician, Heiser had kept detailed records of all his operations using his own revolutionary new method – a herbal paste whose composition he kept secret but which stimulated the uterus into contractions, eventually expelling the foetus. This was both safe and comfortable for patients. It was in fact the only really significant new development in abortion technology during the inter-war period and it was adopted, even before it was patented, by most leading gynaecologists in Germany and abroad.[27]

Another good example of impressive skill and care is that of Frau Johanna A. of Hindenburg, Silesia in 1930. A chance discovery of a buried foetus led to criminal investigations. These revealed that Frau A., a 36-year-old miner's wife, a socialist free-thinker and ardent campaigner for women's reproductive rights, had helped no less than 150 women. She had kept records fully and conscientiously. There was not a single case of complication or injury and the few testimonies from her clients which have been located express gratitude and praise. Like Heiser she behaved with extraordinary care and also displayed great scientific interest, procuring medical instruments, providing aseptic conditions and even preserving a foetus as a specimen in spirit on her desk.[28]

A third example is the carpenter and his wife from a village near Limburg in Hesse. Frau K., was tried for 50 abortions induced on her own and another seven with the help of her husband. In this case there is also no evidence of mishap or death. Frau K. performed each operation in the same way: she carefully inserted a speculum which she had previously boiled, then she injected alum into the cervix with the help of a syringe. She always wore rubber gloves which she had previously boiled. At the trial the patients, who came from the immediate vicinity, expressed great satisfaction with the assistance they had received.[29]

There are many more examples of non-doctors displaying conscientiousness and skill, though naturally there are also cases where lay abortionists caused injuries and deaths. It was clear that the area of abortion practice was pressing and lucrative enough to attract a multitude of practitioners with a wide range of expertise or lack of it. But compared to the accounts of doctors' blunders revealed in judicial files and medico–legal tracts, the impression remains that lay operators were by no means a worse alternative to doctors.[30] Medical blunders were especially disturbing because they reveal a worrying degree of abuse of patients' trust and reckless disregard for the patients' welfare, particularly when little was done to save women injured or infected by the operation.

What is most shocking, is that some serious cases of medical negligence went unpunished. Take the case of the 30-year-old Berlin physician Dr Kurt M., who in 1926 terminated the pregnancy of a 17-year-old dancer by inserting a laminaria tent (*Quellstift*). His colleague, Dr L., completed the operation by curettage. Both acts, however, caused severe injuries – a perforated cervix and a lacerated uterus – which ended in death. It was also found that both doctors lacked proper concern. They dispatched their young patient home by taxi only two hours after the operation; Dr M. left the following morning on his honeymoon and did not inquire after the patient for a month. Despite the horrific injuries they had inflicted, neither doctor was convicted of manslaughter because the expert medical witness asserted that 'the incidence of such injuries . . . was well within the accepted level of surgical errors' and 'there was no reason to assume the doctor had acted negligently'.[31] There are many other examples which demonstrate lack of skill and professional conduct among doctors.[32] Moreover, the case in 1923 of the 33-year-old general practitioner Dr M. who, together with his fiancé Fräulein M. and the help of many midwives, ran a thriving abortion practice, shows that greed, dirt and disorder was by no means confined to lay practitioners.[33]

It would be wrong, however, to suggest that these stories of blunders, subterfuge and malpractice were the medical norm. The numerous medical terminations performed in teaching hospitals suggest that medical know-how under the supervision of leading gynaecologists was adequate, even if it was true that many abortions were carried out by medical students.[34] The point is that, at a time when abortion techniques were rarely taught in medical school, it is not surprising that many general practitioners embarked on this activity ill prepared and often secretly, nor that when things went wrong they failed to send patients to hospital, attempting to save their own skin rather than the health and life of their clients.[35] Lay practitioners with extensive abortion experience can probably be said to have been a safer bet than doctors who had the theoretical knowledge but lacked practice.

## THE COST OF ABORTION

Lay abortionists also offered lower-class women a good deal because they charged substantially less than doctors. After the inflation of 1923 doctors charged between 80 and 200 Reichsmark (RM) even for women from the poorer sections of society. Non-doctors usually only asked between 5 and 30 RM, or they expected the patient to give what she could.[36] Some were also happy to receive payment in kind. For example, in 1921–22 the carpenter's wife from Limburg received a small cash sum or 'a few pounds of flour', 'sausages and meat', 'a jug of Schnapps', 'a sack of oats' or even 'help with ploughing her field'.[37]

Their relative cheapness and reasonable success rate were not the only reasons why so many women turned to lay practitioners. Many doctors were not prepared to help because of their professional or religious convictions or because they feared the consequences, even though the number of those who did was probably growing.[38] A more important reason was a greater sense of equality between patient and lay healer. Payment and negotiation of it was an important guarantee of this. Whereas the legal and medical profession condemned it as a sign of 'commercialism', the exchange of money established a contract between the healer who sold a service and the pregnant woman who paid for the fulfilment of her request. Nowadays we are suspicious about attempts to make individuals feel responsible for their own health and pay for treatment, and see it as a veiled attack on the principle of free access to health care. But at a time when termination of an unwanted pregnancy (unless medical grounds could be demonstrated) was officially regarded as criminal and health insurance funds therefore refused to pay for it, the exchange of money or payment in kind empowered women in need of help. In fact, it increased the status of both parties. Payment to the abortionist was in recognition of services rendered and of a definite skill. In this spirit some wise women described their services matter of factly as 'work' and *Broterwerb*, a means to earn their living for which they naturally expected to be paid. This also explains why so many referred to their activities quite openly, even to their own children who discussed their mother's work in the playground.[39] Some, like the carpenter's wife in Limburg, the free-thinker from Silesia or the chemist Heiser in Berlin, regarded their abortion practice as a kind of 'community service'. They talked of a duty to help; the latter two were socialists and campaigned to reform the abortion law. They received payment which was often simply to cover expenses.[40]

Payment did not just lend status to the activities of lay practitioners; it also increased the power of women patients. Instead of appearing as supplicants before a doctor, who remained expert and arbiter even when charging a fee, and who could easily turn their request down, by paying the lay abortionist women became clients who had to be taken seriously. They could influence the level and conditions of pay, often paying in instalments, delaying payment until after the operation and sometimes not paying the full amount, something that doctors did not permit. Women could often also influence the circumstances of the operation. The carpenter's wife in Limburg, for example, seemed to have performed the operation either in her own or her patient's home, according to the latter's wishes.[41]

## ABORTION METHODS AND ABUSE

Doctors and lay practitioners also used different methods. Most midwives and lay abortionists used a similar technique, of injecting the uterus with either soap or alum or something similar by means of a syringe which had been fitted with a long catheter. Wise women often opted to massage the stomach and they usually chatted to their patient to relax and/or inform her. All this happened while the patient was awake and aware of what was happening. Lay practitioners in fact relied on the cooperation of the pregnant woman. I have not found a single case of lay abortionists having used an anaesthetic, though most doctors did. This was because the normal medical termination consisted of dilatation and curettage: firstly the cervix was dilated with metal instruments or a laminaria tent, after which the foetus was scraped out with a curette (a sharp little knife), an operation which was normally considered to be too painful to endure and also too dangerous to administer without an anaesthetic.[42] Apart from the use of the curette, it was the administration of an anaesthetic which formed the main distinction between doctors' treatment and that of lay practitioners.

Of course, to be unconscious meant less pain but also loss of control by the patient. It exposed her to possible abuse, and might well have been another reason why women preferred to consult non-doctors. While I have so far found only one incident of a 'quack abortionist' abusing a patient, there is plenty of evidence of doctors overstepping their remit. Some doctors, for example, performed operations which had not been requested by the patient. Even if this was done 'in the best interest of the patient' it constituted a serious breach of trust.[43] Abuse of patients' rights was an important issue within the qualitative population policy of the Weimar Republic. When the Depression hit Germany the support for legalized eugenic sterilization gained ground and by 1930 questionnaires revealed a substantial number of hospitals had carried out the operation, some of which were almost certainly without consent.[44] An autocratic attitude towards woman's fertility was rarely found among lay practitioners, who would seldom have possessed the medical know-how to perform such a major operation. According to the judicial files consulted, only one 'quack' offered a woman abortion *and* sterilization.[45]

The unequal power relationship between doctor and patient was particularly damaging to women, since it was nearly always gendered. Although the number of women doctors was rising fast they feature extremely rarely in abortion cases, a situation very different from lay practitioners, where the gender distribution was much more even. As a result it was typically a male doctor in control and always a woman, frequently a young woman on her own, on the receiving end. Although many women had kin and peer support, the number of women seeking an abortion alone, sometimes against the wishes of the child's father, was not insignificant. Moreover, the secrecy surrounding the act protected male irresponsibility or criminality. There are examples of male doctors ignoring their patients' wishes on subjective rather than objective grounds and, worse, displaying misogynist and sadistic tendencies, as when terminations were administered on no other ground than to increase a woman's libido or administered without an anaesthetic to teach a woman a lesson 'to take more care in the future'.[46] But there are other blatant cases of criminal abuse, when women were blackmailed into having sex or simply raped. Although one of the most shocking cases of enforced sex concerned a lay practitioner,[47] the evidence so far suggests that doctors were more frequently guilty of such extreme abuse of their power.[48]

## CLASS DIFFERENCES AND SHARED CULTURE

Women of all classes resorted to illegal abortions in Weimar Germany, but the majority of those tried in cases involving lay practitioners were from the lower classes.[49] For these women, 'quacks' helped to bridge the usual social gap they found when consulting doctors. While doctors were nearly always recruited from the middle classes, lay practitioners came from a similar social background to their patients and shared the same values and attitudes towards life.[50] This was a great bonus for women, especially at a sensitive time when they feared social stigma and needed sympathy and support. Conservative doctors often rejected abortion on moral grounds; Left-leaning practitioners tended to excuse abortion only on medical and economic grounds. Many lay abortionists, on the other hand, agreed with their women patients who linked their physical fate to external forces or simply thought of an unwanted pregnancy as bad luck. Morals did not come into it. They did not judge but simply assisted.[51]

Communication with lay healers was also often easier because they spoke the same language, while medical terminology was often couched in scientific–positivist terms which made little sense to patients, especially those with limited formal education. Doctors referred to curettage or artificial miscarriage while many women and lay practitioners, especially if they were female, talked about unblocking the monthly flow of blood and considered this as a preventive medicine. Popular remedies aimed largely at preventing the onset of diseases were potions or teas made of traditional, often secret, mixtures. It was also natural, therefore, to treat an unwanted pregnancy with teas, potions, hot baths or internal douching. Popular health manuals,[52] journals produced by nature therapy organizations and newspaper advertisements were full of preventive measures for every aspect of physical or emotional ailment, including abortifacients for 'late' periods.

Although some abortions occurred as late as the fifth or sixth month of pregnancy, the case studies suggest that the majority occurred around the third or fourth month.[53] Wise women, in particular, generally shared with their patients the belief that early abortions were neither criminal nor immoral. The old religious doctrine that the foetus had no soul in the first few weeks often lingered on unconsciously even if only in the notion that a child that could not be felt was not alive.[54] Nobody talked of murder or guilt except when the abortion went wrong.[55] The operation was frequently referred to as a natural process; the 'obstacle that hindered the blood from flowing was removed'. It was also a process of cleansing the body of something alien (the term frequently used was *kippen*, that is 'tipping' out what should not be retained).[56]

This shared experience of abortion as a natural, even everyday occurrence and as an accepted form of birth control meant that wise women and quacks were proud of and were admired for their skill, which was sometimes taught to a friend or neighbour as a special favour. It was not rare for neighbours in a working-class community to ask to watch an abortion in order to learn about it for themselves.[57] This also explains why many women talked quite openly about their experience in shops or in the street.[58] Even when wise women asked their patients to return with the aborted foetus to check things were all right – and this suggested the acknowledgement of more than just the 'unblocking of the blood flow' – women did this quite openly and without a sense of disgust.[59] Abortion was often performed in secret but remained nevertheless a public issue discussed within the family, community – particularly the working-class community – and at the workplace. While this kind of gossip sometimes led to denunciation and prosecution, it also ensured an effective flow of information within the community.

## ABORTION IN THE MEDICAL MARKET

Public health policies during the 1920s and early 1930s were inextricably linked with reproduction and eugenics, and control of women's bodies was high on the agenda. However, doctors also pursued their own professional interests in attempting to replace informal networks of self-help with more formal medical care.[60] Doctors attached great importance to gaining more women patients and, through women, access to the rest of the family. Even though doctors seem to have gained the upper hand over midwives and quacks in obstetrics and gynaecology they had failed to medicalize fertility control. In fact, both contraception and abortion, so central to Weimar population planners and social policy, remained to a large extent outside the control of registered doctors.[61] As far as abortion was concerned the medical market remained highly 'pluralist'. It was characterized by low professionalization, high lay participation and a rise of 'medical consumerism'.[62] From the judicial material, contemporary surveys and interviews, there can be no doubt that the abortion market was dominated by lay practitioners and that doctors were the intruders, increasingly tapping new market opportunities, especially since there was an oversupply of doctors during the 1920s which increased the difficulty of gaining a health insurance practice.[63]

Many medical practitioners sought a way into this potentially lucrative field by running their own back-street abortion practice organized on similar lines to the often thriving businesses of their lay competitors. Since the professional code of doctors forbade advertising they did so indirectly using midwives as so-called *Schlepperinnen* (touts). These placed veiled advertisements in local newspapers, examined women initially to confirm their pregnancy and then referred them to the doctor with whom they were in cahoots and who paid them for this service. Once known as willing abortionists, doctors usually attracted enough women of all social backgrounds to specialize in terminations of pregnancy.[64]

The profession as a whole also aimed to appropriate the field of abortion by a war of words. They linked the two issues of lay abortions and 'quackery' (*Kurpfuscherei*) in a vociferous campaign against *Kurierfreiheit* – the liberal principle that healing was a free trade open to all.[65] In Germany, nature therapists and other non-academic health practitioners were generally very well organized. Thus doctors preferred to attack 'quack abortionists', who were generally outside these organizations, in order to boost their anti-quackery campaign.[66] Medical journals made much of each new case of convicted lay abortionists, particularly when injuries or fatalities had occurred. To them, this seemed to provide excellent proof of the dangers of *Kurierfreiheit* to national health and morality.

Yet, if this campaign by doctors was also intended to weaken the standing of the organized popular health movement, this strategy backfired. The nature therapy associations retaliated in their journals by attacking qualified physicians for their 'bungled' abortions every time a trial revealed a medical intervention which had gone wrong. They also condemned illegal abortions, whether induced by doctors or lay persons.[67] Although they insisted on exercising their right of *Kurierfreiheit*, to practice healing in every conceivable form, in this one respect – abortion practice – they were happy to concede the right to their academic colleagues. As one article put it satirically: 'In this area we do not want *Kurierfreiheit*. Each doctor his own abortion!'[68]

Not only did qualified doctors fail to score an easy victory over organized nature therapists, their defamation of quack abortionists was also largely unjustified. When it came to safety in abortion practice, doctors did not turn out to be superior. In fact, in this respect, medical qualifications did not necessarily ensure successful terminations, nor did the lack of medical qualification necessarily mean risk. This had serious consequences for the profession; it effectively blurred the distinction between qualified and unqualified practice or state registered doctors and lay persons in this important field of reproductive health. Put bluntly, most doctors were laymen when it came to terminating pregnancies. In fact, with respect to skill and medical know-how it turned the distinction between academic and non-academic practitioners on its head, since doctors were often inferior to non-doctors. This made nonsense of one of the most important arguments by doctors against *Kurierfreiheit* and explains why the profession was so keen to master this territory in which quacks seemed to reign supreme. If doctors were to displace the non-doctors, they had to remove them with the help of state legislation outlawing all quack abortions, better still all quackery,[69] and at the same time achieve legalization of the medical termination of pregnancy. Or they had to outshine their competitors in skill. Either way they had to acquire experience as quickly as possible, if necessary by trial and error. In the process it is likely that many women became unsuspecting guinea pigs with potentially dire consequences. This, and the perception of academic and lay medicine by ordinary women, challenged the notion of a 'quack' as a dangerous and unscrupulous charlatan, and the claim that the professionalization of medicine had been largely completed by the outbreak of the First World War.[70]

As the sources have revealed, it was not just the expectation of a reasonably safe operation that persuaded so many women to turn to midwives, wise women and quacks when they sought to rid themselves of an unwanted pregnancy. There were clearly other advantages. At the time when most abortions were illegal and publicly frowned upon by the authorities and the medical profession, lay practitioners generally provided an important service to women, particularly from the lower classes, which often saved them from the need for deference, expectancy of humiliation and the lack of control frequently associated with medical consultations. Furthermore, tips about lay abortionists seemed generally to have come from an informal network of communication in the neighbourhood or at the workplace. At a time when many working-class women had only a limited understanding of procreation and fertility control, this might well have been more reassuring and rewarding than consulting a doctor, whose vocabulary was alien and whose interests did not necessarily converge with their own.

## ACKNOWLEDGEMENTS

I am indebted to Gaby Czarnowski, Lara Marks and Willem de Blécourt for their comments and advice. I would like to thank the Wellcome Trust London for a Research Leave Fellowship and the German Academic Exchange Service Bonn for support for this research.

## NOTES

1 Cited from F. Wolf, 'Cyankali: Ein Schauspiel', in *idem*, *Dramen* (East Berlin, 1960). For reviews, see Landeshauptstadt Stuttgart, *Stuttgart im Dritten Reich: Friedrich Wolf: Die Jahre in Stuttgart 1927–1933*, exhibition documentary (Stuttgart, 1983), p. 133ff.

2 See C. Usborne, *The Politics of the Body in Weimar Germany: Women's Reproductive Rights and Duties* (London, 1992); A. Grossmann, *Reforming Sex: The German Movement for Birth Control and Abortion Reform 1920–1950* (New York, 1995).

3 M. Hodann, *Geschlecht und Liebe in biologischer und gesellschaftlicher Beziehung* (Rudolstadt, 1928), p. 128.

4 Usborne, *Politics of the Body*, chap. 3. Other plays included Alfred Döblin, *Die Ehe* and Carl Credé, *Paragraph 218* or *Frauen in Not!* Both playwrights were, like Wolf, socialist physicians.

5 See Usborne, *Politics of the Body*, pp. 181–201.

6 A. Dührssen, 'Die Reform des Paragraph 218', *Sexus* (Leipzig, 1926), vol. 4, pp. 80, 74.

7 For example, L. Klauber, 'Die Abtreibung', in L. Levy-Lenz (ed.), *Sexualkatastrophen. Bilder aus dem modernen Geschlechts – und Eheleben* (Leipzig, 1926). See also *Der Sozialistische Arzt*, the journal of the Association of Socialist Doctors. This was also the view taken by Left-wing pro-abortion reform parliamentarians, for example E. Höllein (KPD), *Gegen den Gebärzwang. Der Kampf um die bewußte Kleinhaltung der Familie* (Berlin, 1928), pp. 174, 179.

8 L. Klauber, 'Geburtenregelung und Sozialismus', in Dr Kappes, 'Bericht von der Dresdener Reichstagung', *Der Sozialistische Arzt*, 39 (1928): n.p.

9 See I. Loudon, *Death in Childbirth: An International Study of Maternal Care and Maternal Mortality 1800–1950* (Oxford, 1992), esp. chaps 13, 26.

10 Usborne, *Politics of the Body*, appendix 2. Within the SPD it was Julius Moses, doctor and member of the Reichstag, who played the crucial role.

11 *Ibid.*, p. 182ff. The estimated abortion rate in England and Wales was put at between only 68,000 and 100,000 in 1935: D. Glass, *Population Policies and Movements in Europe* (London, 1967), p. 54. The estimated German rate was already very high before the war, reflecting the speed of the German demographic transition from large to small families. The socio-economic impact of the lost war

reinforced the trend. The abortion rate was also pushed up by a combination of factors, such as a greater tolerance of family limitation including abortion, an increased desire by women to control their procreation and the economic crisis following the hyperinflation of 1923 and the slump after 1929.

12 For example, H. Jahns, *Das Delikt der Abtreibung im Landgerichtsbezirk Duisburg in der Zeit von 1910–1935* (Düsseldorf, 1938), p. 5. Between 1908 and 1914 about 4 per cent of all detected abortions had been performed by women alone, just over 50 per cent with the help of accomplices and just over 40 per cent by commercial abortionists. During the war as many as one-third of all abortions were self induced, only about 8 per cent with accomplices. After the war the first category decreased to 20.2 per cent, while the number of 'commercial abortions' increased steadily, outstripping all other forms.

13 D.V. Glass, 'The effectiveness of abortion legislation in six countries', *Modern Law Review*, II: 2 (1938): p. 99ff.

14 *Ibid.*, pp. 97–125, esp. pp. 101, 117.

15 For example, Prof. Henkel of Jena University was accused of serious medical malpractice and negligence as well as carrying out unlawful abortions and sterilizations, but was successfully defended by the medical expert, a personal friend (Bundesarchiv Koblenz (BAK), R 86, 2379, vol. 1). Dr J. of Berlin who was tried for 24 illegal abortions, one of which ended in death, was defended by the medical expert and eventually acquitted (Landesarchiv Berlin (LAB), Rep 58, 2138).

16 BAK, R 86, 2379, vol. 1. Henkel was tried by a medical tribunal not by a law court.

17 For example, B. Herrmann, 'Else Kienle (1900–1970) – Eine Ärztin im Mittelpunkt der Abtreibungsdebatte von 1931', in E. Brinkschulte (ed.), *Weibliche Ärzte: Die Durchsetzung des Berufsbildes in Deutschland* (Berlin, 1993), pp. 114–22; M. von Oertzen, ' "Nicht nur fort sollst du dich pflanzen, sondern hinauf": Die Ärztin und Sexualreformerin Anne-Marie Durand-Wever (1889–1970)', in *ibid.*, pp. 140–52. Neither addresses the problem. A. Bergmann, *Die verhütete Sexualität. Die Anfänge der modernen Geburtenkontrolle* (Hamburg, 1992), pp. 185–7 largely adopts the contemporary medical and legal views. An exception is E. Shorter, *A History of Women's Bodies* (London, 1983), p. 207ff.

18 This is based on judicial files which have survived in the following state archives, in Protestant and Catholic, urban and rural regions: Landesarchiv Berlin (LAB), Geheimes Staatsarchiv Preuß. Kulturbesitz (GSAB Dahlem), Bundesarchiv Potsdam (BAP), Brandenburgisches Landeshauptarchiv Potsdam (BrLHAP), Bundesarchiv Koblenz (BAK), Landeshauptarchiv Koblenz (LHAK), Nordrheinwestfälisches Hauptstaatsarchiv Düsseldorf and Kalkum (HSADü), Stadtarchiv Cologne (StadtAK), and Staatsarchiv Munich (SAM). I have also used cases in legal dissertations: W. Köhler, *Das Delikt der Abtreibung im Bezirk des Landgerichts Gera in den Jahren 1896–1930* (Jena, 1935); W. Krieger, 'Erscheinungsform und

Strafzumessung bei der Abtreibung dargestellt an Hand von Gerichtsakten des Landgerichts und Amtgerichts Freiburg i.Br. in den Jahren 1925–1951', unpub. diss., University of Freiburg i.Br., 1952; Jahns, *Abtreibung in Duisburg*; K. Inderheggen, *Das Delikt der Abtreibung im Landgerichtsbezirk Mönchen-Gladbach in der Zeit von 1908–1938* (Jena, 1940).

19 For instance, in Duisburg a third of all commercial abortionists were midwives and they also had the largest abortion practices (Jahn, *Abtreibungen in Duisburg*, p. 65), in Freiburg two out of the seven commercial operators were midwives (Krieger, 'Abtreibungen in Freiburg', pp. 42–3).

20 In Gera no midwives are listed amongst 146 commercial operators, but some simply called 'married women' might well have been deregistered midwives: Köhler, *Abtreibungen in Gera*, p. 12.

21 In the files of the *Landgericht* Gera, for example, 5 of the 13 convicted lay abortionists were nature therapists or connected to the healing trade in one form or another. In 7 of the cases suspected but not tried, 5 were nature therapists: Köhler, *Abtreibung in Gera*, pp. 44, 48. In Duisburg, 5 of the 15 male abortionists were nature therapists and of the 22 female abortionists 7 were former midwives. On closer inspection some other women had links with the healing trade: Jahns, *Abtreibung in Duisburg*, pp. 63–8.

22 Inderheggen, *Abtreibung in M-Gladbach*.

23 See note 12; L. Levy-Lenz, *Wenn Frauen nicht gebären dürfen* (Berlin, 1928), p. 43; Inderheggen, *Abtreibungen in M.-Gladbach*, p. 27; BAK, R 86, 2371, Bl. 153–65, esp. 157.

24 For example, LAB, Rep 58, 2439; BAP, RJMin., 6233, vol. 2, Bl. 87–97; GSAB Dahlem, Rep 84a, 17109.

25 BAK, R 86, 2371, Bl. 153–65, esp. 157. Inderheggen, who strongly disapproved of all 'quack abortionists', conceded that they were much more prevalent than doctors because women thought them more skilled: Inderheggen, *Abtreibung in M.-Gladbach*, p. 27.

26 For instance, LAB, Rep 58, 2439, case against janitor's wife S., who caused the death of a woman but was then found to have performed at least 31 other abortions without any problems. Another case is that of the widow Fanny H., prosecuted for performing an abortion which ended in death. She was found to have performed many previous successful abortions: GSAB Dahlem, Rep 84a, 17142. Or there are many cases of a chance discovery where a widespread abortion practice was revealed which never produced any problems at all, including the case of the homoeopath Sch. who had helped at least 84 women without any mishap: GSAB Dahlem, Rep 84a, 17158.

27 BAK, R 86, 2379, *Vorwärts*, (20 May 1924), (8 October 1924); *Sexual-Hygiene*, I: 4 (1929): 32; S. Vollmann, 'Die Umfrage der Ärztinnen über das Problem der Schwangerschaftsunterbrechung', *Deutsches Ärzteblatt*, 59 (1932): 68; Frau Dr Prager-Heinrich, report in 'Bericht über die Naumburger Tagung am 6. und 7. Dezember', *Die Ärztin*, 7 (1931): 18.

28 BAP, RJMin., 6233, vol. 2, Bl. 87–97, 'Matter for discussion in the Reichstag', 26 April 1930, proceedings against Frau Johanna A. in Hindenburg.
29 GSAB Dahlem, Rep 84a, no. 17109.
30 For example, P. Hüssy, 'Begutachtung und gerichtliche Beurteilung von ärztlichen Kunstfehlern auf dem geburtshilflichen-gynäkologischen Gebiete', in *Beilageheft zur Zeitschrift für Geburtshilfe und Gynäkologie* (Stuttgart, 1935), vol. III.
31 LAB, Rep 58, no. 850, Dr Kurt M., vol. I, vol. II.
32 For example, LAB, Rep 58, 2494, trial in 1931 against Dr S. in Berlin-Charlottenburg in 1931. He was accused of commercial abortion and manslaughter, negligence and malpractice because he used a discredited method and had not offered aftercare.
33 LAB, Rep 58, 416: Dr M.'s surgery was described as 'filthy, smelly and filled with seven cats and one dog'.
34 BAK, R 86, 2380, statistics of artificial miscarriages in maternity hospitals, 1929; Clara Bender, 'Sozialhygienisches zur Indikation der Schwangerschaftsunterbrechung', *Klinische Wochenschrift*, 19 (1925): 933.
35 See the doyen of German gynaecologists Georg Winter's complaints in, 'Strittige Punkte in der Behandlung des fieberhaften Aborts', *Medizinische Welt* (20 Aug. 1927): 1040; Hüssy, 'Begutachtung', p. 8, reports many examples of 'horrifying mistakes' by doctors which 'demonstrate ignorance, lack of technical skill and gross negligence'.
36 Jahns, *Abtreibung in Duisburg*, pp. 66–8; Inderheggen, *Abtreibung in M.-Gladbach*, pp. 106–13; LAB, Rep 58, 2349, midwife S. 1927–1929 and 2064 homoeopath S., 1928.
37 GSAB Dahlem, Rep 84a, 17109.
38 See Carl Credé, *Volk in Not! Das Unheil der Abtreibungsparagraphen* (Dresden, 1927), p. 15.
39 Jahns, *Abtreibung in Duisburg*, p. 67. The case of a miner's wife, whose four-year-old daughter told her playmates: 'My mummy does not need to carry any more babies in her tummy and your mummy does not either if my mummy wants it.'
40 Heiser charged 20 RM which was for syringing and supplying his own cream: LAB, Rep 58, 2453, vol. IX, 1928; Frau K. of Limburg also charged 20 to 30 RM, even at the height of inflation: GSAB Dahlem, Rep 84a, 17109.
41 GSAB Dahlem, Rep 84a, 17109.
42 Winter, 'Strittige Punkte', p. 104, warned that a manual curettage needed a deep anaesthetic but that many GPs did not use one because they had no trained person at hand to do it. Either a second doctor, or even better, a midwife should be called. It was quite wrong to use the help of an untrained 'wife' (clearly assuming doctors to be usually male).
43 For example, SAM, St.anw.Mü I, 1834, Dr Hope Bridges Adams-Lehman, 1914, revealed that aborting women underwent sterilization without consent. See B. Duden, ' "Keine Nachsicht gegen das schöne Geschlecht." Wie sich Ärzte die Kontrolle über Gebärmütter

aneigneten', in S. v. Paczensky and R. Sadrozinzki (eds), *Paragraph 218: Zu Lasten der Frauen* (Hamburg, 1988), pp. 114–33.

44 Usborne, *Politics of the Body*, p. 151ff.

45 Inderheggen, *Abtreibung in M-Gladbach*, p. 111.

46 A. Grotjahn (ed.), *Eine Kartothek zu Paragraph 218: Ärztliche Berichte aus einer Kleinstadtpraxis über 426 künstliche Aborte in einem Jahr* (Berlin, 1932), introduction and p. 17, case 19.

47 Inderheggen, *Abtreibung in M-Gladbach*, pp. 110–11: case no. 15, a 46-year-old printer who forced his patient to have sex because she was 'too cold' for the operation.

48 One family doctor, for example, who practised in a small town in the Rhineland, regularly offered termination of pregnancy in exchange for sex. In most cases the women involved were very young and terrified; intercourse took place immediately and without prophylactics: HSADü, Staatsanw. Kleve, Rep 7, 896.

49 By contrast doctors tried for abortion also catered for middle-class women: for example, LAB Rep 58, 416, 2137–9, 2453, 2494; see also GSAB Dahlem, Rep 84a, 17108, 17112, 17114, etc. The one notable exception was the chemist Heiser whose clients included women of all classes: LAB, Rep 58, 2453.

50 Jahns, *Abtreibung in Duisburg*, p. 63; 'Über die Mißstände auf dem Gebiete der Kurpfuscherei und Maßnahmen zu ihrer Beseitigung', *Veröffentlichung aus dem Gebiet der Medizinalverwaltung*, XXV: 3 (1937): 34. Among all lay practitioners in Berlin in 1926 most had previous occupations as artisans (275) and state officials were in second place (102).

51 See M. Chamberlain, *Old Wives' Tales: Their History, Remedies and Spells* (London, 1981), pp. 145–8.

52 For example, F.E. Bilz, *Das neue Naturheilverfahren* (Dresden, many editions, here 1938).

53 This contrasts with abortions in the Third Reich: see G. Czarnowsky, 'Crime by women – crime by the state: abortion in Nazi Germany', paper given at the conference *Gender and Crime in Britain and Europe, Early Modern and Modern*, Roehampton Institute London, April 1995.

54 BAK, R 86, 2371, Bl. 158, Max Hirsch; See A. Ryter, 'Abtreibung in der Unterschicht zu Beginn des Jahrhunderts: Eine empirische Untersuchung von Strafgerichtsakten des Staatsarchivs Basel-Stadt', unpub. MA diss., University of Basle, 1983, pp. 62–6; *idem*, 'Abtreibung in Basel', in Wiener Historikerinnen (eds), *Die ungeschriebene Geschichte* (Vienna, 1985), pp. 289–97, 294–5; Duden, ' "Keine Nachsicht gegen das schöne Geschlecht" '; J. Mohr, *Abortion in America* (New York, 1978), pp. 4–6, 131; B. Brookes, *Abortion in England 1900–1967* (London, 1988), p. 132; *idem*, 'The illegal operation', in London Feminist History Group (ed.), *The Sexual Dynamics of History* (London, 1983), p. 167.

55 Stadt AK, Abt. 424, 412, Bl. 66. When the abortion procured by midwife K. was not successful she returned her fee.

56 NRWHSA Dü, Reg. Dü 38892, report by judicial doctor. M. Marcuse, 'Zur Frage der Verbreitung und Methodik der willkürlichen

Geburtenbeschränkung in Berliner Proletarierkreisen', *Sexualprobleme*, 9 (1913): 752–80; Ryter, 'Abtreibung'.

57 NRHSA Dü, Reg. Dü, 38892, public prosecutor Dü, 10.12.1914; Inderheggen, *Abtreibung in M.-Gladbach*, p. 166.

58 For example, NRHSA Dü, Reg. Dü, 38892; STAM, Staatsanw. Mü I, 1834, the abortion of a butcher's wife was openly discussed in her own shop.

59 LAB, Rep 58, 2439.

60 Usborne, *Politics of the Body*, p. 142ff.

61 *Ibid.*, chap. 3.

62 See R. Porter, 'Before the fringe: "quackery" and the eighteenth-century medical market', in R. Cooter (ed.), *Studies in the History of Alternative Medicine* (London, 1988), pp. 1–26, esp. p. 3.

63 P. Weindling, *Health, Race and German Politics between National Unification and Nazism 1870–1945* (Cambridge, 1988); LAB, Rep 58, 2138, for an example of a doctor performing abortions because he failed to obtain a panel practice.

64 For example, Dr J., a Berlin gynaecologist, used the services of many midwives since 'the way to the gynaecologist often is via the midwife'. Dr M. used more than ten midwives and several wise women as touts: LAB, Rep 58, 2137 and 416.

65 This was introduced into the Trade Laws of the newly unified Reich in 1871, but after the turn of the century had increasingly come under attack by the medical profession and some politicians. See R. Spree, *Soziale Ungleichheit vor Krankheit und Tod* (Göttingen, 1981), p. 140ff and *idem*, 'Kurpfuscherei-Bekämpfung und ihre sozialen Funktionen', in A. Labisch and R. Spree (eds), *Medizinische Deutungsmacht im sozialen Wandel* (Bonn, 1989), pp. 103–22.

66 See G. Stollberg, 'Die Naturheilvereine im Deutschen Kaiserreich', *Archiv für Sozialgeschichte*, 28 (1988): 287–305.

67 For example, the Central Association for the Parity of Healing Methods called doctors guilty of abortion injuries 'state-registered botchers': *Medizinalpolitische Rundschau*, XVIII (1925): 31–2 and XIX (1926): 51, 52.

68 'Neues von der Abtreibung', *Medizinalpolitische Rundschau*, XIX (1926): 65–6.

69 Only the Nazi regime managed to abolish *Kurierfreiheit* and introduced, with the help of the medical profession, a tightly controlled population policy which was both racist and anti-feminist, granting doctors the upper hand. But even then an important underground abortion network of midwives and lay practitioners continued to exist. See Czarnowski, 'Crime by women', note 57; and *idem*, 'Frauen als Mütter der "Rasse". Abtreibungsverfolgung und Zwangseingriff im Nationalsozialismus', in Deutsches Hygiene Museum (ed.), *Unter anderen Umständen. Zur Geschichte der Abtreibung* (Dresden/Berlin, 1993), pp. 58–72.

70 See the excellent discussion in Spree, *Soziale Ungleichheit vor Krankheit und Tod*, p. 138ff.

Chapter 10

# Healing alternatives in Alicante, Spain, in the late nineteenth and late twentieth centuries

*Enrique Perdiguero*

This chapter seeks to illustrate the variety of healing alternatives in the city and province of Alicante, south-east Spain, during two periods – the final quarter of the nineteenth century and the 1990s. Information on the earlier period has been mostly taken from the local press. Between the mid- and late nineteenth century, newspaper circulation grew considerably and became increasingly relevant for our purposes, giving us some insight into the range of alternatives open to the Alicante population when they fell ill.[1] Data on the present-day situation have been obtained from recent field studies[2] and the fact that we are dealing with two historical periods allows us to make diachronical comparisons. Some aspects of the healing activities under consideration were found to be similar – at least in form – in both periods.

The framework of this essay is that delineated in recent years by the medical historiography which has shifted the emphasis from renowned doctors and orthodox practitioners to the more complex world of medical practice, to include all manner of healers involved in confronting illness.[3] This stance means abandoning the traditional tendency to take 'orthodoxy' as the standard, implicitly or explicitly, when analyzing 'alternative' or 'irregular' treatments or cures.[4]

We shall focus on two groups of healers with two specific ways of treating illness, the *curanderos* and the 'local specialists'. The term *curandero*[5] is used to distance this group from the phenomenon of 'charlatanism' or 'quackery'.[6] 'Quackery' certainly existed in Spain at the end of the last century, and to this day the media are full of advertisements for panaceas and products devised by 'quacks' which promise to cure ailments of every kind. Analysis of this phenomenon requires detailed study and is beyond the scope of this paper.[7]

The *curanderos* treated, and still treat, all manner of illness and thus compete with qualified doctors for patients. The second group, the local specialists, are different because they only deal with 'culture-bound syndromes',[8] ailments that are not usually classified as 'medical' and which are recognized as distinct illnesses in the Alicante region. The most common of these are 'evil eye', 'sun in the head' and indigestion, known as *l'enfit*. Local specialists differ little from the rest of the population; nor did they in the previous century. We call them local specialists because they are specialized in healing one or two 'culture-bound illnesses' and their sphere of action is always local. However, the sources are unclear in defining the borderline between *curanderos* and local specialists. Occasionally *curanderos* act as local specialists and vice versa.

## HEALING ALTERNATIVES IN ALICANTE AT THE END OF THE NINETEENTH CENTURY

During the last part of the nineteenth century doctors observed that *curanderos* and local specialists abounded in the city of Alicante, although the sources do not allow us to make exact calculations of their number and distribution. In 1875 the city of Alicante had 35,000 inhabitants, rising to 50,000 at the turn of the century. By 1900, 30 doctors[9] were working in the capital besides an unknown number of other 'regular' health workers.[10] As in the rest of the country, there were no general medical insurance schemes of any kind, though there were many projects and attempts to implement such schemes before the end of the Civil War in 1939.[11] There was, however, a public medical service. Like all other cities and the majority of towns, the 'municipal beneficence' of Alicante contracted doctors who were to look after the poor in return for a small salary.[12]

On one occasion when city doctors were being contracted, one of them was asked to comment on the possibilities of building up a profitable practice in the city. He replied that the post lacked appeal; although the contracted doctors could dedicate part of their time to private practice, there was a dearth of private patients, due mainly to the innumerable *curanderos* and local specialists.[13] Two other factors which also heralded a bleak economic future for the young doctor just arrived in Alicante were the friendly societies, which provided medical cover to a high proportion of the population,[14] and the popularity of homoeopathic cures.[15] Whatever the case, and allowing for exaggeration – after all the newspapers provided information on only four homoeopathic doctors – it is clear that the *curanderos* and local specialists were regarded as a real threat to regular practitioners. It is difficult to gauge from current research whether this 'threat' shaped the medical market of the period. Yet the testimonies of doctors, many of whom were attracted by the population growth of Alicante before their expectations of having a good clientele were dashed, tended to confirm that competition existed and had its effect.[16] It can be deduced too that population growth and the absence of health cover for many families (though, for example, more than 4,000 families were insured through the main friendly society at the tobacco factory) encouraged the activities of other healers, particularly the *curanderos*.

From the doctors' point of view, this threat was such that Sánchez Santana, editor of the first professional medical periodical to be published in Alicante, *La Fraternidad Médico–Farmacéutica* (1886–88), launched a campaign denouncing all irregular healers who were practising in the city and province.[17] The main aim of this campaign was to secure a position of pre-eminence for the 'orthodox' practitioners in all domains of medical provision. To achieve this, Santana established a section in his periodical entitled 'The Gallery of the Famous Unqualified'. From this section we learn about the variety of unorthodox healing alternatives available to the inhabitants of Alicante and about the colourful characters involved in these practices. Among these are the *curanderos* and local specialists, though descriptions of these two groups are not very detailed. Sánchez Santana ridiculed and railed against the specialists who claimed the ability to cure 'culture-bound illnesses' such as *l'enfit*,[18] and against all spiritualist healers, mediums and seers, such as Consuelito Quiquets. This particular *curandera* was one of the most famous in Alicante, and Sánchez Santana quoted her as an example of the kind of practitioner a mother turned to when her child was suffering from indigestion. She was renowned for being able to see and talk to spirits from the other world and for having healing powers; she also seems to have used magnetized water from time to time. Such was her reputation for healing children that she even rivalled 'El Baldaet', the *curandero* whose activities will be discussed below.[19] From other articles we learn of another healer who used magnetized water to cure, an ex-stonemason who abandoned his trade to cater for people's health needs, a half Moor, Gasparito, who prepared remedies for all kinds of ailments in his own home,[20] and

'Uncle Motherkiller', the '*saludador*' from Rafal, who specialized in the cure of rabies.[21] Besides these healers, who were natives of the province of Alicante, Sánchez Santana also kept tabs on those who came from other regions. These included the 'Circle of Apostles', a famous group of *curanderos*,[22] who were eventually imprisoned for their activities after having established themselves in Alicante.[23]

If the editor of *La Fraternidad Médico–Farmacéutica* is to be believed, there was hardly an inhabitant in Alicante who had not at one time or another consulted an alternative healer.[24] How did these healers operate? Records of their activities are usually scarce and without them it is difficult to gauge the methods they used, who they attended, why people went to them and how successful their cures were . In Alicante these difficulties have been somewhat reduced thanks to a test case which took place in the late nineteenth century and had repercussions at national level. It is interesting to look at this case in more detail because the accused is at the same time typical and unique. Typical, because he shared many of the features common to the *curanderos* operating in Alicante at the end of the century, and unique because – unlike most of the *curanderos* mentioned – there is a wealth of information about this individual owing to the great publicity surrounding the court case.

## The case of 'El Baldaet'

On 26 September 1879 the High Court made public its verdict on an appeal presented by José Cerdá y Baeza, otherwise known as 'El Baldaet', 'against the sentence passed by the court in the first instance, in Alicante, for offences committed through practising a profession without the necessary qualifications'.[25] The verdict claimed among other things

> that at the petition of the sub-delegate of medicine and surgery in the city of Alicante a case had been brought against José Cerdá y Baeza for practising a profession without qualifications claiming that about one hundred patients went to his house every day and that the accused, by placing his right hand on bottles or earthenware vessels full of water that had been brought by the patients, moved his fingers claiming he was magnetizing the water. He then told them to drink it and apply wet cloths to the painful areas. For this he received no remuneration whatsoever.

The outcome of the first court case was that the Alicante judge decreed that an offence had been committed and the guilty party was ordered to pay 10 pesetas fine and costs. Baeza then lodged an appeal which was finally dealt with by the public prosecutor, after having been rejected as inadmissible by three lawyers. The High Court annulled the sentence as only being 'applicable when a person who had no qualifications to heal did it using the medicine which science had provided' and 'José Cerdá Baeza never applied any such medicine to the many patients who came to him'.

This verdict was a blow to the doctors. The case of 'El Baldaet' became a symbol because it showed not only that 'unorthodox' medicine could stand on its own merits but also that the courts were not necessarily going to support the regular doctors. Such was the outcry that Salcedo Ginestal, another qualified doctor, in a book which attempted to expose this kind of 'error', pointed to Baeza as being representative of the worst examples of charlatanism and practice under false pretences.[26]

The repercussions of this case and the fact that José Cerdá Baeza was considered a *curandero* who cured with magnetized water provoked great interest and has enabled us to learn more about his practice. He learnt to magnetize water while involved in an Alicante spiritualist group, which also carried out hypnotic procedures. A number of these groups were set up in Alicante and other centres during the second half of the nineteenth century.[27] In the 1870s these groups were coordinated by the 'Alicante Society of Psychological Studies', directed by the head of the department of natural sciences at the local grammar school, Manual Ausó y Monzó.[28] In 1872, the society began to publish the magazine, *La Revelación*, which was in print well into the twentieth century. Members of the society revealed themselves to be followers of Allan Kardec, the worldwide ideological leader of the movement, who supported the notion of harmonizing spiritualist ideas with the teachings of the Bible.[29]

It was in this atmosphere that Baeza made his appearance. He was known as 'El Baldaet', 'the cripple', because of his hump, his paralyzed legs and left arm and his difficulty in articulating whole sentences when speaking.[30] Alicante spiritualists were divided over the extent of his skills, as was the population in general. This gave rise to a controversy which raged in the pages of *La Revelación*, reflecting above all the views of Ausó y Monzó and his group.[31] To resolve this controversy Dr Anastasio García López, lecturer at the school of medicine at the University of Salamanca, and also a leading homoeopath and spiritualist, was sent to Alicante.[32] At the instigation of the Spanish Spiritualist Society, he made a report on the healing abilities of 'El Baldaet' which was published in *La Revelación*.[33] Through this report we learn a great deal about the illnesses of those attended by 'El Baldaet' and his practice techniques.

It is obvious that in Alicante 'El Baldaet' was considered to offer a genuine therapeutic alternative. Patients could consult him at his home between 9.00 am and 1.00 pm, and from 3.00 pm until dusk. On an average day he attended between one hundred and several hundred patients. His clientele came not only from the city of Alicante, but also from towns and especially villages in the province. They came not only for treatment, but also to collect his therapeutic resource – 'magnetized water'.

All this popularity came after years of constant movement, not only on the edges of the city but also through provincial villages where, on more than one occasion, he had been attacked and told to leave. His income was whatever those who came to him for help chose to give him – and it seems that he earned a good living, though the reports reiterate that his care was entirely without charge and there was not even a hint of 'good will' or the receipt of presents of any kind, something which is hard to believe. The extent of his success can also be judged by the fact that he originally settled on the outskirts of the city but later relocated his practice to the city centre, a reflection of his success and firm financial position.

We know little of those who consulted 'El Baldaet'. Allusions are made to all classes of men and women. Some of his more high-ranking clients refused to admit to their visits, while others who were less reticent allowed their names to be quoted freely, despite their wealth and position. According to the records of Anastasio García López, the kinds of ailments afflicting those who went to 'El Baldaet' in search of relief varied greatly: neuralgia, rheumatism, gastritis, dyspepsia, bronchitis, peripneumonia, endocarditis, anaemia, edema, epitheliomas and so on. His patients included adults as well as children who were often still being breastfed. In the opinion of García López, many of the illnesses were everyday complaints while others could be considered incurable, including cases of blindness. Many of the cases refer to aches and pains which are catalogued by Garicía López as arthritic or rheumatic. All this tells us that José Cerdá Baeza was an alternative to regular practitioners in the broadest sense; he claimed to understand all forms of illnesses and was not limited to any one pathology or the treatment of 'culture-bound syndromes'.[34]

His way of attending the sick was always the same. 'El Baldaet', in García López's opinion, had a method for finding out what was wrong by asking about the symptoms but not stating them himself. According to García Lopez, Baeza detected a way of finding out about the patient through his questioning, which appeared to follow a standard formula but actually varied according to the illness.[35] The editors of *La Revelación* even suggested that he had acquired his approach to healing while apprenticed to his blacksmith father which, during this period, would have also involved dabbling as a vet.[36] 'El Baldaet' would make a diagnosis (an extremely poor one, according to García López) without employing 'technical terminology', neither homing in on the cause nor the nature of the illness though he sometimes managed to locate the sick organ.[37] This absence of 'technical terminology' seems to have been of great importance – it certainly would have bridged a cultural gap – and meant that his diagnosis was comprehensible to the patients he attended. So, for example, when he was confronted with symptoms that resembled gastro-enteritis in a child, 'El Baldaet' diagnosed dribbling caused by teething.[38] This illustrates the importance he put on the 'nosology' of teething as the cause of the illness. He reflected popular conceptions, which rated teething as one of the most frequent causes of infant death in the late nineteenth century,[39] and it is easy to see how this could be classed as an 'illness'.[40] Other diagnoses like 'swollen gut', 'humour of the blood' and 'loose nerves' were all fully understood by his patients and this, at least partially, explains 'El Baldaet's' popularity.

Baeza's healing technique was always the same. First he 'magnetized' the patient and then the water by shaking it at regular intervals, giving instructions for the patient either to drink the water or to apply it to the painful area. He did everything with his right hand, using both the palm and the upper side.[41]

What was 'El Baldaet's' therapeutic success rate? From patient testimonies given to García López, nearly everyone claimed an improvement or a complete cure. García López admitted improvement in some cases, though never a cure; in other patients no change was recorded at all. According to García López, many people went to consult 'El Baldaet' with such trifling ailments that they would have disappeared without his intervention. The consultation was free and, perhaps because of this, many children were taken to him who were not very ill. They cried a lot, were not breastfeeding well, or they had a cough. Many of his patients had followed unsuitable allopathic regimes for some time or had taken patented remedies which, instead of curing them, had actually made them worse. According to García López, these people found relief and even a cure with 'El Baldaet' simply by suspending treatment, allowing nature to take over and bring about a spontaneous cure.[42]

'El Baldaet' carried on with his work after being absolved in court. He even won a privileged place in the 'Gallery of the Famous Unqualified' as 'The Great Apostle'.[43] Esteban Sánchez Santana saw in 'El Baldaet' the incarnation of all the evils which, according to the expression of the day, threatened the 'medical class' – by which he meant qualified doctors. To combat the competition that *curanderos* and local specialists represented in the fight for control and dominance over all aspects of health care in the province, Sánchez Santana proposed the formation of a professional association and advocated the need to keep a close eye on the most famous of these healers. Following the death of two tubercular patients, one in the home of 'El Baldaet' and the other in the house of a visiting German citizen who was accused of trying to pass as a doctor, Sánchez Santana published an article on their activities.[44] The public prosecutor took this as a pretext to take the two to court.[45] Both the German and Baeza were found not guilty and the pained editor of *La Fraternidad Médico–Farmacéutica* called his campaign of aggression to a halt.[46]

The grudge which this medical periodical expressed against such healers shows that they were considered serious rivals to regular practitioners. Economic considerations could greatly influence ordinary people; even when they paid Baeza, it would probably be less than regular medical fees. Moreover, the understanding of illness and belief in the curative properties of magnetized water was shared by healer and patients.

## Healing and the Catholic Church

The Catholic Church was also influential in Alicante. It was keen to uphold the general belief in the possibility of healing through the intervention of the Virgin Mary or the saints, a strategy resorted to by the Alicante population on a regular basis, sometimes in combination with other healing alternatives. The press illustrate this situation very clearly. *La Correspondencia de Alicante*, for example, gave news of cures worked by the Santa Faz, a revered local relic.[47] In the 1880s *El Semanario Católico*, the diocesan newspaper, published stories about the cure of serious illnesses which defied explanation. In many of these stories an openly hostile tone is adopted to reproach those refusing to accept the possibility of miraculous cures.[48] Proof was produced in the form of medical testimonies which invariably certified the impotence of science to cure the person in question.[49] In dramatic accounts the Virgin of Lourdes was most often presented as being responsible for these cures.[50] Other divine intercessors also had a role: San Vicente Ferrer, San Gerano, Santa Teresa de Jesús and others.[51]

Yet it seems the *curanderos* and local specialists did not represent a break with Catholicism, as the pages of *La Revelación* liked to remind its readers. The church, however, did not share this opinion and the claims of the spiritualists were answered systematically by *El Semanario Católico* and *El Alicantino* which, referring to church doctrine, condemned spiritualism as a dangerous fraud.[52] These articles maintained that magnetist, spiritualist and hypnotic practices could cause physical and mental harm, but above all they equated spiritualism with satanism. In 1882 the reading of *La Revelación* was forbidden to Catholics.[53] *El Semanario Católico* denounced a medium who operated in Crevillente, in the province of Alicante, primarily because he gave Protestant publicity leaflets to those who came to consult him.[54]

From José Cerdá y Baeza's case, which was regarded by contemporaries as representative of the practices of *curanderos* and local specialists, it can be concluded that such healers were considered as an important healing alternative in late nineteenth-century Alicante; they were accessible and cheap, and their perceptions of sickness and health were shared by the community. They were, for regular practitioners and the church, a serious force to contend with.

## HEALING ALTERNATIVES IN ALICANTE AT THE END OF THE TWENTIETH CENTURY

In this century conceptions of sickness have moved closer to those of orthodox medicine, which has in turn become increasingly effective. Health care became more accessible in Spain following the setting up of the national health service in the 1940s, which was further built upon during the subsequent three decades. Nowadays, most people have access to medical care through regional health centres and hospitals.[55] The medical market has changed substantially and we might expect that *curanderos* and local specialists would have lost much of their former importance.

Since the beginning of this century such predictions have been made for all places where western scientific medicine has taken hold. It was assumed that a more structured and accessible health service would cause more people to use it more effectively, health would improve immeasurably and the old inequalities caused by socio–economic differences, which only enabled the wealthiest to consult a doctor, would disappear.[56] Yet research carried out in the social sciences – above all by medical sociologists and medical anthropologists – has shown the inaccuracy of such predictions and has revealed the continuing importance of a population fighting illness in its own way.[57] It has also shown continuing use of alternative forms of healing.[58]

Unpublished data on health diagnostics taken from the Department of Public Health at the University of Alicante on towns in the Alicante province, including the capital, Benidorm, and Elche, another major city, reveal that on average 10 per cent of the population use 'complementary medicine', and between 5 and 8 per cent visit *curanderos*. With reference to the recorded incidence of 'culture-bound syndromes', and therefore resort to local specialists, this was especially extensive in the south of the province and involved a third of the population.[59]

What is the explanation for the presence and success of these healing alternatives today? To get closer to an answer we should briefly examine the characteristics of the *curanderos* and local specialists that we have found at work in the city and province of Alicante.[60] The 'culture-bound syndromes' treated by local specialists are illnesses with a special meaning for the population. They have to be cured without the help of regular practitioners who deny their existence. Vague children's illnesses, gastric pains or headaches are commonplace ailments. Relief is offered by local specialists, usually women, who diagnose and cure through rituals which usually do not differentiate between the moment of diagnosis and therapy. The predominance of women is not surprising, given that such ailments are typically treated at home. Rituals used by local specialists usually consist of a series of movements accompanied by an incantation recited in a low voice which has the strength to cure and which normally refers to religious figures – the Virgin Mary, Jesus Christ or various saints.

Those carrying out the rituals acquire their skill when a specific incantation (there is one for each culturally-defined ailment) is communicated to them on a particular day, usually Maundy Thursday or Good Friday. These incantations cannot be transmitted to anyone else except on the days indicated. The transmission is usually from mother to daughter or niece, or from grandmother to granddaughter, and typically takes place when the youngest has reached maturity or is about to leave home. Some have knowledge of incantations for several illnesses, others only for one – usually indigestion, which is the most frequent ailment. Unlike *curanderos*, these local specialists are hard to distinguish from the rest of the population. They are typically housewives or have occupations other than healing and normally treat only a small number of people, including their family and neighbours. They do not practise professionally and do not charge for their help, not even in the form of 'good will'. Some accept presents, but that is unusual. They are, therefore, financially a very accessible alternative for commonplace ailments.

The case of the *curanderos* is rather different. There is no predominance of either sex. Though each *curandero* has special characteristics, they share some general features.[61] Let us first look at a specific case and then go on to highlight the features which they all more or less have in common.

One of the *curanderas* we found holds her practice, according to the sign outside her house, three days a week from 10.00 am to 2.00 pm. The reason for these limited hours is that she felt very weak if she saw her patients on a daily basis. When she is not working, she is just like any other housewife in the lower and lower-middle class district of Alicante where she lives. She uses water that she 'makes' and gives it to the sick. The word 'magnetize' is not mentioned but the procedure is very similar to the one used by 'El Baldaet'. She also makes a cream, 'to cure all kinds of ailments' and sometimes uses rituals like those performed by the local specialists in cases of indigestion or '*l'enfit*'. It is not necessary for the person who is ill to be present; the method used in diagnosis and cure relies on consultation with 'brothers and sisters' about the patient. These 'brothers and sisters' are the spiritual protectors which all *curanderos* claim to have. In this particular case they are saints and diverse religious figures who are represented by figurines in wax and earthenware and in pictures which fill the room where she practices. The meeting is usually very cordial and during it the *curandera* may pass her hand over the patient's head, perhaps to find out how the person is feeling or to diagnose or relieve discomfort. When the aim is diagnostic, it is the 'brothers and sisters' who 'suggest' the diagnosis while the hand of the *curandera* passes over the patient.

In a typical session the *curandera* was consulted mainly by women who needed help with their own ailments or with those of their children who sometimes accompanied them. She dealt with a wide range of problems, including what the *curandera* called 'depression' and 'inflammation'. The symptoms varied a good deal, but were often related to stress: insomnia, fatigue, anorexia and the like. After passing her hands over the patient, the *curandera* would then ask her patient the kind of questions which showed that they already knew each other. She then recommended the water and, in some cases, the cream. She charged for them, but at no time did the price exceed 3 or 4 pesetas. She also stressed that she never recommended ceasing with a treatment prescribed by a doctor and looked upon herself as offering a complementary service. Generally, she gave her patients a diagnosis, and there were also constant references to personal problems throughout the interview.[62]

This *curandera* is an example of those practising in Alicante today. They claim to possess a 'gift', a special blessing or power which comes from a superior being which, in the cases we examined, is usually God. This power is not discovered by accident. These people have suffered a multitude of problems or have been very ill; they have visited doctors and later *curanderos*. Finally someone tells them that to improve their own state of health they need to cure others, thus channelling their 'energy'. The discovery of and the maturation of this faculty is usually achieved with the support of another experienced *curandero* who helps them to understand and handle this 'gift'. Nearly all *curanderos* claim to have a spiritual protector through which they can cure. These protectors, saints or religious figures – the 'brothers and sisters of light' – indicate what the patients are suffering from and what has to be done to cure them.

The way *curanderos* practice nowadays can help us to understand some of the reasons why the population turn to them for help. They do not generally have strict practice hours, though if they do, these are long. They are easily accessible and consultations take place in a 'domestic' environment – often the *curandero*'s own home – which gives a feeling of comfort and familiarity. The *curanderos* also make home visits. The type of conversation they have with those who visit them is not as focused as a consultation with a doctor, since *curanderos* need less information to make their diagnosis. Little medical jargon is used and *curanderos*' healing is normally done by placing their hands on certain points of the patient's body, or simply through the powers they claim. *Curanderos* give advice and often highly moralistic verdicts, they recommend herbs with medicinal properties and prepare 'blessed' water and amulets to prevent illnesses. 'Clinical encounters' with a *curandero* could uncover psychological or social problems as well as organic conditions, and family and social circumstances are often discussed.

Although there are no systematically gathered data on the patients, they appear to share the same socio–demographic characteristics as those resorting most often to the national health service, with the elderly and women predominating. 'Culture-bound syndromes' affect children more often, which explains why so many of them are patients of the local specialists. The process of seeking a consultation normally starts when the grandmother, after pointing out that the doctor cannot find out what the child is suffering from, convinces the mother to use this alternative. If the efficiency of the local specialist is proved, on the next occasion it will be the mother herself who opts to take her children to the local specialist.

There is no doubt that both the *curandero* and the local specialist are readily available and receive their patients in an atmosphere that is more appealing than that offered by regular doctors. The consultation itself reflects the eclecticism of their 'clinical practice'. They resort to concepts, practical beliefs and elements which we would place in the realm of 'tradition' and combine these with characteristics of modern western scientific medicine. They consequently achieve a functional practice that answers the needs of ordinary people. The treatment is often lengthy and is given within the social framework of familiar cultural values and religious beliefs predominant in their socio–economic group. This is especially so in the case of the 'culture-bound syndromes', the existence of which makes sense only in a setting where communication is relaxed and flows freely.

From the remarks of the *curanderos*, it appears that they do not see themselves as working against regular doctors. Rather, they feel that they are integrated in the therapeutic network and are resorted to as one 'alternative' by those looking for a cure for their ills. It should also be borne in mind that many of the people who end up consulting a *curandero* do so simply as a last resort after experiencing the failures of western medical science.

However, these healers are perceived differently now compared with a century ago. Regular doctors no longer feel threatened by them and systematic campaigns like the one Sánchez Santana mounted are unthinkable today. Regular practitioners are now much more certain of their pre-eminence in a medical market which has substantially changed, with the health service theoretically encompassing the whole community. Some of them were surprised when one field study demonstrated that between 20 and 35 per cent of their patients also visited *curanderos* and that many of them found it quite normal to go to a local specialist from time to time.[63]

There is also a notable difference in the church's position today. Occasionally the church issues a communiqué denouncing a particular healer who is organizing some kind of religious celebrations, but silence is the usual tactic. Miracles, though possible, are considered by the Catholic Church to be unlikely and signs of miracles are no longer publicized in the way they were at the end of the last century.

## CONCLUSION

It may be concluded that, in the two periods under study, the healing alternatives offered by *curanderos* and local specialists were and still are available to the Alicante population seeking to resolve their health problems. They act in similar ways, from an external point of view, but they fulfil very different functions. At the end of the nineteenth century the *curanderos* and local specialists were a serious option, used frequently by the population and thus a threat to the aspirations of the regular medical profession. Their accessibility made them a very important alternative. The absence of medical insurance and expensive doctors fees meant that *curanderos* and local specialists were attractive and affordable.

Nowadays their presence seems to fill the gaps left by the medical profession who no longer feel that their dominance is threatened. The sometimes poor organization of the health service which makes access difficult, the failure of western medical science to cure many chronic illnesses and the impersonal treatment given by regular doctors push people towards the *curanderos* and local specialists. The efficiency of modern medicine has been brought into question with regard to many illnesses that, although not fatal, result in long periods of suffering. Moreover, the very often impersonal and scientific approach taken by health professionals towards their patients means that psycho–social problems which the patients themselves want to include when explaining their illness are excluded. Here, again, a consultation with *curanderos* and local specialists offers the opportunity to talk about issues that are not normally part of the relationship with the regular doctor; religion, family problems and hopes and anxieties are not often touched upon in the context of modern medicine.

## NOTES

1 E. La Parra López, 'La Restauración: IV. el clima religioso, cultural y educativo durante la Restauración. La prensa periódica', in A. Mestre Sanchis (ed.), *Historia de la Provincia de Alicante* (Alicante, 1985), vol. V, pp. 328–36.

2 E. Balaguer (ed.), 'El modelo médico no institucionalizado en las comarcas del sur del País Valenciano', unpub. MS, Universidad de Alicante, 1987; *idem*, 'La Medicina popular', in J.Mª. López Piñero (ed.), *Historia de la Medicina Valenciana* (València, 1992), vol. III, pp. 197–209; R. Ballester (ed.), 'Caracterización de las alternativas sanadoras no ortodoxas en la ciudad de Alicante', unpub. MS, Universidad de Alicante, 1994.

3 See, among others, W.F. Bynum and R. Porter (eds), *Medical Fringe and Medical Orthodoxy 1750–1850* (London, 1987); N. Gevitz (ed.), *Other Healers. Unorthodox Medicine in America* (Baltimore, MD, 1988); M. Pelling and C. Webster, 'Medical Practitioners', in C. Webster (ed.), *Health, Medicine and Mortality in the Sixteenth Century* (Cambridge, 1979), pp. 165–235; R. Porter, *Health for Sale: Quackery in England 1660–1850* (Manchester, 1989); M. Ramsey, *Professional and Popular Medicine in France, 1770–1830: The Social World of Medical Practice* (Cambridge, 1988).

4 Porter, *Health for Sale*, pp. 14–15. See also J.H. Young, *The Toadstool Millionaires: A Social History of Patent Medicine in America before Federal Regulation* (Princeton, NJ, 1961); *idem*, *The Medical Messiahs: A Social History of Quackery in Twentieth-Century America*, 2nd edn (Princeton, NJ, 1992); *idem*, *American Health Quackery* (Princeton, NJ, 1992).

5 The term *curandero* does not translate easily into English. Most dictionaries suggest the use of the term 'quack', but this differs greatly from our understanding of the word. The term 'healer' is also inadequate and the expression 'faith healer' too restrictive. Although it is true that most *curanderos* in Spain and Latin America healed through faith, the name *curandero* also comprises all those practising medicine without having a formal qualification, their healing methods being

very diverse. We have therefore opted to leave *curandero* untranslated: *Enciclopedia Universal Ilustrada Europeo Americana* (Madrid, 1905–30), vol. XVI, p. 1196. For further discussion on *curanderos* at the end of the nineteenth century, see A. Albarracín Teulón, 'Intrusos, charlatanes, secretistas, curanderos', *Asclepio*, 24, (1972): 323–66.

6 Porter, *Health for Sale*.

7 But see E. Perdiguero Gil, 'La oferta de medicación a la población en la España de la Restauración a través de la prensa periódica: el caso de Alicante (1875–1879)', in J.L. Carrillo and G. Olagüe (eds), *Actas del XXXIII Congreso Internacional de Historia de la Medicina* (Sevilla, 1994), pp. 729–51; *idem*, 'Las alternativas sanitarias extra-académicas en Alicante (1880–1889) a través de la prensa periódica', in H. Capel Sáez, J.Mª. López Piñero and J. Pardo Tomás (eds), *Ciencia e Ideología en la Ciudad* (València, 1994), vol. II, pp. 221–7.

8 R.C. Simons and C.C. Hughes (eds), *Culture-Bound Syndromes: Folk Illnesses of Psychiatric and Anthropological Interest* (Dordrecht, 1985).

9 J.L. de la Vega Gutiérrez, *Medio siglo de medicina en Alicante (Historia del Ilustre Colegio de Médicos, 1894–1936)* (Alicante, 1984), pp. 212–18.

10 A. Albarracín Teulón, 'La titulación médica en España durante el siglo XIX', *Cuadernos de Historia de la Medicina Española*, 12 (1973): 15–80.

11 J.M. de Miguel, *La sociedad enferma (Las bases sociales de la política sanitaria española)* (Madrid, 1979); M.D. Gómez Molleda (ed.), *Los seguros sociales en la España del siglo* XX (Madrid, 1988), 3 vols; J.Mª. López Piñero, 'La colectivización de la asistencia médica: una introducción histórica', in J.M. de Miguel (ed.), *Planificación y Reforma Sanitaria* (Madrid, 1978), pp. 21–47; E. Rodíguez Ocaña, 'La asistencia médica colectiva en España hasta 1936', in *Historia de la acción social pública en España. Beneficencia y Previsión* (Madrid, 1990), pp. 321–61.

12 E. Perdiguero Gil and J. Bernabeu Mestre, 'La asistencia médica pública en el Alicante del siglo XVIII: los médicos de la ciudad', *Canelobre*, 29/30 (1995): 163–76; A. Albarracín Teulón, 'La asistencia médica en la España rural durante el siglo XIX', *Cuadernos de Historia de la Medicina Española*, 13 (1974): 133–304.

13 Dr Zechnas, 'Nuestro parecer', *La Fraternidad Médico–Farmacéutica*, 8 (1887): pp. 113–15. Dr Zechnas was the pseudonym for Esteban Sánchez Santana, MD (1853–1918).

14 E. Balaguer and R. Ballester, 'Desigualdades sociales y en salud en funcion de la ocupación y el sexo: El ejemplo de la Fábrica de Tabacos de Alicante (1875–1936)', in R. Huertas and R. Campos (eds), *Medicina social y clase obrera en España (Siglos XIX y XX)* (Madrid, 1992), vol. I, pp. 49–66.

15 For homoeopathy in nineteenth-century Spain, see A. Albarracín Teulón, 'La Homeopatía en España: Una aproximación a su historia', *Acta Homoepathica Argentinensia*, 11 (1990): 25–50; *idem*, 'Estética, ética y política en la Homeopatía española del siglo XIX', *Acta Homoepathica Argentinensia*, 11 (1990): 51–66.

16 E. Manero Mollá, *Estudios sobre la Topografia Médica de Alicante* (Alicante, 1883), pp. 125–6.
17 Dr Zechnas, 'Cuestión Vital', *La Fraternidad Médico–Farmacéutica* (hereafter *FM–F*), 10 (1887): 145–7.
18 *Idem*, 'Variaciones', *FM–F*, 11 (1887): 161–3; *idem*, '¿Quién es el responsable?', *FM–F*, 11 (1887): 176; *idem*, 'Fenómeno de transparencia', *FM–F*, 19 (1887): 304.
19 *Idem*, 'Uno de tantos', *FM–F*, 12 (1887): 177–8.
20 See n. 18.
21 Dr Zechnas, 'Cuadro número tres', *FM–F*, 14 (1887): 209–12.
22 *Idem*, 'Hidrofobia', *FM–F*, 16 (1887): 255–6.
23 Albarracín Teulón, 'Intrusos, charlatanes, secretistas, curanderos'.
24 Dr Zechnas, 'Siempre lo mismo', *FM–F*, 16 (1887): 241–2.
25 The sentence was published by a national journal, *El Siglo Médico*, 24 (1880): 27–8 and by the local press, *La Unión Democrática*, 7 Oct. 1879, 17 Dec. 1879. It was based on the law of 1855 which regulated the medical profession; this commissioned doctors in each city (the sub-delegate of medicine, under the orders of the Civil Governor) to denounce those practising medicine without the appropriate title. On these laws, see L. Sánchez Granjel, 'Legislación sanitaria del siglo XIX', in *idem* (ed.), *El Ejercicio médico* (Salamanca, 1974), pp. 87–136.
26 E. Salcedo y Ginestal, *Madre e Hijo. Doctrina científica y errores vulgares en Obstetricia y Ginecología* (Madrid, 1898), p. 4.
27 E. La Parra López, 'El clima religioso, cultural y educativo durante la Restauración: El espiritismo', in A. Mestre Sanchís (ed.), *Historia de la Provincia de Alicante* (Alicante, 1985), vol. V, pp. 316–18.
28 Naturalist, medical doctor, homoeopathic practitioner and author of a work on homoeopathy: M. Ausó y Monzó, *La Homeopatía* (Alicante, 1881).
29 A. Castiglioni, *Encantamiento y Magia*, 2nd edn (Mexico, 1972), pp. 293–4.
30 'Baldat' in Catalan, the language spoken by the population of Alicante during the nineteenth century, means disabled. 'Baldaet' is a diminutive of 'Baldat'. For a complete physical description of José Cerdá y Baeza, see A. García López, *La Revelación*, 8 (1879): 115–16.
31 See *La Revelación*, 6 (1877): 249; 6 (1877): 264; 6 (1877): 276–80; 7 (1878): 17–24; 7 (1878): 48; 7 (1878): 120; 7 (1878): 144; 7 (1878): 171–5.
32 He was an exceptional character who combined regular orthodox practice with homoeopathy and spiritualism. He was also a member of parliament and chairman of the Spanish societies of hydrology, spiritualism and homoeopathy. See C. Albarracín Serra, 'Homeopatía y espiritismo: la obra del Dr Anastasio García López', unpub. MD diss., Universidad Complutense de Madrid, 1988.
33 This report is divided into two articles which I henceforth refer to as one work: A. García López, 'Informe dado a la Sociedad Espiritista Española en el mes de Marzo de 1878 por D. Anastasio García López sobre las facultades medianímicas del curandero de Alicante, llamado José Cerda (a) "El Baldaet" ', *La Revelación*, 8 (1879): 115–18, 133–8.

34 The best known was the evil eye: R. Salillas y Panzano, *La fascinación en España. Estudio hecho con la información promovida por la Sección de Ciencias Morales y Políticas del Ateneo de Madrid* (Madrid, 1905). This has never been recognized as an illness by doctors and is considered as a curse by many.
35 García López, 'Informe dado a la Sociedad Espiritista Española'.
36 *La Revelación*, 7 (1878): 17.
37 García López, 'Informe dado a la Sociedad Espiritista Española'.
38 *Ibid.*
39 Ortí Lucas, 'Análisis semántico–documental y estudio epidemiológico de Pego (Alicante)', unpub. MD diss., Universidad de Alicante, 1988, 2 vols; V. Orts Buchón, 'Evolución de los diagnósticos de defunción en Villajoyosa (Alicante)', unpub. MD diss., Universidad de Alicante, 1988.
40 E. Perdiguero, 'Causas de muerte y relación entre conocimiento científico y conocimiento popular', *Boletín de la Asociación de Demografía Histórica*, XI: 3 (1993): 67–88.
41 García López, 'Informe dado a la Sociedad Espiritista Española'.
42 *Ibid.*
43 Dr Zechnas, 'El Gran Apostol', *FM–F*, 13 (1887): 193–4.
44 *Idem*, 'Ni en Africa', *FM–F*, 16 (1887): 273–4.
45 *Idem*, 'Nuestra Denuncia', *FM–F*, 21 (1887): 321–4.
46 *Ibid.*
47 *La Correspondencia de Alicante*, 5 March 1877.
48 *El Semanario Católico*, 31 Jan. 1880, p. 60.
49 *Ibid.*, 31 Jan. 1880, p. 64; 8 Jan. 1882, p. 384.
50 *Ibid.*, 15 April 1876, pp. 175–8.
51 *Ibid.*, 28 April 1883; 'El Milagro de San Genaro juzgado por un librepensador', *ibid.*, 29 Oct. 1881, pp. 433–6; 'El corazón de Santa Teresa de Jesús, su transverberación y sus espinas', *ibid.*, 14 Oct. 1882, pp. 552–7; 'Aparición y milagros en Irlanda', *ibid.*, 10 April 1880, pp. 173–5; 'Las apariciones de Knock en Irlanda: Descripción de las apariciones', *ibid.*, 10 June 1880; 'Acontecimento milagroso', *ibid.*, 7 Nov. 1885, pp. 550–1; 'Noticia', *ibid.*, 6 Feb. 1886, pp. 64–7; 'Curación milagrosa en Cangas', *ibid.*, 2 July 1887, pp. 356–7; *La Unión Democrática*, 24 Sept. 1880; 'La aparición de Nuestra señora de Lourdes', *El Semanario Católico*, 2 Oct. 1880, pp. 498–505; 'La fuente de Lourdes según el abate Pedro Richard', *ibid.*, 2 Oct. 1880; 'Gloria a Dios y a María Santísima de Lourdes', *ibid.*, 2 Oct. 1880, p. 509.
52 See, for example, 'El mundo de los espíritus', *El Semanario Católico*, 12 Nov. 1881, pp. 586–92; 'Los espiritistas delante de los Tribunales de Justicia', *ibid.*, 2 Dec. 1882, pp. 636–40; 'El Espiritismo', *ibid.*, 6 Jan. 1883, pp. 5–10, 13 Jan. 1883, pp. 15–20, 20 Jan. 1883, pp. 28–32, 27 Jan. 1883, pp. 37–41, 3 Feb. 1882, pp. 53–5; 10 Feb. 1883, pp. 66–9.
53 *Ibid.*, 30 Dec. 1882, pp. 688–9.
54 *Ibid.*, 26 May 1883, pp. 307–8.
55 The national health service is funded in three main ways: through

employers, employees and government support. For Alicante and its region, the Comunidad Valenciana, see P. Rodríguez Martínez and M.D. Murria Mele (eds), *Libro Blanco de la Salud de la Comunidad Valenciana* (València, 1991); F. García Benavides, *La Salud en la Comunidad Valenciana* (València, 1992), p. 61.

56 M. Calnan, *Health and Illness. The Lay Perspective* (London, 1980), pp. 1–14.

57 J.Mª. Comelles, 'El papel de los no profesionales en los procesos asistenciales', *Jano*, 29 (1985): 375–62; *idem*, 'La importancia creciente de los no profesionales en los procesos asistenciales', *Canelobre*, 11 (1987): 12–18; E.L. Menéndez, 'El modelo médico hegemónico: transacciones y alternativas hacia una fundamentación teórica del modelo de autoatención en salud', *Arxiu d'Etnografia de Catalunya*, 3 (1984): 83–119.

58 In the different countries in the European Community it has been observed that 'complementary medicines' are used by between 10 and 40 per cent of the population: G. Lewith and D. Aldridge (eds), *Complementary Medicine and the European Community* (Essex, 1991). For a social and political perspective, see K. Bakx, 'The "eclipse" of folk medicine in western society?', *Sociology of Health and Illness*, 13 (1991): 20–38. In Spain data show that about 9 per cent of the population turn to 'alternative' therapies: 'Las terapias paralelas y la medicina clásica', *OCU-Compra Maestra*, 134 (1991): 24–9.

59 E. Perdiguero, 'El mal de ojo de la literatura antisupersticiosa a la Antropología Médica', in A. Albarracín Teulón (ed.), *Misterio y realidad: estudios sobre la enfermedad humana* (Madrid, 1988), pp. 47–66.

60 For a complete account of these surveys, see E. Perdiguero and C. Serrano, 'El curanderisme a l'Alacantí', *Quaderns de Migjorn*, 1 (1993): 169–81. For *curanderos* in Spain today see P. Rodriguez, *Curanderos. Viaje hacia el milagro* (Madrid, 1992).

61 X. Granero, 'La ideología dominante en los estudios de curanderismo urbano', in *Primeres Jornades d'Antropologia de la Medicina* (Tarragona, 1982), vol. 2:1, pp. 69–89.

62 Perdiguero and Serrano, 'Curanderisme a l'Alacanti'.

63 Ballester, 'Caracterización de las alternativas sanadoras no ortodoxas', pp. 17–19.

Chapter 11

# Bosom serpents and alimentary amphibians

## A language for sickness

*Gillian Bennett*

In December 1989 a sensational American newspaper printed a story about a 29-year-old French woman, Marianne Koss, who 'began suffering from an odd illness'.[1] No matter how much she ate she got weaker and weaker, as if she was being deprived of food. 'Meanwhile', she is reported as saying, 'I was getting a very unhealthy looking paunch and hearing strange growling sounds from my stomach. All day long, I'd have a terrible queasy feeling as if something was wriggling round inside of me.' Her doctor decided she must be operated on and the surgeon got to work. The report goes on: 'Stunned, the surgeon watched in horror as the largest frog he ever saw leapt out of Marianne's stomach onto the operating room floor.' Marianne made a full recovery and the frog is said to be at Arles zoo.

Such accounts are not, of course, confined to twentieth-century America. The notion that the human body may be invaded by a noxious creature has been incorporated into a number of different belief systems and is the structuring motif of a wide variety of stories, moral as well as sensational, from many times and places. Such stories can be found in the Puritan literature of Divine Providences, where the events are represented as wonders sent by God;[2] they were used in medieval exempla as cautionary tales about spiritual sickness,[3] in European witchcraft accusations as evidence of the operation of diabolic powers[4] and in the American Deep South as aspects of 'hoodoo'.[5] Among Mexican–American women they may be presented as evidence of the sexual danger men pose to women,[6] among male Indians of women's threat to men[7] and doubtless in many other ways according to the context.

During the past three years, I have compiled a list of over 130 accounts of invading creatures. The latest is the story of Marianne

Koss and the earliest dates from 1612.[8] From even earlier times, there is an apparent allusion to frogs in the stomach in 'The Flyting of Dunbar and Kennedy' (c. 1508) by the 'Scottish Chaucer', Dunbar[9] and an eleventh-century reference to the case of a young monk whose skin was said to be discoloured by worms lodged in his throat.[10] There are accounts from the sixteenth, seventeenth and eighteenth centuries, and from every decade since 1800. I have no doubt that this is still a very partial list which could well double as my researches continue.

My data are all in story form. One is an oral story recorded in 1984. The others have been collected from a variety of written sources – correspondence, newspapers, compilations of folklore and urban legends, collections of medical curiosities, regional magazines, journals of anomalous phenomena, folklore journals and medical journals. Eighty of these stories are reasonably full narratives and come from not too diverse times and places – the northern United States, the United Kingdom and Southern Ireland during the period 1720–1990.[11] What is particularly noticeable about these is that they are all presented as accounts of sickness naturally acquired and, however sensational, show a serious interest in the aetiology, symptomatology and treatment of disease. These characteristics have led me to explore an aspect of stories about bosom serpents and alimentary amphibians that, so far as I am aware, has not been previously documented – their presentation as medical discourse.

Clearly, the narrators of most of these 80 stories consider the happenings they relate to be *medical* events. They may be framed as explanations of a death, or else the narrator may say that the protagonist was 'attacked by various complaints' or 'gradually sickened', or perhaps the events are contextualized in terms of hospitals, doctors and remedies. All the stories share three plot elements: a preoccupation with the sufferings and symptoms, a vivid description of the creature and a story climax in which the victim's sufferings are explained and/or brought to an end. They centre on the concept that illness may be caused by a creature getting into the human body and taking up residence there, feeding either on the host's food or on his or her body so that they become weak, anorexic (though often bloated), pain wracked and tormented by the noises and movements of the creature within their body.

These traditions, though nowadays reduced to the status of 'folklore' by official western medicine, may once have been a part of received medical and zoological knowledge. Extant medical works of fourteenth-century England, for example, list remedies to cope with such emergencies as 'gif an addere oþere eny ouþer evel worme be y-cropyn in-to a manys body, oþer to breyde þer-in' [if an adder or any other evil worm has crept into a man's body in order to breed therein],[12] and Edward Topsell, in his *History of Four-footed Beasts and Serpents* (1658) states that 'Serpents do sometimes creep into the mouths of them that are fast asleep . . . and then is the poor man miserably and wretchedly tormented'.[13]

Fashions of explanation having changed, the symptoms so carefully described in the stories would nowadays probably be put down to gastro–intestinal disorders. However, patients today still commonly utilize animal imagery as a means of visualizing or talking about their disease. A handbook for nurses and social workers, for instance, draws attention to a patient's description of cancer as 'an animal creeping through the body and devouring flesh on the way'.[14] The concept of disease I shall be discussing here can be seen as a literal reading of this sort of visualization, which not only serves as a language to describe symptoms, but is a complete explanatory system, allowing patients to understand how they came to be ill and, as a logical next step, what they must do to be well.

In this essay I look at what the 80 accounts can show about patients and their healers as they wrestle for remedies within this conceptual framework. The story-like nature of this material means that detail such as persons, places or dates should not be interpreted too literally; as one folklorist has memorably said, 'storytellers will tell stories as they damn well please'.[15] We should also remember that there is no independent evidence for their status as fact or fiction. Nevertheless, stories have one advantage which, it seems to me, outweighs these disadvantages. Because they are constantly adjusted to the world view of tellers and hearers, they will reflect contemporary ideas about what is interesting and believable as well as, or better than, apparently more factual and reliable material.

In the following section, I outline the patterns of expectation the stories reveal about patients, healers and the nature and cause of disease. Thereafter I look at the traditional means of ridding oneself of an invading creature, and in the penultimate section I discuss how the stories provide a means of debating the relative efficacy of regular and irregular medicine.

## BOSOM SERPENTS AND ALIMENTARY AMPHIBIANS IN STORY AND TRADITION

> When I was a boy at home, there was a big man in the union house [poor house] who could not work because he had a toad in his stomach. He said it ate the victuals he swallowed, preventing his deriving any nourishment from them, and keeping him continually hungry. When he could get out for a day he used to come to our house to beg a basin of milk, which he said 'quietened' the toad better than anything. He was a tall, large-framed man, with a gaunt, hollow face, like one pined [starved]; and I shall never forget the ravenous way in which he swallowed the milk, and the big lumps of bread and bacon which my mother ordered the servants to bring him. It was of no use trying to persuade him of the impossibility of a toad living in his stomach. His reply was always, 'My mate seed 'is hint legs go down when I was drinkin' watter outen a dyke'.[16]

### The creatures

The story above is typical in the way it implicates amphibians or snakes in human disease. Though a minority of stories refer to tapeworms, octopi, eels and other creatures,[17] over two-thirds refer to snakes, serpents, worms, toads, frogs or newts. Within this general framework of expectation, different places produce their own 'dialect'. In Ireland, for example, there seems to have been a particular dread of newts (variously termed 'man leppers' or 'dark lookers'),[18] and West Yorkshire has a tradition of 'waterwolves',[19] which may also perhaps be newts, though this is by no means certain (dialect dictionaries are not very helpful on this score).

Changing times also produce changing emphases. For example, bosom serpents – snakes lodged in the heart – are mentioned only in the older sources, though snakes and worms crop up throughout the seventeenth and eighteenth centuries in other organs and account for just over half the incidents reported. Alimentary amphibians are particularly numerous in nineteenth-century stories. Twentieth-century narratives feature the most eclectic range of animals.

Special circumstances have also produced distinct variations over time. For example, since the western world became obsessed with fear of obesity there have been persistent rumours that diet pills contain tapeworm eggs which hatch out inside the body.[20] Similarly, from the 1920s onwards the fashion for sea bathing combined with the expansion of the overseas holiday market seems to have produced fears of accidentally swallowing octopus eggs,[21] while the increasing importation of foods from abroad appears to have provided a context for various food panics,[22] including a rumour in the 1920s that a batch of specially large eggs were crocodile eggs which would hatch out once eaten.[23]

The invading creatures share some common features. First and most obviously, they are 'interstitial', that is they do not belong unambiguously to received cultural categories but either cross boundaries or fall between them. They are thus both defiled and dangerous according to Mary Douglas's persuasive analysis[24] and have long been associated in western traditions with evil or magic, or both.[25] But their ambiguity is not the only thing about them that makes them natural candidates for disease causation. Their life cycles, habitats and body shapes also seem to play a part. The overwhelming majority of them belong to egg-laying species and many are (or are thought to be) aquatic for at least part of their life cycle. This makes them obvious candidates for accidental ingestion, especially in areas where people are likely to drink out of natural watercourses or where water quality is poor. In addition, the human digestive organs being popularly conceived of as winding sewers and pond-like sacs, few creatures would seem to be more naturally adapted to this environment than amphibians. Similarly, popular sexual imagery might also play a part in stories where snakes are said to invade the female body.[26]

The creatures are said to get into the body via two routes. Snakes apparently crawl into the mouth and slither down the gullet of sleeping persons, while other creatures are said to be accidentally ingested (often in the form of eggs), in water or on wild foodstuffs. In six stories a doctor demonstrates, to his own satisfaction at least, that there is no creature in the patient's body, but generally its existence is unequivocally proved when it emerges, nearly always alive, from the patient's body. In some stories, the audience is not told exactly why this happens, but usually there is an explanation. Very occasionally it is said to leave voluntarily when its victim is sick or dying, and sometimes it is discovered in the body during an autopsy. In one story the creature is 'hatched' in a woman's body and in another a woman gives birth to it. In most stories, however, there is some sort of medical intervention. Occasionally the patients are cured after dosing themselves with proprietary medicines and sometimes they use traditional methods on themselves (for example, starving or luring the creature out), and in three cases they stumble on the remedy accidentally. In about a quarter of the stories, a member of the regular medical profession gets rid of the creature by means of surgery or purging, and in another quarter quacks or folk healers tempt the creature out using one of the traditional methods.

Interestingly, what storytellers have to say about how the creature was taken from the victim's body appears to be influenced by prevailing medical fashions. Twentieth-century narrators tend to favour surgical removal and nineteenth-century ones usually claim that the creature was vomited. Before the nineteenth century, the preferred exit route seems to be the anal one. Stories in which the creature is tempted out by traditional means, however, come from almost all periods and places.

## The patients

The patients are generally said to be female, young, rural and, in the overwhelming majority of cases, uneducated. There are a number of ways of interpreting these trends. It is possible, for instance, that they may be an artefact of the types of source from which the stories were collected. Almost half come from compilations of legends and folklore made between 1850 and 1950. As the prevailing folklore theory at that time led collectors to focus almost exclusively on the rural poor,[27] this may account for at least some of the dominance of these groups in the stories. To a lesser degree, the influence of the popular concept of folklore as 'old wives' tales' may also account for the high proportion of women patients. However, if the folklore sources were unduly influencing the age, sex and social class ascribed to patients in the stories, one would expect old people to outnumber young ones, for nineteenth-century folklorists valued the old above all other informants. As it happens, however, the patient is said to be old in only five stories.

An alternative explanation for these tendencies is that they are products, not so much of the context in which they were printed, as the world view of the narrators who told them. It is rare for storytellers to remember a story in every detail or to pass it on exactly as they heard it themselves. What they forget will be made up from their stock of cultural assumptions and their personal prejudices. These may include, among other things, sexual metaphors (penile snake imagery that would encourage them to present the invaded person as female), medical and social prejudices (the belief that women are literally the weaker sex) and perhaps class biases that would lead them to ascribe what they see as 'ignorant superstitions' to less well-educated groups of people.

A more literal reading could be that, in the past, these groups made up the bulk of the irregulars' patients and that the presence of an invading animal was a diagnosis favoured by quacks and folk healers. But again, the stories provide little evidence for this reading. The irregulars' patients do not seem to be necessarily either poor or female. There are five stories, for example, where the patient is plainly well to do. In one of these stories the creature exits spontaneously, but in three out of the remaining four the patient is attended by an irregular practitioner. Similarly, out of 35 stories featuring irregular healers, the sexual balance is roughly equal, the patient being said to be a man in 14 cases and a woman in 16 (in the remaining ones, the sex of the patient is not given). More interestingly, regular doctors are not necessarily portrayed as being outside the tradition: seven stories show regular doctors using traditional means to tempt the creature out of their patients' bodies. And, of course, this interpretation does not account for modern stories in which surgeons, with all the resources of scientific medicine at their disposal, relieve patients like Marianne Koss of their unwelcome guests, or a story in which the American Government, no less, advises people to use the traditional cure to rid themselves of tapeworms ingested in diet pills.[28]

It is possible, therefore, to read the stories even more literally; to see them as reflecting the real-life circumstances of the storytellers and their audiences. The fact that women feature in the stories more often than men may simply mean that they are more likely to have an interest in health, to tell medical tales and feature their own sex as protagonists. Similarly, the fact that large numbers of the patients are said to come from rural, remote or disadvantaged areas could simply mean that people from these sorts of background frequently fall prey to digestive disorders. In particular, it could very well be that fears about the quality of the drinking water are an essential part of the context of the tradition. 'No wonder that people think they sometimes swallow frogs', said a contributor to the correspondence magazine *Notes and Queries*,

> there is no doubt that they often do, for the kind of water which poor people are obliged to drink in many country places . . . is dreadful–liquid mud out of ponds trampled up by cows I have

seen standing in tubs to settle, preparatory to being boiled for drinking.[29]

### The healers

In contrast to the predominance of female patients, the healers are principally male. The sex of the practitioner is not always mentioned, but where it is they are said to be men in twenty-one stories, female in only eight. Moreover, whether regular or irregular, healers are nearly always accredited with high social status – so long, that is, as they are successful in finding a cure. In the stories in which the successful removal of the invading creature is achieved by a third person, regular medical attendants are invariably called 'doctor', but so are several practitioners who would appear to be outside the medical establishment. Many of these are referred to by name as if well known ('Doctor Ban', 'Dr Fred Wild', 'Reverend Dr Hankins', and so on), and in two stories apparently irregular practitioners are called 'eminent physicians'. Among the remainder of the irregulars, one is a Patriarch of the Mormon Church and one is a Prince. Two healers are called 'wise women' and one is a 'mum', both terms used approvingly.[30] One is called a 'passing peddlar' but the term is used non-judgmentally and might, in fact, reflect the almost cosmopolitan status of packmen.[31] Of 35 irregular practitioners, only two are referred to disparagingly as 'old women' and only three are called 'quacks'. The impression is therefore that little or no distinction is made between regular and irregular practitioners' status, and that both traditional therapies and traditional healers are well regarded.

## TRADITIONAL THERAPIES

The picture of the popular approach to therapy is given in some detail in 20 stories and in comments on two others, and the picture is independently confirmed in an authoritative article about the folklore of newts.[32] The remedies rely on somehow tricking the creature out of the body. The assumption is that, as the creatures are ravenous and feasting on the hosts' food and drink (if not on the hosts themselves), they can be starved and tempted out by offering them tasty nourishment outside the body. The earliest reference to this belief I have found in story form is from Rabelais's *Quart Livre* (c. 1548), though there is a woodcut from Hieronymous Brunschwig's *Cirurgia* of 1497 which shows a worm being extracted from a patient by holding him upside down over a bowl of milk.[33] In Rabelais's version the giant Bringuenarilles 'fell ill with convulsions of the heart so horrific and dangerous, as if serpents had entered his stomach via the mouth'. The giant's brother recalls that he has 'heard said that a snake, having entered the stomach, suddenly emerges back out if one holds the patient by his feet and places a bowl of milk near his mouth'.[34]

Almost four hundred years later, in 1982, the American Government is said to advise people infested with tapeworms after having taken 'diet pills' to starve for several days:

> Then they set a bowl of hot milk in front of the person. He had to keep his mouth open. After a while the tapeworm began to come up his throat 'cause he smelt the milk. They kept moving the bowl further away until the tapeworm was completely out.[35]

As in this example, the patient is usually forbidden drink for several hours or starved for several days. Alternatively he or she is forced to eat an inordinately large meal but forbidden drink. The food is usually strong tasting and salty bacon is the prime favourite. Salt beef, salt herring and toasted cheese are also frequently mentioned, and 'a pound of salt' and 'a strong solution of salt and water' are advised in two stories. The aim here is to make the creature unbearably thirsty. Sometimes the victims are taken to a stream to await the effects of the remedy; sometimes the cure takes place at home where patients go to bed with a basin of milk or water at hand, or hold their heads over a bowl. Elsewhere the food (roasted meat, onions or milk) is set out in front of the patient to tempt the creature out, the vessel being placed far enough away to make it entirely leave the victim's body. Great care must be taken to shut the mouth promptly so it does not jump back in, and an alternative method is to grab the creature as it comes out of the mouth or to lasso it. A couple of examples will show some variations of the technique.

> A 'worm with legs' ran down a man's throat as he slept in a field, and he pined away [i.e. became very thin], with an ever-increasing appetite, until he was persuaded to consult a 'wise person'. He was kept from drinking for two days by the expert, and then fed on bacon and taken to a stream. The patient's mouth was fastened open, and a freshly toasted piece of bacon put near it. The thirsty 'worm' heard the running water, and

> came out into the man's mouth, where it smelt the meat and sprang on it, fixing its claws in it. The 'wise man' then threw the bacon into the water, and the man rapidly recovered.[36]
>
> Now snakes adore fresh milk, and the only way to save somebody suffering from a snake inside, is to bend the sufferer's head over a bowl of new milk and at the same time to hold a strong band tight against the person's mouth like a noose. When the snake puts its head out to drink the milk, the noose must be suddenly drawn tight behind the snake's head until it is throttled. Then the snake can be drawn out of the sick person's mouth.[37]

Surprisingly, very few deaths are recorded as a result of these procedures; there are only two. In one a nurse is bitten by a hungry snake inside her – one assumes that she was starving the snake before trying the traditional remedy;[38] and in the other, a doctor puts a piece of cheese on his patient's tongue, but when a frog comes up to eat it, it chokes her.[39]

There are also, of course, instances where medical attendants are exposed when they set out to deceive their patients. An account from 1854, for example, reports the prosecution of a 'female quack' for assaulting a young woman by pretending to pull worms from her body (the creature is actually an eel kept for the purpose).[40] There are also 'well known medical stories' in which a regular physician attempts to cure what he believes to be a 'hysterical illness' by pretending to remove frogs or other creatures from a patient. Interestingly enough, the victim in these cases is often unconvinced and persists in being ill, accusing the doctor of having left a breeding female inside.[41]

Despite these exceptions, the consistency of the picture of traditional cures, and the way that they address the cause of disease as seen by the patient, suggests that the majority of patients and healers share a world view and belong to the same community of belief as far as medical matters are concerned.

## DEBATING MEDICAL ALTERNATIVES

When the unanimity of this world view began to crumble, stories about bosom serpents and alimentary amphibians became the vehicle for some very lively debate. The sturdy independence of patients who chose to prescribe their own treatment became anathema to an increasingly professionalized medical establishment.

The regular doctors' position, stated or implied, was that they and they alone were the authority on matters of health.[42] Within this context, tales about invading creatures were useful propaganda for both sides. Told by one group of people, they could be adapted to show the ignorance and incompetence of regular doctors and the validity of popular conceptions. Told by others, they could be used to demonstrate the superstitious ignorance of the average patient and the danger of irregular treatment.

Two well-told stories exemplify the different approaches. The first is a typical, though elaborate, Irish tale.[43] A farmer becomes ill after falling asleep in his hayfield. After a restless night, the doctor is sent for.

> The doctor stripped him and examined him well, but saw nothing out of the way with him. He put his ear to his side and to his back, but he heard nothing, though the poor man himself was calling out: 'Now! now! don't you hear it? Now, aren't you listening to it jumping?' But the doctor could perceive nothing at all, and he thought the man was out of his senses, and there was nothing the matter with him.

Eventually 'there was not a doctor in the county . . . that they had not got'. A passing beggarman then makes his entrance and diagnoses the farmer's trouble as being due to his swallowing an 'alt pluachra' (*lissotriton punctatus*, Ireland's only species of newt).[44] He advises the sick farmer to consult Mac Dermott, Prince of Coolavin, 'the best doctor in Connacht or the five provinces' and this he eventually does. The story ends with the farmer – successfully delivered of 12 baby alt pluachras and their old mother by the traditional method – giving thanks:

> He was for three hours before he could speak a word; but the first thing he said was: 'I am a new man' . . . As long as he was alive he never lay down on green grass again; and another thing, if there was any sickness or ill-health on him, it isn't the doctors he used to call in to him.

The anti-doctor theme is elaborated with considerable emphasis as the story unfolds. The man's wife, for instance: 'could hardly keep in her anger . . . "That doctor *braduch*", says she. "He's not worth a *traneen* [that thieving doctor . . . he isn't worth a straw]; . . . he said himself he knew nothing about anything . . . he'll cross this threshold no more" '. The sick farmer, too, has harsh words for the doctors:

> The doctors, is it . . . My curse on them . . . they know nothing . . . There isn't a medicine man in the county that I hadn't in this house with me, and isn't half the cattle I had on the farm sold to pay them. I never got a relief no matter how small from a man of them.

Thus the story is a powerful advertisement for traditional ways of dealing with health problems.

Its mirror image is a tale taken from the notebooks of an American country physician, written in 1870 and later published by a fellow doctor.[45] This story is framed as a polemic against traditional medicine and in favour of the new 'scientific' approach to disease. It tells how, as a young man, the physician overhears a 'horse doctor' telling how his daughter at the age of 14 was 'drinking out of a . . . spring in the back lot and accidentally swallowed a very tiny snake'. The family find an 'old Indian doctor' who begins 'dosing her with all sorts and kinds of nostrums and concoctions'. Meanwhile, the physician leaves the area and becomes one of the new breed of scientific doctors and makes 'an exhaustive study' of 'anything pertaining to living creatures in the human organs'. Twenty-five years later, having moved back to his home town, he is called in to a mysterious case and finds it is none other than the horse doctor's daughter. 'Her 25 years', he says, had been spent in bed 'telling people of her condition'. 'No doubt', he observes, 'during all the strenuous treatments to which she had been subjected, her life had been put to the test and even laid low from the harsh remedies which had been employed without doing her a particle of good'. His treatment is to persuade her to get up from her bed and return to normal life. The patient is not convinced, and asks, 'Yes, but what about the snake? How will you get him?' 'Martha', he says. 'You haven't any snake'. He reflects that:

> It was a case that didn't need medicine . . . Instead of whimsical notions from her father, she should have been told the truth about her hysterical condition. This would have saved her twenty-five years of suffering and a fortune spent on her without help or relief.

The patient gradually recovers some of her strength and marries her childhood sweetheart. After her death shortly afterwards, an autopsy is performed. Her lungs are shown to have been 'almost entirely consumed' with tuberculosis.[46]

The second story is thus a mirror image of the first: the failure of the regular doctors in the Irish story is matched by the failure of the 'old Indian doctor' and a host of other empirics in the American story. In the Irish story the family are almost bankrupted by the expense of the regulars and in the American story they are almost ruined by the irregulars; in the Irish story all the regulars fail while in the American all the irregulars fail; in the Irish story traditional concepts of illness are triumphantly justified when no fewer than 12 little alt pluachras and their mother come from the patient's body, and in the American one scientific medicine is justified when the autopsy proves that the patient is suffering from a common disease not a bizarre infestation.

An English perspective on this debate can be seen in the columns of *Notes and Queries*. Between 1852 and 1854, just before the establishment of the General Medical Council and at a time of active contention between regular and irregular practitioners, there was a lengthy correspondence on the subject of 'Newspaper folklore'. This had been initiated by a person calling himself 'A Londoner' who, deploring the inhumanity of an age which could allow a child to suffer so, had sent in a story about a little girl who had a snake lodged 'just above her diaphragm'.[47] Two correspondents reply to 'A Londoner's' letter. The first remarks that he has often read such stories in the provincial press and has always thought them 'to be emanations from the brains of that highly imaginative class of persons, the village correspondent';[48] the second is a Birmingham surgeon who regards all such cases as hypochondria and sends in two personal experience stories illustrative of the ignorant superstitions of his patients.[49] Two years later 'A Londoner' revives the subject, enclosing a newspaper account of the 'Escape of a snake from a man's mouth'.[50] A correspondent promptly writes to correct his account. The creature was a worm not a snake, he says, and was swallowed in the East Indies where 'such things are common enough'.[51] Five other correspondents now join in. Three people send factual letters discussing the phenomenon and alleging that no creature could survive in the acidic environment of the human stomach and two people send in amusing little dismissive anecdotes.[52]

The tradition is so vital, however, that the discussion is spontaneously renewed almost 50 years later in 1901.[53] Matters were still so far undecided, however, that in 1903 a correspondent calling himself 'Dubious', apparently unaware of the previous controversy, writes to the magazine in some perplexity:

> I have several times met with remarkable stories in the newspapers of men and women vomiting newts, frogs, eels etc . . . which have developed in the stomach of the patient. I have always regarded it as impossible . . . but in some of these newspaper reports the names of the persons concerned have been given, and the stories have been vouched for by medical men. I should be obliged if any reader . . . could say definitely what truth (if any) there is likely to be in such stories, and whether there is the slightest danger in swallowing (say) the egg of a newt.[54]

## CONCLUSION

The 80 stories that I have discussed in this essay are dramatic codifications of a coherent body of medical information. Though we must be careful to keep in mind that they represent a 'storified' version of a medical tradition, the picture seems to be a naturalistic one and I would argue that it can be taken seriously as the medical discourse of lay persons and (more cautiously) as evidence of medical practice.

I have suggested that the stories are likely to reflect ordinary people's lives and physical conditions fairly accurately. The circumstances described appear to be just those that would foster traditions attributing disease to the predations of evil or defiled creatures in the human body. These traditions have probably been particularly popular in times and places where the condition of the drinking water would give rise to fears of pollution and where creatures might be easily ingested by accident. Though they are all interstitial, the creatures that are said to get into the body are real animals appropriate to the locations in which they are said to lurk and in which the story events are set. They get into the body by natural, not supernatural means, and the cure is to get them out.

The image of the invading creature fits the symptoms the patients describe very well, helping them to visualize their sickness and discuss their sufferings with others. In turn, the explanation suggests the cure. This may be effected by force or trickery. Regular physicians usually resort to force; irregulars tend to prefer trickery. Both may be successful – as long as the diagnosis is accepted. It is up to the patients to choose their healer or their therapy, and the stories frequently show patients engaged in the exercise of that choice. The stories give no indication that irregular practitioners and traditional methods were regarded as second rate by those who used them, and no indication of any secrecy or shame attached to either. Though, according to the stories, women are more likely than men to seek medical advice, men are almost equally likely to consult an irregular or adopt unorthodox treatment for their ills. Men also provided the bulk of the medical attendants – all the regular ones and the majority of the irregulars too.

There are two aspects of the stories that are especially interesting. The first is that the stories provide evidence of a very specific approach to therapy which does not reveal itself so clearly elsewhere, as far as I am aware. The remedies might even have been attempted on occasion. Certainly, they are a logical next step from the diagnosis. They have other very persuasive advantages too; they take the patient's description at face value and work *with* it. In particular, they potently address the folk belief that 'disease is an entity which is "in" until it is brought "oot" ', as Scottish physician David Rorie has memorably said.[55] The more recalcitrant the disease, the more obdurate the creature within, so the more complex the procedure for getting it out. The theatrical show put on for, or by, the patient – the starvation, the tying up, the lassoing and so on – is expertly geared to this conception of sickness and cure.

Then again, traditional therapies are low-technology, inexpensive options. They do not involve 'medicine' and they do not require patients to be 'ill', to stop work or hand over their autonomy to the healer. Once known, they can be self-administered and they rely only on the self-discipline of the patient and on the utilization of homely foodstuffs – mainly salt or milk. Best of all, they contain a built-in explanation of failure. If the patient continues to be ill, then obviously one of the creatures has got back in or been left to breed, hence the number of stories that insist that the alt pluachras, or whatever, emerge in family groups accompanied by the mother, who is always the most difficult and most wily of them all.

The second significant aspect of stories about bosom serpents and alimentary amphibians is their ability to be a vehicle for dialectic debate. Thus they may become a *cause célèbre* through which popular ignorance may be deplored or the failures of doctors exposed. On the one hand, telling 'well-known medical stories' about credulous patients demonstrates the scientific superiority of the regular medical profession and asserts doctors' authority on medical matters. Conversely for the patient, telling stories about doctors' ignorance and the triumph of their own diagnosis gives them the confidence to defend their right to know what is wrong with them.

Stories of bosom serpents and alimentary amphibians are thus a complete language for talking about sickness. They are a metaphor-come-true which allows a rational aetiology to be deduced from the central image and a logical cure devised. But they are also a means whereby lay persons may talk informedly to each other and to their therapists about the nature and course of their sufferings. Best of all, they are a means through which the efficacy of the various medical alternatives may be debated. The doctor need never have the last word (though he often does even here). The stories are there to be told, to demonstrate that no matter how many times patients are told that their sufferings are imaginary, in the end the scoffers will be confounded and the patient will be dramatically vindicated.

## NOTES

1 Dr Bruno Gosse, 'Docs nearly croak when 4lb frog is removed from woman's stomach', *Sun*, 12 Dec. 1989, p. 15.

2 See, for example, Increase Mather, *Remarkable Providences Illustrative of the Earlier Days of American Colonization* (Boston, MA, 1684), n.p.

3 Jacques Berlioz, 'L'Homme au crapaud: Genèse d'un exemplum médiéval', in Centre alpin et rhodanien d'ethnologie (ed.), *Tradition et histoire dans la culture populaire* (Grenoble, 1990).

4 See, for example, the trial of Julian Cox in 1663: Alan C. Kors and Edward Peters, *Witchcraft in Europe 1100–1700: A Documentary History* (Philadelphia, PA, 1972), p. 306.

5 See, for example, Richard M. Dorson, *Negro Folktales in Michigan* (Cambridge, MA, 1956), p. 108; Harry H. Hyatt, *Hoodoo, Conjuration, Witchcraft, Rootwork* (New York, 1970–78); Newbell Niles Pucket, *Folk Beliefs of the Southern Negro* (Chapel Hill, NC, 1926), pp. 249–53; Frances Cattermole-Tally, 'The intrusion of animals into the human body: fantasy and reality', *Folklore*, 106 (1995): 89–91.

6 See, for example, Rosan A. Jordan, 'The vaginal serpent and other themes from Mexican–American Women's Lore', in Rosan A. Jordan and Susan J. Kalčik (eds), *Women's Folklore, Women's Culture* (Philadelphia, PA, 1985), pp. 26–44.

7 Verrier Elwin, 'The vagina dentata legend', *British Journal of Medical Psychology*, 19 (1943): 443.

8 J.G. Wallace-James, 'Animals in people's insides', *Notes and Queries*, 9 (viii) (1901), quoting Calderwood's *Historie of the Kirk of Scotland* (no further details given).

9 Priscilla Bawcutt, *Dunbar the Maker* (Oxford, 1992), p. 37. My thanks to Jacqueline Simpson for this reference.

10 Pierre-André Sigal, *L'Homme et le Miracle dans la France médiévale (XIe–XIIe siècle)* (Paris, 1985), p. 43. My thanks to Jean-Bruno Renard for this reference.

11 The others come from widely different times and places or are paraphrases, summaries or otherwise incomplete. For the purposes of discussion I have left these to one side in order to concentrate on the fuller and more homogeneous group of stories.

12 George Henslow, *Medical Works of the Fourteenth Century* (London, 1899), p. 18.

13 Quoted in Robert D. Arner, 'Of snakes and those who swallow them: some folk analogues for Hawthorne's "Egotism; Or, The Bosom Serpent" ', *Southern Folklore Quarterly*, 35 (1971): 337.

14 Phyllis H. Williams, *South Italian Folkways in Europe and America: A Handbook for Social Workers, Visiting Nurses, School Teachers, and Physicians* (New Haven, CT, 1938), p. 167.

15 Keith Cunningham, 'The Vanishing Hitchhiker in Arizona-Almost', *Southwest Folklore*, 3 (1979): 48.

16 R.R., 'Frog folk-lore', *Notes and Queries*, 6 (i) (1880): 392.

17 There are also single accounts involving a centipede, a slug, beetle larvae, a 'beast', a 'nest of insects' and a mouse; also, rather more idiosyncratically, a 'live creature', 'something wick', 'two uncommon creatures', 'live animals about the size of a sixpence' and 'something . . . like a monkey'.

18 Douglas Hyde, *Beside the Fire: A Collection of Irish Gaelic Folk Stories* (London, 1890), p. 183.

19 Ian Dewhirst, 'The Haworth water-wolf, and others', *Transactions of the Yorkshire Dialect Society*, part 62, vol. 11 (1962): 25–7; *idem*, 'T'watter-wolf', *The Countryman* (Spring 1966): 105–8; *idem*, 'In search of the water-wolf', *Lore and Language*, [1] (4) (1971): 12–14.

20 Ronald L. Baker, *Hoosier Folk Legends* (Bloomington, IN, 1982), p. 226; Jean-Loïc LeQuellec, *Alcool de Singe et Liqueur de Vipère . . . plus quelques autres recettes* (Vouillé, 1991), pp. 59–61; Elizabeth Tucker, 'The seven-day wonder diet: magic and ritual in diet folklore', *Indiana Folklore*, 11 (1978): 141–50, esp. p. 144.

21 'Sorry about that, myth!', *Daily Mirror* ('Live Letters' column), 15 April 1986; Jan Harold Brunvand, *The Choking Doberman and Other 'New' Urban Legends* (New York and London, 1984), pp. 110–11. See also Stith Thompson, *Motif Index of Folk Literature* (Helsinki, 1932–36, revised and enlarged edition Bloomington, IN, 1955–58), motif B784.1.4.

22 See, for example, Gary Alan Fine, 'Mercantile legends and the world economy: dangerous imports from the Third World', *Western Folklore*, 48 (1989): 153–62; William M. Clements, 'Catflesh in Mexican food: meaning in a contamination rumor', *Studies in Popular Culture*, 14 (1991): 39–51.

23 See 'A crocodile scare. An amusing hoax over Egyptian eggs', *IP News*, 15 April 1920, p. 8.

24 Mary Douglas, *Purity and Danger: An Analysis of Concepts of Pollution and Taboo* (London, 1966). See also William M. Clements, 'Interstitiality in contemporary legends', *Contemporary Legend*, 1 (1991): 81–91.

25 See, for example, Harry H. Hyatt, *Folklore from Adams County, Illinois* (New York, 1935), nos 1580–91; George Ewart Evans, *The Horse in*

*the Furrow* (London, 1960), pp. 260–71; E. and M.A. Radford, *The Encyclopedia of Superstitions*, ed. and revised by Christina Hole (London, 1980), pp. 341–3.

26 Indeed, the sexual content is quite overt in some stories from areas other than the northern United States, the United Kingdom and Ireland. Tales of vaginal serpents are told by Mexican–American women (see Jordan, 'The vaginal serpent'). In other accounts from the southern states of America the presence of an invading creature is mistaken for an out-of-wedlock pregnancy: see Dorson, *Negro Folktales*, pp. 150–1. The current discussion, however, focuses only on stories told in the northern United States. Note, too, that in stories from these regions snakes are just as likely to invade the bodies of males as females.

27 Gillian Bennett, 'Folklore studies and the English rural myth', *Rural History*, 4 (1993): 77–91.

28 Baker, *Hoosier Folk Legends*, p. 226.

29 R.R., 'Frog Folk-Lore'.

30 Other neutral terms used are (once each) 'apothecary', 'gentlemen', 'druggist', 'chemist', 'herbalist', 'surgeon' and 'they'.

31 See, for example, Margaret Spufford, 'The pedlar, the historian and the folklorist: seventeenth-century communications', *Folklore*, 105 (1994): 13–24.

32 Edward Peacock, 'Superstitions relating to the newt', *Folk-Lore*, 10 (1899): 251–2.

33 My thanks to Matthew Ramsey for this reference. The woodcut is reproduced in D.G. Guthrie's *History of Medicine* (London, 1945) facing p. 129.

34 Quoted in LeQuellec, *Alcool de Singe et Liqueur de Vipère*, p. 65. My translation.

35 Baker, *Hoosier Folk Legends*, p. 226.

36 Thomas J. Westropp, 'A folklore survey of County Clare', *Folk-Lore*, 22 (1911): 454.

37 Comment following story in Martin Hughes, 'Strange tales of Lincolnshire: the adder', *Lincolnshire Life*, 8: 7 (1958): 46.

38 Rodney Dale, *The Tumour in the Whale: An Hilarious Collection of Apocryphal Anecdotes* (London, 1978), pp. 74–5. Needless to say, readers are strongly advised not to attempt any of these methods.

39 J.B. Partridge, 'Notes on English folklore', *Folk-Lore*, 28 (1917): 311–15.

40 C. Mansfield Ingleby, 'Newspaper folklore', *Notes and Queries*, 1 (ix) (1854): 276–7.

41 *Ibid.*, 1 (vi) (1852): 466.

42 Roy Porter, *Health for Sale: Quackery in England 1660–1850* (Manchester, 1989), p. 201.

43 Hyde, *Beside the Fire*.

44 *Ibid.*, p. 183.

45 Donald J. Sawyer, 'The lady with the snake in her', *New York Folklore Quarterly*, 25 (1969): 299–305.

46 Cynics will note the irony. The sceptical regular doctor, by using the term 'consumed', unconsciously echoes the language and assumptions of the tradition he criticizes. They might also note that, despite his triumphant air, the physician failed to diagnose her condition.
47 A Londoner, 'Newspaper folklore', *Notes and Queries*, 1 (vi) (1852): 221.
48 KPDE, 'Newspaper folklore', *Notes and Queries*, 1 (vi) (1852): 338.
49 Ingleby, 'Newspaper folklore', *Notes and Queries*, 1 (ix) (1854): 276–7.
50 A Londoner, 'Newspaper folklore', *Notes and Queries*, 1 (ix) (1854): 29–30.
51 Mackenzie Walcot, 'Newspaper folklore', *Notes and Queries*, 1 (ix) (1854): 84.
52 See the remaining correspondence under the title of 'Newspaper folklore', in *Notes and Queries*, 1 (ix) (1854): 276–7, 523–4.
53 See the correspondence about 'Animals in people's insides', *Notes and Queries*, 9 (vii) (1901): 222–3, 332–3, 390–2; 9 (viii) (1901): 89–90, 346; 9 (xii) (1903), 414–15, 471.
54 Dubious, 'Animals in people's insides', *Notes and Queries*, 9 (xi) (1903): 467–8.
55 David Buchan (ed.), *Folk Tradition and Folk Medicine in Scotland: The Writings of David Rorie* (Edinburgh, 1994), p. 100.

Chapter 12

# Women as *Winti* healers

## Rationality and contradiction in the preservation of a Suriname healing tradition

*Ineke van Wetering*

The survival of 'magic' in a group that has been in contact with the modern world for centuries is generally looked upon as a sign of cultural conservatism. Moreover, resistance to the ideology of a dominant stratum has often been noted as a strong force that will keep 'tradition' alive. This is certainly true of so-called *Winti* beliefs and practices as found among the urban lower classes of the Creole population in Suriname, many of whom migrated to the Netherlands in the 1970s. The Creoles, descendants of slaves brought from Africa to the Caribbean, have long been exposed to a civilizing campaign against 'idolatry' and 'quackery', launched by both the Dutch colonial state and the Christian churches. These efforts have been partly successful as most Creoles profess a Christian creed and turn to modern western medicine whenever the need for treatment arises. This, however, does not prevent some of them from cherishing the African cultural heritage, so they will add rituals to modern medical practices for the promotion of health and well-being, and consult traditional healers – both in Suriname and the Netherlands.

Data on the *Winti* cult in the Netherlands have been gathered in one of Amsterdam's new suburbs, Bijlmermeer. A large number of Creole migrants from Suriname, who feared for their future when Suriname gained independence in 1975, have settled there. The high ethnic population density of the suburb – about 25 per cent of Bijlmermeer's inhabitants are Surinamese, and in some apartment buildings the percentage is considerably higher – has enabled the residents to maintain a community life that in many ways is reminiscent of Paramaribo, Suriname's capital. Many inhabitants are unemployed and have received little schooling. The elderly and the numerous single women mostly live off social security benefits, as do many of the young. A great number of households are female headed. The newcomers show allegiance to various 'traditional' institutions related to kinship and religion, and the specific mixture of beliefs and practices, mostly referred to as *Winti* – after the belief in possessing spirits that is one of the characteristics of the belief system – contains distinct ideas about healing with magical connotations.[1]

In looking for explanations for a lingering traditionalism we do well to pay attention to what the adepts have to say. We may safely assume that they see a rationale in their behaviour. Whether they entertain the *Winti*-related complex of beliefs consciously and express these in so many words is another matter. People are often only partly aware of their motivation and will express their views in chance remarks or in symbolic language. Direct questioning on the part of the researcher rarely produces unambiguous results. Most adherents will cling to an appeal to 'tradition'.

Anthropologists look for an interpretation in their own way, which more often than not turns out to be different from the insiders' view. The very language in which the interpretation is stated is different. As a rule anthropologists will not see *Winti* as purely or mainly 'African', as some adherents do.[2] Rather, they see the religious system as syncretic, in which African, Christian and other elements have been blended during more than three centuries of colonial domination, resistance and accommodation. It has also been suggested[3] that *Winti* is part of the survival strategies employed by a marginal population segment; the ethics of kinship are invoked as a buttress against the vicissitudes of migration and life in a periphery.

The issue to be addressed here is the logic of social reproduction. World views will only survive when actively reproduced by a human group.[4] In the process, more than one reason, motive or mechanism may be involved. Among Creoles, solidarity among kin is a significant incentive. Those who have an interest in the support of a kin group, mostly lower-class women, will make an effort to promote solidarity by sponsoring rituals. Thus the enhancement of well-being – the express and manifest goal of a *Winti* ritual – is one reason behind the efforts to keep tradition alive. In the home country the recruitment of kin used to be a demanding task and in the Netherlands it is even more difficult. Forms of entrepreneurship are required to bring relatives and other members of an ethnic community together. Entrepreneurship, however, has a dynamic of its own and is liable to create conflicts between aims and means. Here we shall discuss the mobilizing efforts and strategies of women who embark on careers as informal healers, and see how they deal with such conflicts.

## MEDICAL AND RELIGIOUS PLURALISM

The efficacy of the civilizing policy mentioned above, implemented energetically for about a century, is borne out by the fact that most Creoles regard themselves as Christians and consult doctors. The offensive set in too late, however, to dislodge a cultural complex that was formed on the plantations and had survived in secret. The result has been ambiguous[5] but has hardened into a social code. In formal settings, any allegiance to African–American beliefs and practices is denied, yet it is fully understood that the realities of private life diverge from the formal model. All who cherish aspirations to rise in the social hierarchy – and on the whole, men had greater opportunities to realize these than women – would stress membership of a church or one of the many associations like the Freemasons. Nevertheless, many Creoles view 'the culture' as part of their identity.

A similar pluralism is found in medical matters. All Creoles will turn to the institutions of western health care which are available. Whenever these fail to provide relief, however, or when it is felt that other forces are involved, a traditional healer will be consulted. A distinction between 'doctor's disease' and 'Negro's illness' – complaints to be submitted respectively to medical or ritual specialists – has for a long time been part and parcel of popular culture.[6] Although middle-class Creoles will look askance at most manifestations of *Winti*, in cases of emergency this is one of the alternative traditions they may turn to.

Some of the embarrassment has disappeared since the administrative repeal in Suriname of all prohibitions on *Winti* rituals in 1971. Young intellectuals in search of a new identity and 'roots' stress the positive side of the cultural heritage.[7] This does not imply, however, that all the stigma attached to *Winti* has been removed. As an ideology that underpins solidarity between kinship groups, *Winti* touches sensitive issues. Poor relatives can apply to those more fortunate by defining distress in terms of the supernatural, thus illness and misfortune present an occasion to activate the struggle between social classes and their respective world views.

The cultural heritage is, like all forms of culture, not an unchanging corpus of belief and practice. In *Winti* there has always been ample space for personal interpretations and initiatives and this certainly holds true in the Netherlands, but has been equally applicable in Suriname. On the one hand, there are factors that make for continuity. There is much social activity among Creoles and great efforts are made to keep networks intact. This facilitates a reinforcement of shared assumptions. Social control is often experienced as tight and gossip is much feared. On the other hand, opportunities for changes in lifestyle are great. The brittleness of kin ties plays a part and the social organization of *Winti* beliefs and practice are also conducive to change. The private character of ritual therapy, and the fact that one's personal guardian spirit may provide a legitimate inspiration (even if not in accordance with tradition), result in further fragmentation. The ensuing freedom for *bricolage* makes it easy to use ritual measures as a supplement to medical treatment.[8] 'Even if it is to no avail, no harm is done' often seems to be the motto, and it is a view shared by many Surinamese general practitioners in Bijlmermeer. However, the symbolic use of herbal remedies and paraphernalia can bring people to carry out actions that are contrary to modern western assumptions.

Much of *Winti*'s appeal is in its magical ritual. In a holistic world view, the adepts see a connection between a disruption of physical functioning and the relations between human beings and the preternatural. Illness, misfortune and failures in the social field are attributed to the wrath of the spirits. Only by appeasing the unseen powers can one hope for health, success and well-being. In concrete cases, this attitude is put into practice at different levels of sophistication. Attempts are made to escape police arrest and detention by placing offerings close to the court building. When in fear of losing a social security benefit the same may be done near the welfare office. Such action was not unusual in Suriname. As a corollary of a style of thinking this may be called 'rational', but it is usually not accepted as such by modern observers.

In some practices a rationale can be detected which is acceptable to western minds. As in many other therapeutic systems from Africa or other parts of the world, *Winti* rituals open up ways to induce changes in those involved that would be hard to bring about by secular means only. Expressed in symbolic language, participants may be confronted with aspects of their attitudes and behaviour which are harmful or a barrier to optimal functioning. By means of ritual, attempts can be made to bring conflicts into the open, to remove psychological blocks and mobilize inner forces for perseverance or a new start. As these aspects have been discussed elsewhere,[9] there is no reason to go into detail here. For a marginal section of the population, among whom many have dropped out of the race for social success, these practices can be a valuable source of support.

## *WINTI* HEALERS

Whoever looks for recognition as a *Winti* healer or *bonuman* should be able to present some credentials. An intimate knowledge of 'tradition' is a first requirement, gained by participation in the social life of a district where *Winti* is practised, and personal contact with elder kin who have been active as healers. These are accepted as guarantees against malpractice. Rural communities, in particular those of the plantations from which most Creoles trace their descent, are part of a mythical image of true religion and social harmony. The kin group, originating from a specific plantation, used to be the cult group.[10] This is no longer so, but the myth of the plantation is still valid.

This implies that those who have moved to the city in search of education and a job cannot boast of the right qualifications for the healing role, so the openings for an alternative career as healer are reserved for people who are underprivileged in other ways. As a creed of one-time slaves and of rural communities in later days, *Winti* beliefs could uphold patterns of equality for a long time. These views are well attuned to relations within an urban fringe and a *Winti* spirit is regarded as free to select a medium. Apart from the elderly, to whom special connections with the unseen powers are attributed, women and children are often looked upon as their vessels, and this offers women an opportunity to exert influence.

This is accepted not only by common believers but also by the middle classes, who are equally inclined to attribute therapeutic potential to those who control few secular resources.[11] Moreover, the well-off and educated who have not grown up with *Winti* have only vague notions of what it entails. Many Creoles openly state that their attempts to gain a better understanding of their background have been in vain and the complaint that any search for the roots of their own culture was fruitless is an almost standard reply. What people remember is the doings of a grandmother in traditional clothing who busied herself with herbs and other things children should not be inquisitive about. Thus knowledge about traditional ritual healing is a scarce resource, to which the disadvantaged have privileged access. Furthermore, this type of knowledge is constructed in a way that implies a challenge to middle-class notions. It is not the kind of learning received at school which counts, but the knowledge only life itself can bring. Apart from this, the supernatural beings are the only reliable source of authority. A medium of a high-ranking spirit who makes a pronouncement in a state of trance, speaks *ex cathedra*. When a serious problem presents itself, an interpretation offered by a spirit must be accepted. Human beings are liable to dissimulate, but 'the dark is sincere'.

Those aspiring to perform a healing role are numerous and rivalry is intense, especially among men. They will often play the 'bigger fish' game, each having guardian spirits with sporting names like *Man moro man* ('man overcomes others') and may gain favour in that way.[12] But the risks are great. Men are often suspected of practising *Winti* for financial gain only, and to commit fraud.[13] Tall stories about swindling male healers are common, a stigma that is not attached to female *bonuman*. To this day, women often look for other women when in need of a ritual expert. In the ethnic community the interests of patients, often one's children and other relatives, are regarded as safe when entrusted to a maternal figure.

## Women and healing rituals

As Herskovits and Herskovits already noted in the 1920s, women act as the guardians of traditional culture.[14] This is related to their mediating role in family, kin group and society, and is the outcome of a historic process. Sexual relations used to be the main links between the dominant group and slaves, and later between the dominant group and the lower strata.[15] During the slavery period, women's chances of manumission were larger than those of men and children were likely to be emancipated with their mothers.[16] Women's position as intermediaries has deeply influenced both the kinship system and religion.

In the relations with the out group, women have adhered to this role. In the period after the Second World War, lower-class women also gained opportunities for power exertion in the public domain. In Suriname politics, the branches of the main Creole party on a ward level were in women's hands.[17] Politicians looked for support among potential voters and women supplied this, gaining some advantages as a result. This is partly to be regarded as no more than the defence strategy of a marginal sector (the benefits reaped by men were usually bigger), but still these tactics were not unsuccessful. As with other 'black' groups in the western hemisphere, women are active in maintaining networks of kin and other relations.[18]

A primary religious domain is the home, where the mother and maternal grandmother are in charge. Unskilled men, unable to offer security, often remained unattached to their partners' household or to that of other kin. This pattern, common in Paramaribo, is retained in the Netherlands.[19] Women expect to be self supporting; they greatly value a position as main tenant of their apartment and their independent authority over the children. The home serves as a basis for an outward thrust and, by ritual means, is converted into public space. Whenever situations arise that demand ritual action, women are the first to assist each other in the venture. It is hard now to get a kin group together for communal rituals but as a rule, the members of a household, relatives that can be recruited at short notice, and others who belong to a personal network, form the impromptu social units that keep tradition alive.

The organization of festivities, secular and sacred, figures largely in the mobilizing efforts of this ethnic group.[20] Healing rituals are part of informal ethnic politics. This aspect is of interest for discussion in the field of feminist studies about women's opportunities for playing a part in public life. The generalization, that the sphere of activity allotted to female healers is restricted to the domestic space,[21] is not applicable to the Creole group. To embark on a career as healer, which becomes possible after the menopause, means to engage in a form of entrepreneurship. Lower-class women who strike out on this market are up against the dominant, modern western notions and practices of the middle class and elite.

## Healers and entrepreneurship

Apart from kinship networks, the relation between healers and patients is one of the links that affiliates potential adherents. This tie is usually a personal one; it is often honoured after concluding the treatment proper. A healer will try to muster a stable following beyond the confines of his or her kin group. It is far from easy, though, to start a cult group on bases other than kinship relations. As indicated above, suspicion is always rife that personal gain is the ultimate aim. On the other hand, ritual experts are much in demand, so aspiring healers see many opportunities. However, a change in organizational form, from family cult to leader–follower model, can hardly be without consequences. Although intended to maintain or even save 'tradition', the change in reproductory mode may have some unforeseeable effects.

There is a manifest difference between the chances that male and female healers have to achieve a position on the healing market. The opportunities for men to establish contacts with formal institutions in Dutch health care, social work and control systems are better than those of women. Some male specialists can boast of a training in social work, nursing or anthropology, and speak a language understood by functionaries in hospitals, institutions and prisons. This is not to say that such strategies are without risk. As mediators between cultural worlds, the entrepreneurs are forced to enter into negotiations with the outside world and develop a defence strategy to make their own approach acceptable. These manoeuvres often undermine a healer's reputation among his peers. In the eyes of potential followers, an orientation to western middle-class norms discredits their magical powers.

Women who entertain hopes of gaining a foothold as healers mostly lack the cultural assets and do not fulfil other requirements for successfully making such contacts. Their resources in terms of time, money and energy are restricted. The social base for a female healer's role, that of mother and grandmother, demands investments which can only be used on one occasion or for one goal and are thereafter useless in maintaining relations with the outside world. Material resources are deployed and absorbed by events in the inner circle. Contacts between kin and other relevant relations, essential for credibility and reputation, demand full personal attention and do not carry those involved beyond the ethnic community. A disadvantage is that the circle of potential clients is narrow, but a positive effect is that this strategy does not detract from one's religious charisma.

Disappointments in life, experiences of powerlessness and failure – almost inevitable for people in this social sector – count as conditional for acceptance as a healer. It is argued that, without personal acquaintance with life's vicissitudes, empathy with the problems of others would be impossible. Suffering which has left its traces yields dignity and authority. As a result, the behaviour of healers in the semi publicity of group life is usually calm and reserved. This is regarded as befitting all persons of senior age, but is pre-eminently expected of ritual experts. A certain aloofness also gives ample occasion to observe what is going on and this engenders 'capital' – in the form of information – for a diagnosis of current problems. This attitude is useful for the type of complaints presented to healers for treatment as these matters are often related to interpersonal conflicts.[22] As in most circles, where religion and healing are linked a definition of illness or symptoms is a general or broad one; all forms of physical and psychic affliction, misfortune and bad luck are thought fit to be dealt with ritually. Expected successes that fail to materialize are also an occasion to look for therapy: 'not doing well' or 'not prospering' is a frequently heard complaint.

## The ups and downs of a female healer – the case of Orsyla

Orsyla's life history is well suited to illustrate the career of a female healer who ventured into entrepreneurship. Although she grew up in the city and lacked healers among her relatives and, as a consequence, was not predestined for the role, she did belong to the disadvantaged. The course of her life – a micro history – can be taken as typical for that of numerous women of her class. Her story shows to what extent a career as a healer comes naturally and is intertwined with both the routine of a woman's daily life and notions of ritual. At the same time it shows that it is perfectly possible for the venture to come to nothing. In that case the healer ends as one among the many maternal figures in her social circle.

Orsyla was born during the economic recession of the early 1930s. She grew up in a lower-class neighbourhood in Paramaribo as the eldest daughter in a female-headed household. Orsyla hardly knew her father, having met him once, by coincidence, in a shop when she was eight years old. Her mother, who had a number of children to keep, had married later but had to compete with her husband's 'outdoor wife'. The stepfather, however, had recognized Orsyla. Her mother added to the meagre finances by taking in laundry and at a relatively young age Orsyla had to lend a hand, first of all with a house-cleaning job. Although, in retrospect, it caused amazement to realize how low her and her peers' wages were in those days, Orsyla still feels proud of the contribution she made. She was her mother's support and stay. She had also been instrumental in upholding norms of propriety, recalling that her younger brother would only wear one pair of socks to school, so she would wash them every night. In the Caribbean, clothes and public appearance matter greatly as signs of social status and respectability. In recognition of this, Orsyla made good use of her employer's cast-off clothes and learned to sew in order that she could present herself well.

Although her relatives were members of the Moravian church, Orsyla's curiosity about *Winti* was aroused at an early age. Her mother strongly opposed 'heathen practices', so Orsyla had to search for information elsewhere. This was not hard as the sound of drums and *Winti* songs could frequently be heard in the neighbourhood. Adults will not discuss ritual with children (though their conversations are full of allusions), so along with other children, Orsyla pried over fences and through hedges whenever a party gradually changed into a ritual, most usually at birthday celebrations and wakes. Gradually, she imbibed *Winti* lore.

Later, as a young woman, Orsyla joined clubs that strove to preserve tradition. There was plenty of choice in the 1950s and 1960s. Popular theatre and choirs were formal organizations to which the informal *Winti* interests could be attached, and in this way she was recruited to the retinue of a traditional healer who needed a choir to accompany the rituals. Music is of great importance, even essential, to call up the spirits. As a rule, men play drums and most of the singers are female. A healer should pay his assistants for their part in making a ritual a success, and women are content with a smaller remuneration than men. But participation offers other advantages. Women like Orsyla, who have not been familiar with *Winti* since childhood, have ample opportunity to get acquainted with the cult and to observe healers in action. Orsyla was fully aware that ritual knowledge is a scarce resource and that healers regard their co-workers as potential rivals, but she was also quite conscious of the fact that this offered her a chance to make a start on realizing an aspiration.

Orsyla's ambition gradually took form in the shape of a possessing spirit. In this world view a model is manifest containing various self images, expressing various aspects of a personality. The pluriformity of the cosmology, in which the spirit pantheon is divided into sub-types and several mixtures and crossbred varieties are recognized,[23] offers ample scope to define one's identity. Every human being is regarded as harbouring, within the soul or self, a pair of parent figures – the *dyodyo* – who are representatives of the higher spirits. Mother Earth is present in all human beings, in one of her many forms, but most noticeably in women in the second half of their life. Male principles, in African or Amerindian form, are also present in each person. They lie dormant and the cult furthers the articulation of these personal forces. Next to these ideal images, lesser spirits manifest themselves, also in different forms, and particularly among the young and active. As a rule, they are imagined as forest spirits. As in many other cosmologies, the forest or wilderness is pictured as civilization's antipode, symbol of untamed and capricious forces that may thwart the higher purposes of the *Winti* cult. The Creole lower classes, especially, uphold the view that each person entertains a spirit of the wild or a demon and this power is regarded as dangerous but also as an indispensable source of support.[24] To make use of these powers and keep them in control are among the foremost goals of a ritual.

At an early age spirits had manifested themselves in Orsyla. When she was about 12 years old, she dreamt of a manifestation of Mother Earth or *Aisa*, a plain type of earth spirit – a 'granny' wearing a blue cotton skirt. The old woman wore a necklace of pyrope beads and said that Orsyla should also wear such a necklace, which she eventually did. Later, Orsyla would dream of other jewels, in honour of other spirits, and she often bought such items. When she was about 15 or 16 years old, she realized that she would one day be a medium of a sky spirit, a *Kromanti*.

Orsyla had no difficulty at all to discern in her aspirations the expression of a forest spirit, and a male one at that. The spirit grew and thrived, it seems, on her personal circumstances. The way her stepfather treated her long-suffering mother aroused a deeply felt indignation; a reaction Orsyla interpreted in a frame of reference familiar to her, that 'of another world'. She regarded her mother's husband as an unworthy partner, even as a rival. The leader of the cult group she had joined also offended her as, in this company, she met with patent male chauvinism and exploitation which was most obvious in money matters. *Winti*, as such, is not a religion that disparages women; women earn prestige and authority as sponsors and mediums, though financial compensation for efforts made is often slight. Personal experience supported Orsyla in the conviction that men are not to be trusted and that solidarity among women is essential for survival.

Orsyla sees her inner demon as a force that has gradually grown into maturity, though on the other hand she also allows for the view that the spirit has been forced upon her, 'sent' by an ill wisher. A son of her stepfather's 'outdoor wife' was suspected of having bribed two bush sprites, *bakru*, or demons, to invade her. The distinction between benign and evil spirits is often hazy when powers of the wilderness are involved and the evil only surfaced later. The diagnosis was only made when misfortune had already struck.

Orsyla's ritual practice started by coincidence and haphazardly. She was 27 years old and married to a man who had a steady job at a bauxite company. In the compound where they had found lodgings lived a woman who started to behave in a strange way. In the late afternoon, when the pace of social life in the tropics quickens, the woman withdrew into her house and closed her door and shutters. The woman was under great strain and one day she smashed a flat iron that broke into pieces. Orsyla overheard the noise and took action. She picked up a calabash and some leaves from shrubs in the compound, and addressed the spirit that had invaded the woman. She simply asked the spirit what was the matter and why it had come over her, after which the woman calmed down. Familiarity with this form of symbolic language made contact possible. Orsyla took this as a good omen and attributed her successful intervention to the power of her guardian spirits. At that moment, their exact nature had not yet been revealed. Divination to ascertain this would only take place later.

Orsyla also became involved by misfortune, another way that is current among non-specialists. Her first pregnancies ended in miscarriages, and these were attributed by herself and others to envy. From the outset, Orsyla had been highly conscious of other people's jealousy. Although her own situation had been far from rosy, she had been able to present herself in public as an attractive, confident young woman. The envy deeply angered her: 'I have worked hard enough to earn my money and my clothes'. Some people in the neighbourhood had even threatened to physically harm her. She had managed to escape, but the incident had left a deep impression. Now, years later, she remembered the names of these neighbours and the alley from which they came. They returned in dreams where she had to crawl through the alley and wriggle out of a heap of dirt. Once, when she was pregnant again, she had walked through the alley and met a man who recalled her former mishaps and confirmed her interpretation. However, this time the pregnancy went well and she bore a son, the happy outcome being attributed to the ritual measures taken in time.

Until the miscarriages, conflicts between Orsyla's mother and her stepfather's concubine had been in the background, but the evil witchcraft called up by the rival party was a threat to Orsyla's mother's descent group. After Orsyla's repeated reproductive troubles, her mother cast aside her reluctance to call upon a traditional healer and a friend of the family, called 'grandfather' by the children, was asked to perform a protective ritual. He obliged and managed to stave off further mishaps that way. Afterwards, Orsyla gave birth to several children without problems.

When her children were young, Orsyla had little chance of participating in clubs, let alone of venturing out to do other things. She had a job and took care of her home. Apart from common-or-garden dealings with ritual, she had little occasion to be involved on a regular basis. But the spirits do not rest for such a reason. It gradually dawned on her that another spirit was with her, an African sky spirit. This was brought out in her dreams and by other signs. The spirit strongly objected to women's magical devices of 'tying' a man, an action which might have been suggested and incited by Orsyla's husband's many infidelities. This type of witchcraft is much feared by men and many women in comparable circumstances reputedly resort to it, but the sky spirit objected. It was also repelled by the menstrual and post-partum taboos that she had to observe after her many confinements. Furthermore, Orsyla increasingly realized that she was not only host to this high spirit, but also to a forest power. These little sprites are represented as gnomes that like to tease and kick up a row when offended, though they are 'workers' and indispensable for a healer.

In 1975, when Suriname gained political independence and many of its inhabitants fled the country, Orsyla hesitated. Her mother left and acquired an old age pension, but Orsyla felt tied to the home country because of her children, even though they were grown. Kin and friends lived on both sides of the Atlantic. The final decision to leave was perhaps prompted by estrangement from her husband. She had not been spared the disappointments experienced by her mother and many other women, her husband having spent his earnings with lovers around town rather than bringing them home. Unskilled, Orsyla had little chance of earning a living for herself through gainful employment. Pressures from kin made themselves felt and the opportunity of obtaining a social security benefit in the Netherlands undermined the sense of responsibility towards elderly kin, which inspired fear for the future in Orsyla.

Her experience of employment in the Netherlands was not positive. As a moonshiner she was underpaid and national insurance was not paid for her by her employer, and legal assistance proved inadequate to obtain redress. The firm she worked for went out of business and documents could not be found or had never been drawn up. So Orsyla was on welfare. Because she, as a mother and grandmother, wished to live up to the expectations of those back home, the allowance was not sufficient.

At this stage she started to explore the prospects of generating additional income as a healer. She was actively involved in Creole community life in Amsterdam and was appreciated for her cheerful character, liveliness and sense of humour. In this circle, she could expect to meet potential clients. Orsyla found these initially within her kin group; young nieces who had fallen victim to envy, had conflicts with partners or wished to protect a pregnancy or a newborn baby against evil influences. There were children's illnesses to deal with and family quarrels to be made up, and friends also called upon her for assistance. The ritual remedies applied were the usual ones – a herbal ablution to wash off evil and strengthen the beneficial effect.

It was not easy for Orsyla to move beyond this small circle. Most of the women she met lived off a modest allowance, just as she did. They also followed the strategy of enlarging their spending potential by incurring debts,[25] a practice which is taken for granted as part of motherhood. The strategy enables women to enlarge collective funds or credit and fall back on supportive networks in turn. An informal security system has incorporated the assets of the formal system so that the latter are seen as one resource among others, though ready money to meet a suddenly arising need for a purificatory ritual is often lacking.

Orsyla made a trip to Suriname in connection with family affairs and returned full of stories about her successful performances as a healer. She had found two of her sisters bogged down in difficulties, but had taken ritual action which clearly did them good. Of course, money to pay her properly was not available, but her reputation was growing. This was also due to the rituals she had performed in Amsterdam. Her name was on everybody's lips now. She had carried a supply of fresh herbs from the home country and was buoyant with expectations.

At the same time, Orsyla realized the dangers involved. She felt that these were particularly imminent when one's name is banded about by people who fail to pay up. One is exposed to jealousies and all the evil forces evoked thereby. As a precaution, she did not refer to herself as a *bonuman* (healer), but as *yepiman* (helper), to ward off envy. A healer incurs great risks. Confronted with many forms of evil, he or she is liable to be contaminated or saddled with these burdens and as a result, one's own soul force is likely to diminish. A healer should be careful to strengthen all supportive guardian spirits by ritual means, which implies financial costs because spirits should receive offerings and jewels. Orsyla made sure of pleasing them by investing in a jewel as soon as she had a windfall. This is a well-known savings system because jewels count as nest eggs.

Finances were Orsyla's greatest problem. In her opinion, her services were both undervalued and underpaid. Her 'own people', the Creoles, rated lowest in her estimation when money matters were at issue. She preferred to have Hindustani or native Dutch people as clients. What hurt her most was that many clients, who had told her that they had no money to pay, suddenly turned to male healers and produced hundreds of guilders. Even one of Orsyla's nieces deserted her to squander her money on a good-for-nothing ritual performed by a swindler. Those clients who felt that ordinary, trustworthy ritual therapy was inadequate to meet their often exalted expectations tended to make such a desperate move. In these situations, female healers like Orsyla put up a good fight. They try to 'break' competitors, both male and female, speaking disparagingly of rituals performed by others and supporting these allegations by contrived arguments accepted as valid in this particular school of religious thinking. For instance, they might suggest that spirits have been offered the wrong type of drink, or that they have been offered in the wrong sequence. This behaviour is more or less accepted as part of a social routine and will not unduly influence public opinion.

Apart from her activities as a healer, Orsyla also made some money on the side with her knowledge of traditional culture. She was familiar with the wishes of the various spirits and was often invited to dress other women for festivals where specific costumes were required. She prepared the traditional starched head scarves for birthdays and other occasions and could earn anything between two and a half to 25 guilders. As part of a multicultural manifestation, Orsyla was once asked to introduce traditional songs and games from Suriname to a play group of children at a neighbourhood centre. It brought her 100 guilders. For the rest, however, opportunities were limited. Once, a *bonuman*, looking for female assistants to prepare ritual offerings and meals, offered her this task, but she was furious upon hearing the fees: 'He earns thousands of guilders and he wants to fob me off with a few tenners'.

Once in a while, Orsyla withdrew from public life. This did her good because, when relaxing peaceably on her couch, she received all sorts of intimations, about the correct use of herbs for instance. She also had dreams about things that went awry in her circle. On the other hand, these periods of quiet caused her a sense of frustration, of being deadlocked. This was connected with her material situation and also with her own strategies. She had pawned most of her jewels and was usually unable to redeem them on time and this made her guardian spirits, to whom the jewels were dedicated, very angry. To pacify them, she bought new ones as soon as the occasion presented itself. Orsyla also ran into difficulties with the rent so that the telephone and electricity were occasionally cut off. The opportunities in cultural entrepreneurship are limited and her ambitions exceeded them. 'It is either sink or swim' she used to say, and she feared things would turn out badly.

To attract more clients she started to stretch tradition. The familiar boundary between 'doctor's disease' and 'Negro's illness' was shifted in favour of the latter. Making use of her charisma, Orsyla would diagnose complaints in an authoritative manner, pointing out 'spiritual' causes of diseases in a way the accepted formula would not allow. She found response as, in her circles, it is considered normal to use two or even three interpretations at the same time. Orsyla certainly is not the only one who is keen to see *Winti* interpretations make headway in diagnoses of disease.

The same can be observed in current diagnoses of a feared disease like cancer. One is expected to see a doctor for all serious ailments, but this does not rule out the belief in medicinal herbs or wrathful spirits. Other common disorders like diabetes and high blood pressure are incorporated into traditional lore as well; these are also attributed to angered reptile spirits. Diseases are explained in accordance with a world view which underpins the maintenance of kinship ties with relatives back home. Although the variety of interpretations is large and a proliferation of ideas is to be noted – no justice to the variety has been done here – a pattern can be recognized.

## RATIONALITY AND CONTRADICTION

One of the central questions in the study of a therapeutic system is that of rationality. In this paper different factors have been mentioned that make for a survival of belief in the healing powers of ritual. The well-being of clients is one. Although no instances of successful treatment in Orsyla's practice have been cited here, many patients expressed their satisfaction. It is clear that healers like Orsyla, through their insight into human nature, their life experience and dedication, prove their worth as therapists.

Another rationale discussed here is that of the relation between healing symbols and social ethics. *Winti* religion – including interpretations of illness and recommended therapies – gives expression to trust in the inner circle's informal leaders, the mothers and grandmothers. This worldview also helps to maintain ties between a peripheral group which has migrated to another part of the world with an equally peripheral set of kin in the home country and enhances the latter's chances of survival in this way. Apart from creating a meaningful role in the second half of life as well as social security and satisfying ambition, this ethic moves women like Orsyla to be active in the reproduction of 'culture'.

*Winti*'s informal organization marks out entrepreneurship as one of the most significant modes of social and cultural reproduction. Although solidarity with the underprivileged is important, an enterprise calls for more than social sensitiveness. Assertiveness, symbolized as an inner demon, is an indispensable personal quality required of an entrepreneur. The dangerous side of demons is recognized by the adherents of the *Winti* worldview. The risks involved are only partly charted. Economic behaviour is based on speculations about opportunities for expansion that are not always realistic. This intensifies competition and jealousy. Some healers, a large majority male, who are bent on material gain and short-term success, resort to bungling. But the healers who act in good faith, like Orsyla, are also tempted to expand their range of action, whenever an opportunity presents itself. This is a hazardous strategy which may sometimes be successful but which, in the long run, imperils the reputation of both *Winti* and its practitioners. Moreover, such manoeuvres may prove inadequate to keep the healers afloat. Also, the rationality of entrepreneurship is liable to clash with the rationalities of social ethics and therapy. A number of male healers try to resolve the predicament by opting for fraud.

Bona fide healers are the ones who are weighed down under the burden of a social conflict they are unable to solve.

It has been argued here that there is no intrinsic lack of rationality in *Winti* therapy which would explain an ongoing process of drift into marginality. This world view, formerly maligned as backward or idolatrous, and at present the object of attempts at revaluation, has not been fully and publicly accepted in the Creole community as yet. The difficulties in reproducing *Winti* – rather than any inherent deficiency – tempts its practitioners to use tactics that undermine their reputation. In particular, entrepreneurship as a necessary but problematic reproductory mode can be singled out as a discrediting factor.

## NOTES

1 The representativeness of all statements about *Winti* world view and practice, and of the case discussed below, is a pending issue. The investigations upon which this contribution is based have been purely qualitative. The data I have gathered are solely to be regarded as the product of personal relationships and participant observation. This implies that the data presented here are reliable. Whether they are representative is another matter as interviewing a sample of healers active in Amsterdam proved to be impossible. Even the posing of direct questions to participants in *Winti* rituals often caused problems. Participant observation was the option left open.

2 See, for instance, Tijno Venema, *Famiri nanga kulturu: Creoolse sociale verhoudingen en Winti in Amsterdam* (Amsterdam, 1992), p. 83. This is also discussed by H.J.M Stephen, *Winti: Afro–Surinaamse religie en magische rituelen in Suriname en Nederland* (Amsterdam, 1983), p. 29.

3 Venema, *Famiri nanga kulturu*, pp. 33, 98–102. See also Stephen, *Winti*, p. 18, and *idem*, *De macht van de Fodoe – Winti* (Amsterdam, 1986), p. 43.

4 Peter L. Berger and Thomas Luckmann, *The Social Construction of Reality* (Harmondsworth, 1966, 1976).

5 Fred Budike and Bim Mungra, *Creolen en Hindostanen* (Houten, 1986), p. 135. For a general discussion of 'double consciousness' in dominated groups, see James C. Scott, *Domination and the Arts of Resistance: Hidden Transcripts* (New Haven, CT, and London, 1990), pp. 43–4.

6 F.P. Penard and A.P. Penard, 'Surinaamsch bijgeloof', *Bijdragen tot de Taal-, Land- en Volkenkunde van Nederlandsch Indië*, 67 (1913): 157–83; Ch. J. Wooding, *Evolving Culture: A Cross-Cultural Study of Suriname, West Africa and the Caribbean* (Washington, DC, 1981).

7 Jan Voorhoeve and Ursy Lichtveld (eds), *Creole Drum* (New Haven, CT and London, 1975).

8 A term introduced by Claude Lévi-Strauss, *The Savage Mind* (Chicago, IL, [1962] 1976), pp. 18–22, to denote an intellectual activity which

is unplanned and which makes use of available, heterogeneous elements to create meanings.

9 Ch. J. Wooding, *Geesten genezen* (Groningen, 1984); I. van Wetering, 'De magie van de *Winti* genezer', in M. Gijswijt-Hofstra (ed.), *Geloven in genezen, Volkskundig Bulletin*, 17: 1 (1991): 195–217; *idem*, 'Transformations of slave experience', in Stephan Palmié (ed.), *Slave Cultures and Cultures of Slavery* (Knoxville, TN, 1995), pp. 271–304.

10 Wooding, *Evolving Culture*; Peter E. Schoonheym, *Je geld of . . . je leven* (Utrecht, 1980).

11 This is also true of other parts of the world. See, for instance, Michael Taussig, *Shamanism, Colonialism and the Wild Man: A Study in Terror and Healing* (Chicago, IL and London, 1987).

12 Schoonheym, *Je geld of*, p. 74.

13 Venema, *Famiri nanga kulturu*, p. 153.

14 Melville J. Herskovits and Frances S. Herskovits, *Suriname Folklore* (New York, [1936] 1969), p. 9.

15 Sidney W. Mintz, 'The Caribbean as a sociocultural area', in M.M. Horowitz (ed.), *Peoples and Cultures of the Caribbean* (Garden City, NY, 1971), pp. 17–46.

16 R.A.J. van Lier, *Frontier Society: A Social Analysis of the History of Suriname* (The Hague, 1971), p. 100.

17 Rosemary Brana Shute, 'Women, clubs and politics', *Urban Anthropology*, 5: 2 (1976): 157–85.

18 Carol B. Stack, *All our Kin* (New York, 1974).

19 Ineke Gooskens, *Surinaamse en Antilliaanse kliënten van de Gemeentelijke Sociale Dienst in Amsterdam* (Amsterdam, 1976), p. 58; Jenny Hoolt, *De Amsterdammers in zeven bevolkingscategorieën* (Amsterdam, 1982); Maria Lenders and Marjolein van de Rhoer, *Mijn God, hoe ga ik doen: de positie van Creoolse alleenstaande moeders in Amsterdam* (Amsterdam, 1984), p. 4; Joan Ferrier, *De Surinamers* (Muiderberg, 1985), p. 124; Venema, *Famiri nanga kulturu*, pp. 25, 52.

20 W. van Wetering, 'Informal supportive networks: quasi-kin groups, religion and social order among Suriname Creoles in the Netherlands', *Sociologia Neerlandica*, 23: 2 (1987): 92–101.

21 Carol Shepherd McClain, 'Reinterpreting women in healing roles', in *idem* (ed.), *Women as Healers: Cross-Cultural Perspectives* (New Brunswick, NJ, and London, 1989), pp. 1–19.

22 See Venema, *Famiri nanga kulturu*, pp. 83, 91.

23 Wooding, *Evolving Culture*.

24 W. van Wetering, 'Demons in a garbage chute', in Barry Chevannes (ed.), *Rastafari and other African–Caribbean World Views* (London, 1995), pp. 211–32.

25 Lenders and Van de Rhoer, *Mijn God, hoe ga ik doen*, p. 59.

# Index